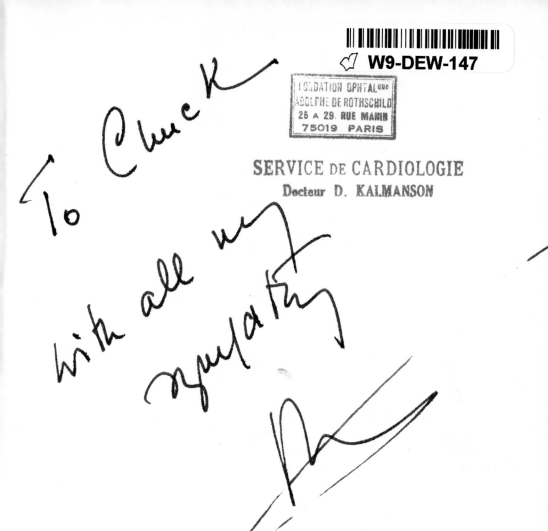

To Chuck

with all my
sympathy

SERVICE DE CARDIOLOGIE
Docteur D. KALMANSON

THE MITRAL VALVE
A Pluridisciplinary Approach

Daniel Kalmanson, M.D., Editor
Fondation Adolphe de Rothschild
Department of Cardiology

Publishing Sciences Group, Inc.
Acton, Massachusetts
a subsidiary of CHC Corporation

Proceedings of the First International Symposium on the Mitral Valve, Paris, May 26–28, 1975, under the auspices of the Fondation Adolphe de Rothschild, Department of Cardiology. Sponsored by the French Cardiac Society and the European Cardiac Society.

Distributed in

Canada
  McAinsh & Company, Ltd.
  1835 Yonge Street
  Toronto, Ontario M4S 1L6
  Canada

Printed in the United States of America.

International Standard Book Number: 0-88416-116-1

Library of Congress Catalog Card Number: 75-17444

PARTICIPANT CONTRIBUTORS

J. Acar, M.D.
Associate Professor, Chief,
  Department of Cardiology,
  Hôpital Intercommunal de
  Créteil, France

W.W. Angell, M.D.
Chief, Cardiac Surgery
  Department, Western Heart
  Associates, San Jose, California

D.W. Baker, BSEE
Associate Professor, Director of
  Center for Bioengineering,
  University of Washington,
  Seattle, Washington

A.C. Beall, Jr., M.D.
Professor of Surgery, Chief,
  Department of Surgery, Baylor
  College of Medicine, Texas
  Medical Center, Houston, Texas

B.J. Bellhouse, M.A., D.Phil.
Department of Engineering
  Science, University of Oxford,
  Oxford, England

V.O. Björk, M.D.
Professor, Department of Thoracic
  and Cardiovascular Surgery,
  Karolinska Sjukhuset, Thoracic
  Surgical Clinic, Stockholm,
  Sweden

D. Borkenhagen, M.D.
Harvard Medical School, Boston,
  Massachusetts

C. Cabrol, M.D.
Professor, Chief, Department of
  Cardiovascular Surgery, Hôpital
  La Pitié-Salpétrière, Paris,
  France

J.P. Cachera, M.D.
Associate Professor, Assistant
  Director, Centre de Recherches
  Chirurgicales Henri Mondor,
  Université Paris-Val-de-Marne,
  Créteil, France

A. Carpentier, M.D., Ph.D.
Professeur Ag. Chirurgie
  Cardiaque, Université Paris IV,
  Head Laboratoire d'Etudes des
  Greffes et Prothèses Cardiaques,
  Hopital Broussais, Paris, France

A. Deloche, M.D.
Associate Professor, Clinique de
  Chirurgie Cardiovasculaire,
  Hôpital Broussais, Paris, France

H. Denolin, M.D.
Professor of Cardiology; Secretary
  of the European Society of
  Cardiology, Brussels, Belgium

H.T. Dodge, M.D.
Professor of Medicine, University
  of Washington, Seattle,
  Washington

Ch. Dubost, M.D.
Professor of Surgery, Director,
  Clinique Chirurgicale
  Cardio-Vasculaire, Hôpital
  Broussais, Paris, France

C.M.G. Duran, M.D., D.Phil.
Professor, Chief, Centro Medico
  Nacional "Marques de
  Valdecilla," Santander, Spain

J.D. Folts, Ph.D.
Associate Professor, Department
  of Medicine, University of
  Wisconsin, Madison, Wisconsin

F. Fontan, M.D.
Associate Professor, Clinique
  Chirurgicale des Maladies
  Cardiovasculaires, Hôpital du
  Tondu, Bordeaux, France

P.G. Hugenholtz, M.D.
Professor of Medicine, Department
  of Cardiology, Erasmus
  Universiteit Rotterdam,
  Thoraxcentrum, Rotterdam, the
  Netherlands

D. Kalmanson, M.D.
Director of Clinical Teaching,
Chief, Department of
Cardiology, Cardiovascular
Research Center A.R.N.T.I.C.,
Fondation A. de Rothschild,
Paris, France

H.P. Krayenbühl, M.D.
Professor, Department of
Cardiology, Kantonsspital
Zürich, Zürich, Switzerland

S. Laniado, M.D.
Chief, Department of Intensive
Coronary Care, Ichilov Hospital,
Tel-Aviv, Israel

H.N. Neufeld, M.D.
Professor of Cardiology,
Department of Cardiology,
Chaim Sheba Medical Center,
Tel-Hashomer, Israel

S.P. Nolan, M.D.
Professor, Chief, Department of
Surgery, University of Virginia,
Charlottesville, Virginia

J.H. Oury, M.D.
Medical Corps U.S. Navy; Chief,
Department of Cardiothoracic
Surgery, Naval Regional
Medical Center, San Diego,
California

J.K. Perloff, M.D.
Professor of Medicine, Department
of Medicine and Pediatrics,
Hospital of the University of
Pennsylvania, Philadelphia,
Pennsylvania

J. Pernod, M.D.
Professor of Cardiology, Chief,
Department of Cardiology,
Hôpital Percy, Clamart, France

R.L. Popp, M.D.
Associate Professor, Department
of Cardiology, Stanford
University Medical Center,
Stanford, California

N. Ranganathan, M.D.
Department of Pathology, St.
Michael's Hospital, Toronto,
Canada

R.S. Reneman, M.D.
Professor of Physiology, Chief,
Department of Physiology,
Medical Faculty Maastrichit,
Maastrichit, the Netherlands

C. Rioux, M.D.
Associate Professor, Chief,
Cardiothoracic Surgery, Hôpital
Pontchaillou, Rennes, France

J. Roelandt, M.D.
Department of Echocardiography,
Erasmus Universiteit
Rotterdam, Thoraxcentrum,
Rotterdam, the Netherlands

W. Rutishauser, M.D.
Professor, Department of
Cardiology, Kantonsspital
Zürich, Zürich, Switzerland

M.D. Silver, M.D.
Professor of Pathology, Chief,
Department of Pathology,
University of Toronto, Toronto,
Canada

W. Somerville, M.D.
Professor; Chief, Cardiac
Department, Middlesex
Hospital, London, England

E.H. Sonnenblick, M.D.
Associate Professor of Medicine,
Department of Cardiology,
Albert Einstein College of
Medicine of Yeshiva University,
Bronx, New York

A. Starr, M.D.
Professor of Surgery, Department
of Cardiopulmonary Surgery,
University of Oregon Medical
School, Portland, Oregon

L. Talbot, Ph.D.
Professor of Fluid Dynamics,
Department of Engineering
Science, University of Oxford,
Oxford, England

D.E.M. Taylor, Ph.D., F.R.C.S.
Professor of Physiology, Chief,
Department of Physiology,
University Medical School,
Edinburgh, Great Britain

A.G. Tsakiris, M.D.
Department of Cardiology, Centre
Hospitalier Universitaire de
Sherbrooke, Sherbrooke,
Canada

C. Veyrat, M.D.
Chargée de Recherches au
C.N.R.S., Hôpital Tenon, Paris,
France

J. Whamond, Ph.D.
Department of Physiology,
University Medical School,
Edinburgh, Great Britain

J.T.M. Wright, Ph.D.
Lecturer, Department of
Bio-Engineering, University of
Liverpool, Liverpool, Great
Britain

M. Yacoub, M.D.
Consultant Cardiac Surgeon,
Chief, Department of Cardiac
Surgery, Harefield Hospital,
Harefield, Middlesex, Great
Britain

E.L. Yellin, Ph.D.
Associate Professor, Department
of Surgery and Physiology,
Albert Einstein College of
Medicine of Yeshiva University,
Bronx, New York

DISCUSSANTS

J. Barlow, M.D.
Professor, General Hospital,
Johannesburg, South Africa

H.F. Bassett, M.D.
Manchester Royal Infirmary,
Manchester, Great Britain

T. Berger, M.D.
University of Alabama Hospital,
Birmingham, Alabama

H. Borst, M.D.
Department of Surgery, Hannover
Medical School, Hannover,
Germany

Y. Bouvrain, M.D.
Professor, Department of
Cardiology, Hôpital
Lariboisière, Paris, France

M. Braimbridge, M.D.
St. Thomas Hospital, London,
Great Britain

B. Branchini, M.D.
Military Hospital, Trieste, Italy

P. Chiche, M.D.
Professor, Department of
Cardiology, Hôpital Tenon,
Paris, France

G. Faivre, M.D.
Professor, Department of
Cardiology, Centre Hospitalier
Regional de Nancy, France

M. Fawzy, M.D.
Harefield Hospital, Harefield,
Middlesex, Great Britain

R. Frater, M.D.
Professor, Albert Einstein
College of Medicine, Yeshiva
University, Bronx, New York

I. Gabe, M.D.
Professor, Department of
Cardiology, Midhurst Hospital,
Midhurst, Great Britain

W. Hancock, M.D.
Professor, Hancock Laboratories,
Anaheim, California

J. Horeau, M.D.
Department of Cardiology, Centre
Hospitalier Regional de Nantes,
France

R. Kaster, M.D.
Medical Incorporated,
Minneapolis, Minnesota

R. Kinsley, M.D.
University Witwatersrand,
Medical School, Johannesburg,
South Africa

K. Lyngborg, M.D.
Rigshospitalet, Copenhagen,
Denmark

D. Mendel, M.D.
St. Thomas Hospital, London,
Great Britain

K. Messmer, M.D.
Kantonsspital Zürich, Zürich,
Switzerland

**P. Peronneau, Ph.D., C.E.T.C.,
C.N.R.S.**
Hôpital Broussais, Paris, France

K. Reid, M.D.
National Heart Hospital London,
London, Great Britain

K. Ross, M.D.
Western Hospital, Southampton,
Hampshire, Great Britain

J.M. Thiron, M.D.
Rouen, France

R. Tricot, M.D.
Professor, Department of
  Cardiology, Hôpital Bichat,
  Paris, France

D. Tunstall-Pedoe, M.D., D.Phil.
Hackney Hospital, London, England

D.W. Wieting, Ph.D.
Head, Department of
  Mechanical Engineering, Tulane
  University, New Orleans,
  Louisiana

CONTENTS

INTRODUCTION

Contribution and Prospects of the Pluridisciplinary Approach

The recent and considerable progress in mitral valve surgery has been an incentive for cardiologists and physiologists to improve their knowledge of the normal and pathological function of the mitral valve, and to perfect their diagnostic techniques in order to make the indications for surgery more precise. Thus numerous original achievements regarding mitral-valve functional anatomy, physiology, hemodynamics, and ultrasonic diagnostic techniques have been performed these last years, along with continuing improvements in surgical techniques.

Unfortunately, most of these studies were carried out on an isolated, "tribal" approach basis. This situation made it desirable to collect and evaluate the latest "hard data" acquired in the different disciplines, and to integrate them into an overall perspective.

Such were the goals of the First International Symposium on the Mitral Valve, held in Paris, under the auspices of the Fondation A. de Rothschild, May 26–28, 1975. This symposium brought together top-ranking cardiologists, surgeons, anatomists, physiologists, biomedical engineers, and fluid dynamicists.

This book represents the Proceedings of the meeting, including papers and discussions. It is divided into ten sections listed in the original, logical order of presentation. It will be seen from the contents that, for obvious reasons, not all of the disciplines involved with the mitral valve were included in the program of the symposium. Such conventional topics as clinical pictures or phonocardiography, which have not considerably evolved in recent years, were deliberately discarded. On the other hand, an unusual emphasis was purposely put on the new data obtained by recent electromagnetic and ultrasonic investigations, as well as on new conceptual orientations.

To start with, the present trend toward a broader and above all more functional concept of the normal and diseased mitral apparatus is illustrated in Parts I and II. An entirely new hemodynamic approach to the mitral valve, both experimental and clinical, is described in Parts III, IV, and V. The paramount importance of the knowledge of instantaneous mitral flow rate and velocity for our understanding of mitral valve physiology, pathophysiology, and surgical correction is clearly demonstrated. In addition, the debate between different research teams about the hemodynamic characteristics of different prosthetic valves is an original and enlightening contribution to persisting controversies, and an incentive for further studies. In Part VI, the valuable results of non-invasive ultrasonic exploration of the mitral valve are reviewed; this should pave the way for a more routine use of ultrasound for diagnosing mitral-valve disease and for disclosing anomalies of implanted prosthetic valves. The role of myocardial, atrial, and ventricular performances, and particularly their clinical implications regarding the time course and optimal timing for operation, is discussed in Part VII. An open forum on the indications and late results of prosthetic valves, grafts, and reconstructive surgery provides the logical conclusion to the book in Parts VIII, IX and X. At the end of each section, there is a discussion of some of the problems presented in the papers, followed by a brief summary by one of the chairmen of the session giving the current status of the topic being considered.

•   •   •

Is it possible, in spite of the wide range of the presentations and the complexity of their topics, to draw an overall conclusion, or at least to suggest general trend?

KNOWLEDGE GAP AND THE PLURIDISCIPLINARY APPROACH. First and foremost, entirely new findings are presented, and recent data have also been collected that previously either went unnoticed or were considered useless or irrelevant to the study of mitral-valve pathophysiology and surgery. One hopes this book will make it clear that the mitral apparatus, contrary to the conventional and restrictive definition, consists of a sophisticated mosaic or puzzle, the reassembling of which demands the close participation of all the involved disciplines. The present meeting has stimulated awareness of the need to air these views still further. One cannot dissociate this result from the thought-provoking contacts and mutual exchanges between scientists of differing specialties. These mutual exchanges appear to be essential for discovering the missing links, for closing the wide existing knowledge gap between various disciplines, and hence for leading to a better understanding and a more effective solution of pending valvular problems.

HEURISTIC GAP AND THE SYSTEMIC, TRANSDISCIPLINARY APPROACH. Nonetheless, if these mutual exchanges are a prerequisite, they are far from being sufficient. Left to themselves, they might well be doomed to what the linguists term a "defeated expectancy." As one progresses through the Proceedings, a more compelling requirement becomes more apparent in order to make pluridisciplinary meetings more effective. It will, in effect, be of no little importance to the reader to notice a number of conflicting appraisals or conclusions of the issues under consideration, most often originating from differing heuristic approaches. For example, the validity of the most recent functional description of the anatomy of the mitral valve is questioned by the surgeons (Parts I and II); the application of model mitral valves to human physiology is seriously doubted by the cardiologists and surgeons (Parts III and IV); and the hydraulic order of merit of the prosthetic valves, as determined by the fluid dynamicists, is by and large flatly denied by cardiologists (Parts, V, VIII, and X).

Such discrepancies reveal and stress the shortcomings of the conventional, analytical, *sequential*—even if pluridisciplinary—approach, which simply does not take into account the multiple feedbacks that the achievements of each discipline are liable to generate. Far from resulting in a stalemate, these should pave the way for a new, simultaneous, transdisciplinary, and above all integrated approach, the so-called *systemic approach*, essential to the study of such highly complex biological problems as those raised by the mitral valve. This is indeed the most important challenge to present-day cardiovascular research, and it can only be taken up by building one or several closely interconnected, nonetheless flexible, pluridisciplinary teams. It is frustrating to note that 30 years after the dramatic launching of the systemic approach proposed by Wiener,[1] with Rosenblueth and McCulloch, for the study of complex neurological problems, later supported and generalized by Von Bertalanffy,[2] such an approach to the cardiovascular system still remains in the realm of wishful thinking.

RELEVANCY GAP AND FUZZY SETS THEORY. No matter how distressing such a delay may appear, it is not solely responsible for the shortcomings of our progress in clinical applications of cardiovascular physiology and pathophysiology. Throughout many articles and discussions of the Proceedings, although it is not always clearly voiced, there is a restless and uneasy sense of our inability to apply numerical data to concrete situations with which the cardiologists and surgeons are routinely faced. The fact nonetheless remains that cardiological practice (as any other medical practice) is finally a *decision-making process*, for which unfortunately even the most sophisticated techniques are far from being adequate. Such a *relevancy gap* appears particularly clearly in Parts V and VII, respectively dealing with the theoretical and clinical confrontation of prosthetic valves, and the assessment and the role of left ventricular performance in mitral-valve disease. It is most likely that it is not so much our technology but our approach which here fails us. The inability of precise figures to characterize, for clinical use, complex biological situations has led Zadeh[3] to imagine a potential way out of this dilemma, based on a new mathematical theory, the Fuzzy Sets Theory.

Fuzzy Sets are sets of elements whose limits are ill-defined and imprecise, the transition between membership and nonmembership being gradual. These sets allow "graded membership" in contrast to classic mathematics, in which the only possible choice for an element is either to belong or not to belong to the set considered. Such a concept clearly applies to cardiovascular data such as calculated mitral-valve area, measured cardiac output, myocardial compliance, ventricular performance, classes of heart failure, etc. Regrettably, it is not possible to include an outline of such a theory here, but perhaps the reader might refer to some publications[3-5] which may clarify many obscure and irritating points left unanswered by the present book.

By way of conclusion, it is the Editor's hope that, aside from providing a wealth of recent and factual data on the mitral valve, these Proceedings might contribute, albeit on a very modest scale, to spread the gospel of a renewed, transdisciplinary, and integrated systemic approach to cardiovascular problems, perhaps supported in some way by the Fuzzy Sets Theory. The Editor would then feel largely rewarded for his efforts, and above all, justified for having demanded such time consuming and painstaking work from all authors, to whom he is so deeply indebted and to whom he here expresses his sincere gratitude. A particular acknowledgment is due for the valuable collaboration of Dr. Colette Veyrat.

Paris, July 1975   Daniel Kalmanson, M.D.

REFERENCES

1. Wiener, N. *Cybernetics*. Hermann Edit: Paris, 1948.
2. Von Bertalanffy, L. An outline of general system theory. *Brit. J. Philos. Science*, 1:139, 1950.
3. Zadeh, L.A. Outline of a new approach to the analysis of complex systems and decision processes. Memorandum ERL-M 342. Berkeley, Calif., Electronics Research Laboratory, University of California, Berkeley, Calif., 1972.
4. Kaufman, A. *Théorie des sous-ensembles flous et ses applications*. Vol. 1, Masson et Cie Edit: Paris, 1972.
5. Kalmanson, D. and Stegall, H.F. Cardiovascular investigations and fuzzy sets theory. *Amer. J. Cardiol.* 35:80, 1975.

PART ONE

ANATOMY AND PHYSIOLOGY OF THE NORMAL MITRAL VALVE

1 Recent Advances in the Knowledge of the Anatomy of the Mitral Valve

N. Ranganathan, M.D.
M.D. Silver, M.D.
E.D. Wigle, M.D.

INTRODUCTION

The mitral valve is a complex unit comprising the annulus, the leaflets, the chordae tendineae, the papillary muscles, and the underlying left ventricular myocardium.[1-8] Recent classification of the chordae tendineae of the mitral valve according to their morphology and site of insertion has made it possible to redefine the valve's anatomy, clarifying some of the controversies regarding the organization of the posterior leaflet.[7,8] In this chapter we will discuss the anatomy of the valve in light of these findings.

The mitral valve consists of a continuous veil of tissue inserted around the entire circumference of the mitral orifice. The basal portion of this veil is attached to a fibromuscular ring, the annulus. The mitral-valve annulus extends along the left atrioventricular sulcus and is fixed medially to the central cardiac skeleton at the aortic root. The

4

free margin of the leaflet veil shows several indentations. Two are regularly placed and permit the division of the veil into anterior and posterior leaflets (Fig. 1). These are the anterolateral and the posteromedial commissures. While the tips of the papillary muscles may be used as a guide to locate the commissures,[1] definitive identification can be made by recognizing a specific type of fan-shaped chordae called the "commissural chordae tendineae"[7] (Fig. 2). These arise as single stems that branch radially like the struts of a fan to insert into the free margins of the commissural regions. The extent of the commissural area can be defined by the spread of insertion of these chordae. Although both anterolateral and posteromedial commissural areas have equal amounts of valvular tissue, the posteromedial commissural chorda has a greater spread than its anterolateral counterpart.[8] This might explain the greater susceptibility of this region to mitral regurgitation.[2,8] Once the commissures are defined, the organization of the rest of the leaflets is easy. All the valvular tissue anterior to the commissures becomes the anterior leaflet, and all the valvular tissue posterior to the commissures becomes the posterior mitral leaflet.

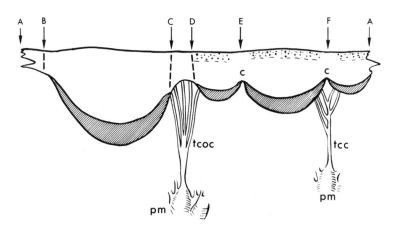

Figure 1. Diagrammatic representation of the mitral valve with fan-shaped commissural and cleft chordae tendineae attached. A-B = anterolateral commissure; B-C = anterior leaflet; C-D = posteromedial commissure; D-A = posterior leaflet; D-E = postero-medial commissural scallop; E-F = middle scallop; F-A = anterolateral commissural scallop; c = cleft; pm = papillary muscle; tcoc = typical commissural chorda; tcc = typical cleft chorda. The dotted area represents basal zone and the rough zone is cross hatched. Intervening areas of the leaflet are the clear zones.

THE ANTERIOR MITRAL LEAFLET

The anterior mitral leaflet is a semicircular or triangular structure. The distal third of the leaflet's surface is rough to palpation and opaque to transillumination, and receives the insertion of the chordae tendineae on its ventricular surface.[8] This is the rough zone of the leaflet. The leaflet surface is clear and membranous proximal to the rough zone (Fig. 1). There is a distinct ridge along the superior margin of the rough zone, this being the line of leaflet closure. During valve closure, the rough zone comes into apposition with its counterpart on the posterior leaflet.

The anterior leaflet has a common attachment to the cardiac skeleton with the left coronary cusp and half of the non-coronary cusp

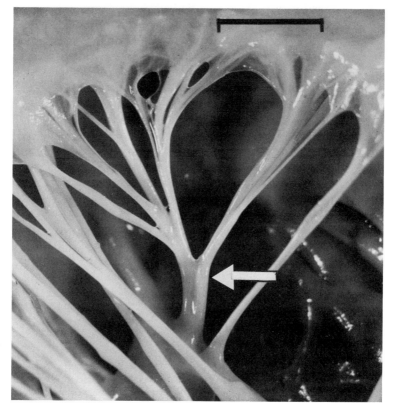

Figure 2. Fan-shaped commissural chorda (arrow) inserting into the wide posteromedial commissural area. Scale indicates 5 mm.

of the aortic valve. Thus it forms an important boundary dividing the in-flow and out-flow tracts of the left ventricle.[8-11] The mitral valve differs from the tricuspid valve in this respect, since the latter does not share a common attachment to the pulmonary valve, which is separated by the infundibulum of the right ventricle. To a certain extent, this relationship limits the degree of dilatation of the mitral ring that would result just from ventricular dilatation. While right ventricular dilatation would necessarily result in a complete tricuspid ring dilatation, this is not necessarily the case with the mitral valve.

THE POSTERIOR MITRAL LEAFLET

The posterior leaflet comprises all leaflet tissue posterior to the two commissural areas. This definition excludes the concept of accessory cusps.[2] Defined this way, the posterior leaflet has a greater attachment to the atrioventricular annulus than does the anterior leaflet.[8] This leaflet often has a number of indentations or clefts along its free margin. In the majority of the normal hearts studied (92%), this leaflet was a triscalloped structure with a large middle scallop and two equal-sized commissural scallops on either side of it (Figs. 1 and 3).[8] Again one can see typical fan-shaped chordae tendineae that insert into and define the clefts between the individual scallops of the posterior leaflet.

Three zones can be identified on the leaflet surface: 1) a rough

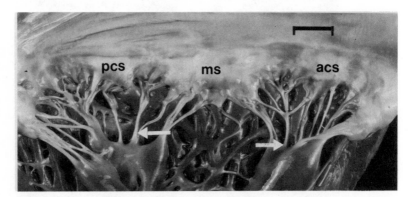

Figure 3. Mitral valve showing the tri-scalloped posterior leaflet with a large middle scallop (ms) and two comparably sized commissural scallops on either side of it. acs = anterolateral commissural scallop; pcs = postero-medial commissural scallop. Fan shaped cleft chordae (arrows) insert into the clefts between the scallops. Scale indicates 1 cm.

zone forming the distal portion of the leaflet; 2) a clear zone proximal to this; and 3) a basal zone (Figs. 1 and 3).[8] The rough zone, similar to that of the anterior leaflet, has chordal insertions on its ventricular surface, is opaque to transillumination, and comes into close contact with the anterior leaflet during valve closure. As in the anterior leaflet, this zone is broadest at the lower-most portion of the scallop, tapering towards the clefts between the scallops. The basal zone between the clear zone and the annulus receives the insertion of basal chordae tendineae that originate directly from trabeculum carneae of the left ventricular myocardium.[7] This zone is most obvious on the middle scallop, because the majority of the basal chordae tendineae tend to insert into this region. The ratio of rough zone to clear zone in the middle scallop of the posterior leaflet is 1.4, while in the anterior leaflet it is 0.6.[8] This implies that a greater portion of the posterior leaflet comes into contact with the anterior leaflet during valve closure. Recognition of the scalloped nature of the posterior leaflet has clinical implications in the prolapsed mitral leaflet syndrome,[12,13] where one or more of these posterior leaflet scallops bulge into the left atrium as assessed by cineangiography.[14-16]

CHORDAE TENDINEAE OF THE MITRAL LEAFLETS

The rough zones of both the anterior and the posterior leaflets and basal zone of the posterior leaflet receive insertion of chordae tendineae.[7] Typically each rough zone chorda splits into three cords soon after its origin from the papillary muscle. One inserts into the free margin of the leaflet, and one inserts beyond the free margin to the line of closure. An intermediate cord inserts between the two (Fig. 4). Occasionally further branching of these cords may be observed, giving rise to secondary branches that insert in the same area as the parent cords. Among the anterior leaflet rough-zone chordae, two are by far the thickest and largest: these are the "strut chordae tendineae." They often originate from the tips of the anterolateral and the posteromedial papillary muscle, inserting between four and five o'clock positions on the posteromedial side and between the seven and eight o'clock position on the anterolateral side (Fig. 5). Strut chordae tendineae were present in more than 90% of the hearts examined.[7] The rough-zone chordae tendineae of the posterior leaflet in general are shorter and thinner than those of the anterior leaflet. The posterior leaflet does not have strut chordae among its rough-zone chordae tendineae. Chordae tendineae inserting into the basal regions of the

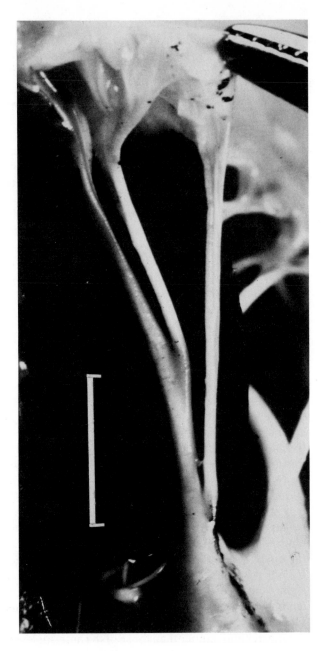

Figure 4. Typical "rough zone" chorda branching into three cords before inserting into posterior leaflet. Scale indicates 5 mm.

posterior leaflet were found in 31 of the 50 hearts examined.[7] In 12 hearts they were only attached to the middle scallop region. These arise as single strands directly from the left ventricular wall or from small trabeculum carneae to insert into the ventricular surface of the leaflet near the annulus.

The chordae tendineae passing to the anterolateral commissure and the adjoining half of the anterior and the posterior leaflets arise from the anterolateral papillary muscle group; the chordae passing to the posteromedial commissure and the adjoining half of the anterior and the posterior leaflets originate from the posteromedial group of papillary muscles. On an average, 25 chordae tendineae insert into the mitral valve. There is no significant difference in the total number between the two sexes. Of the 25 chordae tendineae, 9 are inserted into the anterior leaflet (7 rough-zone chordae and 2 strut chordae) and 14 into the posterior leaflet (10 rough-zone chordae, 2 cleft chordae and 2 basal chordae). Two are inserted into the commissures.

Fleshy and muscular chordae tendineae are occasionally observed in normal hearts, generally arising from the anterolateral papillary muscle.[7] Their clinical significance is yet to be clearly defined. Chordae tendineae inserting into the rough zone may occasionally have less than three cords. Such was the case in 17% of the rough-zone chordae of the anterior leaflet and 16% of those of the posterior

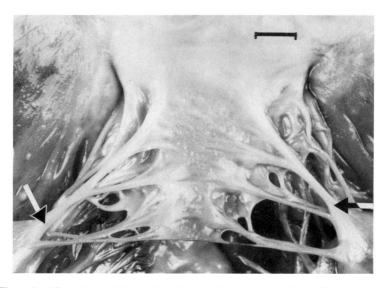

Figure 5. "Strut chordae" (arrows), originating from the tips of the papillary muscles, insert into the anterior leaflet on the ventricular surface. Scale indicates 5mm.

leaflet.[7] Occasionally some of the cords may insert only into the free margin. Such free-edge cords tend to be more common in the tricuspid valve.[17]

The new classification of the chordae tendineae has allowed a clearer definition of the mitral leaflets and in addition has a significant bearing on the syndrome of ruptured chordae tendineae.[7,8] The resultant degree of mitral regurgitation and hemodynamic derangement is related not only to the number of chordae, but also the type of chorda tendinea that is ruptured. In our experience, rupture of strut chordae tendineae often results in severe mitral regurgitation with a flail anterior leaflet; however, rupture of one or more branches of the rough zone chordae, especially of the posterior leaflet, causes only moderate mitral regurgitation.

THE LEFT VENTRICULAR PAPILLARY MUSCLES

There are two groups of papillary muscles in the left ventricle: the anterolateral and the posteromedial. Each group supplies chordae tendineae to one half of both the leaflets. Each group of the papillary muscles may have one or two distinct 'bellies' of muscle, occasionally more than two, especially in the posteromedial group. Often the anterolateral group tends to have one belly.[18] The tips of the papillary muscle usually point to the respective commissures.[1] The left ventricular papillary muscle seems to have at least three recognizable morphologic types, depending on the nature of the attachment to the subjacent ventricular wall and the relative length of the body of the papillary muscle that protrudes freely into the ventricular cavity:[18]

1. They could be either completely tethered, i.e., a papillary muscle fully adherent to the subjacent ventricular myocardium and protruding very little into the ventricular cavity with few trabecular attachments;

2. They could be free and fingerlike, i.e., the papillary muscle with one third or more of the body protruding freely into the ventricular cavity with very few or no trabecular attachments;

3. They could be mixed or intermediate in type with part of the body free, but also with considerable trabecular attachments and tethering in some other parts (Fig. 6).

THE ARTERIAL SUPPLY OF THE LEFT VENTRICULAR PAPILLARY MUSCLES

The anterolateral papillary muscle receives branches from the anterior descending coronary artery and either the diagonal left ventricular arteries or the marginal branches of the left circumflex artery. The posteromedial papillary muscle receives a variable supply from the left circumflex artery and/or branches of the right coronary artery.[18-21] The epicordial branches of the coronary arteries course from base to the apex of the heart, giving penetrating intramyocardial branches. The arterial vasculature of the papillary muscle as studied by stereoscopic arteriography seems to be related to its gross morphologic feature.[18] Two main types of arrangement of long, penetrating intramyocardial vessels are observed (Fig. 6). The fingerlike

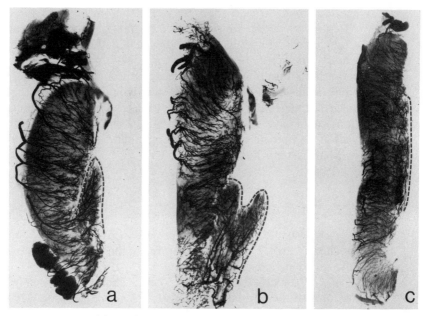

Figure 6. Arterial vasculature of the human left ventricular papillary muscles. Dotted line outlines the papillary muscles. (a) fingerlike papillary muscle with a central artery entering the base to supply the entire papillary muscle, (b) mixed type of papillary muscle with segmental distribution as well as a central artery supplying free medial belly, (c) tethered type of papillary muscle with segmental distribution of long penetrating intramyocardial vessels and rich subendocardial anastomosis.

papillary muscle usually receives a large central artery at its base; this arises from one of the epicardial arteries in that region. The central artery is often long and terminal, and might measure as much as 900 microns at its entry into the papillary muscle. It goes through the muscle mass towards the apex, dividing to form a network of anastomosis. After the fourth or the fifth division, it supplies almost the entire papillary muscle. Such free, fingerlike, papillary-muscle bellies often show very few or no anastomotic connections with the extrapapillary subendocardial plexus. On the other hand, the tethered variety of the papillary muscles often has a segmental type of distribution of the long penetrating intramyocardial vessels. The branches of these vessels not only connect with one another, but also have connections with the extrapapillary subendocardial plexus. A mixed type of arrangement would be found in the papillary muscles of the mixed or the intermediate type. When thick trabecular attachments were noted, one could often demonstrate penetrating intramyocardial vessels coursing through them as well. The variation in the arterial vasculature would have significant effect in occlusive coronary-artery disease in terms of resulting histopathologic damage to the papillary muscles. Tethering and trabecular attachments tend to preserve the integrity of papillary muscle through anastomotic plexus, while occlusion of a large central artery would be expected to result in severe damage to an entire papillary muscle.[18] These anatomic variations could have a considerable influence on functional alterations as well as pathologic changes in the papillary muscles accompanying coronary artery disease.

REFERENCES

1. Rusted, I.E., Schiefley, C.H., Edwards, J.E.   Studies of the mitral valve: I. Anatomic features of the normal mitral valve and associated structures. *Circulation* 6:825, 1952.

2. Chiechi, M.A., Lees, W.M., Thompson, R.   Functional anatomy of the normal mitral valve. *J. Thorac. Surg.* 32:378, 1956.

3. Von Der Spuy, J.C.   The functional and clinical anatomy of the mitral valve. *Brit. Heart J.* 20:471, 1958.

4. Davila, J.C., Palmer, T.E.   The mitral valve. *Arch. Surg.* 84:174, 1962.

5. Du Plessis, L.A., Marchand, P.   The anatomy of the mitral valve and its associated structures. *Thorax* 19:221, 1964.

6. Silverman, M.E., Hurst, J.W.   The mitral complex. *Amer. Heart J.* 76:399, 1968.

7. Lam, J.H.C., Ranganathan, N., Wigle, E.D., Silver, M.D. Morphology of the human mitral valve: I. Chordae tendineae: A new classification. *Circulation* 41:449, 1970.

8. Ranganathan, N., Lam, J.H.C., Wigle, E.D., Silver, M.D. Morphology of the human mitral valve. II. The valve leaflets. *Circulation* 41:459, 1970.

9. Gross, L., Kugel, M.A. Topographic anatomy and histology of the valves in the human heart. *Amer. J. Path.* 7:445, 1931.

10. Zimmerman, J. The functional and surgical anatomy of the heart. *Ann. Roy. Coll. Surg. Eng.* 39:348, 1966.

11. Walmsley, R., Watson, H. The outflow tract of the left ventricle. *Brit. Heart J.* 28:435, 1966.

12. Criley, J.M., Lewis, K.B., Humphries, J.O., Ross, R.S. Prolapse of the mitral valve: Clinical and cineangiocardiographic findings. *Brit. Heart J.* 28:488, 1966.

13. Barlow, J.B., Bosman, C.K. Aneurysmal protrusion of the posterior leaflet of the mitral valve: An auscultatory electrocardiographic syndrome. *Amer. Heart J.* 71:166, 1966.

14. Trent, J.K., Adelman, A.G., Wigle, E.D., Silver, M.D. Morphology of a prolapsed posterior mitral valve leaflet. *Amer. Heart J.* 79:539, 1970.

15. Ranganathan, N., Silver, M.D., Robinson, T.I., Kostuk, W.J., Felderhof, C.H., Patt, N.L., Wilson, J.K., Wigle, E.D. Angiographic-morphologic correlation in patients with severe mitral regurgitation due to prolapse of the posterior mitral valve leaflet. *Circulation* 48:514, 1973.

16. Ranganathan, N., Robinson, T.I., Silver, M.D., Patt, N.L., Wilson, J.K. Angiographic clinical correlation in mitral click syndrome. *Circulation* 48 (suppl. IV):IV. 206, 1973.

17. Silver, M.D., Lam, J.H.C., Ranganathan, N., Wigle, E.D. Morphology of the human tricuspid valve. *Circulation* 43:333, 1971.

18. Ranganathan, N., Burch, G.E. Gross morphology and arterial supply of the papillary muscles of the left ventricle of man. *Amer. Heart J.* 77:506, 1969.

19. Estes, E.H., Dalton, F.M., Entman, M.L., Dixon, H.B., Hackel, D.B. The anatomy and blood supply of the papillary muscles of the left ventricle. *Amer. Heart J.* 71:356, 1966.

20. James, T.N. Anatomy of the coronary arteries in health and disease. *Circulation* 32:1020, 1965.

21. Fulton, W.F.M. The coronary arteries: arteriography, microanatomy and pathogenesis of obliterative coronary artery disease. Springfield, Ill.: Charles C Thomas, 1965.

2 Anatomy of the Mitral Valve Chordae and Cusps

Magdi Yacoub, M.D.

In an attempt to characterize the anatomy of mitral valve chordae and cusps and its relation to function, the mitral valves from 60 cows and 20 human hearts were studied. This was done with the valves in the closed (Fig. 1) and open position (Fig. 2).

The results of this investigation showed that the mitral valve is formed of 4 separate functional units (cusps and chordae) which move independently of each other (Figs. 3a and b). In this study the functional units are referred to according to their position (anterior, posterior, medial and lateral) (Fig. 1). Each functional unit is formed of a leaflet and its own chordae.

The shape of the leaflets is usually semicircular except the lateral and medial cusps which are commonly bilobed. On average the base of the anterior leaflet constitutes 30% of the circumference compared to 25% for the posterior leaflet, 21% for the lateral leaflet and 24% for the medial leaflet.

The chordae to each cusp are arranged in a constant fashion (Figs. 2 and 4), and comprise three sets:

16

1. Two major fixing chordae, arising from separate heads of the same papillary muscle or two different papillary muscles in the case of the anterior and posterior cusps. Each major fixing chorda gives three sets of branches which are termed proximal, intermediate, and marginal. The proximal branches are attached to the ventricular surface of the leaflet near the "annulus," the intermediate to the ventricular surface of the leaflet near the edge, and the marginal to the edge of the leaflet (Fig. 5). The attachment of the branches of each major fixing chorda to the leaflet is along a straight line extending from the free angle of each leaflet towards the midpoint of its attachment to the annulus (Fig. 5).

2. Two lateral fixing chordae which give several branches, which are attached to the lateral border of the cusp at the edge, or just adjoining it.

3. Two commissural chordae attached to the adjoining sides of two leaflets and having a characteristic appearance because of the mode of their branching. This

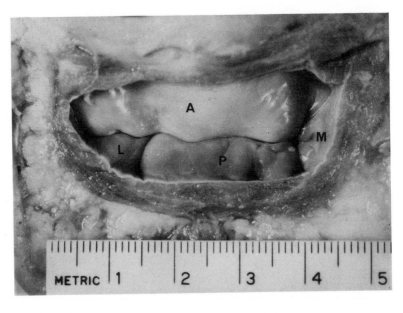

Figure 1. Atrial view of mitral valve in the closed position. A–anterior cusp, L–lateral cusp, P–posterior cusp, M–medial cusp.

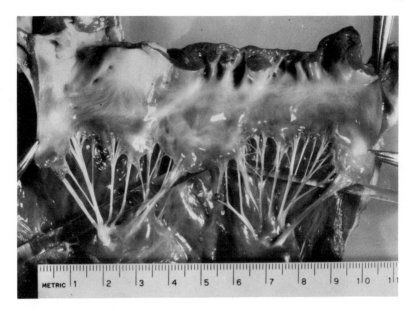

A

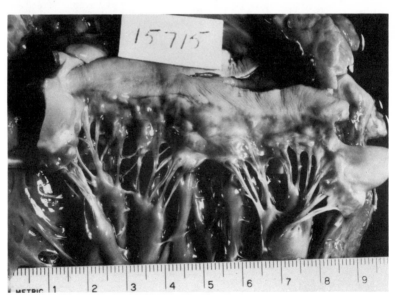

B

Figure 2. Mitral valve apparatus in the open position viewed from the ventricular side after transecting the anterior cusp, A–cow, B–human.

18

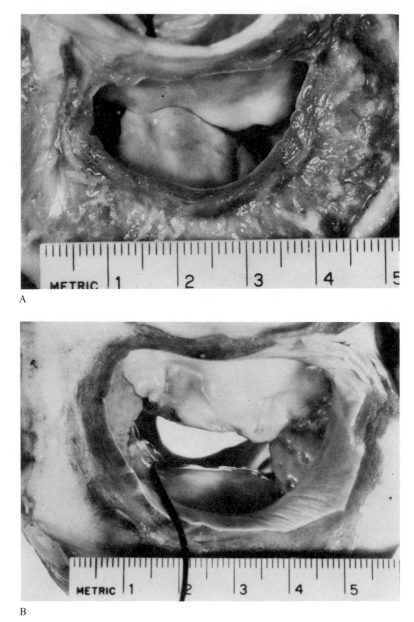

A

B

Figure 3. Mitral valve viewed from the atrial side showing the independent movement of the medial and lateral cusps (A) and posterior cusp (B).

branching is regular with alternate branches attaching to one of the adjoining cusps. The commissural chordae are very easily identifiable and can serve to delineate the different cusps.

The attachment of the chordae to the head of each papillary muscle is constant and is arranged in the form of a semicircle in the following order (Figs. 2 and 4).

1. Major fixing chorda to anterior cusp.

2. Lateral fixing chorda to anterior cusp.

3. Commissural chorda to anterior and lateral cusps.

4. Major fixing chordae to lateral cusp in the case of the anterior papillary muscle, and medial cusp in the case of the posterior papillary muscle.

5. Commissural chorda between lateral or medial cusp and posterior cusp.

6. Lateral fixing to posterior cusp.

7. Major fixing chorda to posterior cusp.

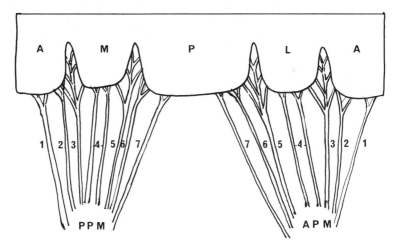

Figure 4. Diagram of mitral valve as in Fig. 2, illustrating the arrangement of the chordae. 1. Major fixing chorda to anterior cusp. 2. Lateral fixing chorda to anterior cusp. 3. Commissural chorda. 4. Major fixing chordae of lateral and medial cusps. 5. Commissural chorda. 6. Lateral fixing of posterior cusp. 7. Major fixing of posterior cusp.

20

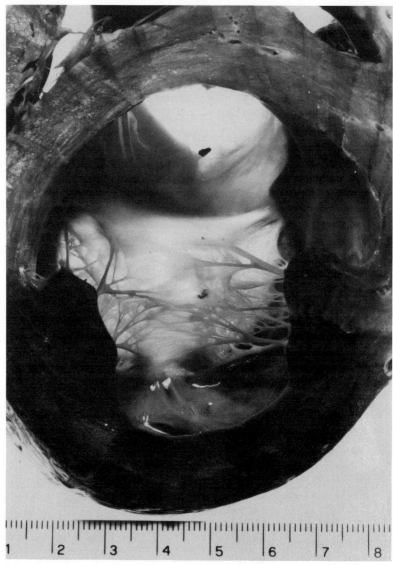

Figure 5. Mitral valve in closed position viewed from the ventricular surface showing the mode branching of the major fixing chordae.

In conclusion, the anatomy of the mitral valve cusps and chordae is constant, fairly easy to identify, and related closely to function.

3 The Physiology of the Mitral Valve Annulus*

Anastasios G. Tsakiris, M.D.

The rings of both atrioventricular valves have been generally considered to be rigid structures, providing the support for the valve cusps. Although, in the past, observations in the isolated heart[1] and in the perfused heart of open-chest animals[2,3] have suggested that the mitral valve annulus does indeed contract, no precise information has been available until recently concerning the magnitude and temporal relationships of changes in the size of the valve ring throughout the cardiac cycle in the intact animal or man.

In order to study this question, detailed measurements of the

* The investigation was carried out in the Department of Physiology, Mayo Clinic and Mayo Foundation, and was supported in part by Research Grants HE-3532 and HE-4664 from the National Institutes of Health, AHA CI 10 from the American Heart Association, MA-4159 from the Medical Research Council of Canada, and by a grant from the Joseph C. Edwards Foundation.

21

dynamic geometry of the mitral annulus were carried out in intact dogs in which the valve ring was rendered "visible" by the insertion of 7 to 11 small radiopaque markers, during cardiopulmonary bypass, 8 to 16 weeks before the studies.[4] On the day of the experiments the dogs were anesthetized. After catheter placement they were positioned, with the aid of a halfbody fiberglass cast, in a biplane videosystem so that in one projection the plane of the mitral annulus was parallel to the central axis of the roentgen beam, while in the other the entire circumference of the valve ring was visualized (Fig. 1). In the course of these experiments, since only minimal rotation of the valve ring was observed throughout the cardiac cycle, the orifice of the mitral valve could be accurately measured in this projection. Observations were made during "control" conditions and during interventions such as changes in heart rate, shortening of the P-R interval, and induced atrial fibrillation.[4]

These studies demonstrated clearly that the orifice of the left-sided atrioventricular valve is not a rigid structure. Figure 2 illustrates

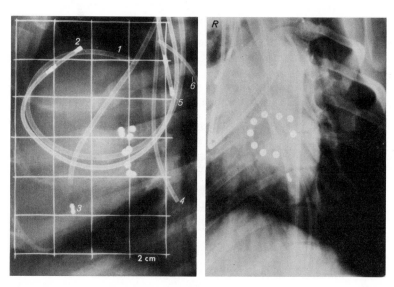

Figure 1. Biplane roentgenograms demonstrating projections of mitral annulus on television screen. In left panel, the nine lead beads inserted in endocardial surface of mitral ring are shown by the vertically oriented videosystem, the central axis of which was parallel to the plane of the annulus. The right panel demonstrates the circumference of the mitral valve ring as visualized by the horizontal-image intensifier system, whose axis was perpendicular to the plane of the annulus. Cardiac catheters were positioned in the pulmonary artery (1), right ventricle (2), left ventricle (3), a pulmonary vein (4), right atrium (5), and aortic arch (6).

the degree and temporal sequence of the changes in the area of the mitral ring during two cardiac cycles, with the atria and ventricles beating in normal sequence. The size of the annulus increased in late diastole until it reached its maximum, which coincided approximately with the P wave of the electrocardiogram. Then a rapid narrowing of the ring was observed during the atrial and ventricular contractions, followed by a rapid increase in size during ventricular isovolumetric relaxation. In the dogs studied, the decrease in size of the mitral annulus under "control" conditions varied between 19 and 34% of the maximal diastolic ring size. It was rather surprising to note that approximately one-half to two-thirds of the total decrease in annular size occurred during atrial contraction, and that the size of the valve orifice was considerably reduced before the onset of ventricular systole. Since a subsequent study of the motion of the tricuspid ring[5] showed striking similarities between the two atrioventricular valves in both the temporal sequence and the degree of annular narrowing during the cardiac cycle, it appears probable that one of the functions of atrial contraction is the reduction in size of the atrioventricular valve orifices prior to the onset of ventricular systole.

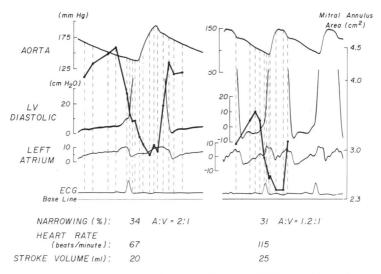

Figure 2. Narrowing of the mitral annulus (heavy solid line) and hemodynamic parameters during "control" conditions (left panel) and during decreased aortic pressure in the same dog. Area of mitral annulus is reduced progressively during atrial and ventricular contractions and approximately 60% to two-thirds of the total narrowing occurs before the onset of ventricular contraction. The size of the ring is different in the two cardiac cycles.

Mitral annular narrowing was eccentric (Fig. 3). The shortening of the segments delineated by beads 1,2,3, and 4 that comprise the ventral margin of the annulus, to which the anterior leaflet is attached, was negligible. The reduction in size was caused by the shortening of the lateral and dorsal portions of the ring delineated by beads 4,5,6, and 7. This shortening tends to appose the posterior leaflet to the larger ventral leaflet and, possibly, to deflect dorsally those parts of the anterior leaflet that are close to the anterolateral commissure.

How are these observations to be reconciled with the presence of a fibrous rigid ring? The relationships at the base of the mitral and aortic valves are best demonstrated when the mitral orifice is viewed from above with the left atrium removed (Fig. 4). The only two fibrous structures that can be found are: a) the right fibrous trigone, which represents confluence of fibrous tissue related to the dorsal aspect of the aortic root, the mitral valve, the tricuspid valve and the membranous septum, and b) the left fibrous trigone, which is composed of fibrous tissue at the confluence of the left margin of the aortic and mitral valves. Between them is the anterior leaflet of the mitral valve in direct continuity with the base of the aorta and the left and posterior aortic cusps. A ring of fibrous tissue does not exist in this region. When histologic sections are cut around the left atrioventricular junction, in a plane perpendicular to the ring, one finds fine tendonlike

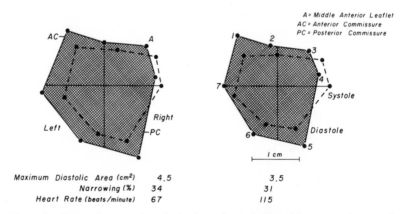

Maximum Diastolic Area (cm²)	4.5	3.5
Narrowing (%)	34	31
Heart Rate (beats/minute)	67	115

Figure 3. Eccentric narrowing of mitral annulus as indicated by greater decrease in length of segments delineated by beads 4,5,6, and 7 situated mainly on dorsal and lateral portions of the ring, as compared to negligible changes in segments 1 through 4 at the base of the anterior leaflet. Shaded area = area of mitral annulus during diastole; area enclosed by interrupted line = mitral annulus during systole. Positions of commissures (AC and PC) and of midpoint of base of anterior leaflet (A) are approximate (same heartbeats as in Figure 2).

structures extending dorsally from both fibrous trigones. These fine collagenous bundles are located endocardially and extend about half-way around the mitral orifice. Therefore, the dorsal one-third to one-half of the mitral ring does not have any fibrous tissue; in this region the base of the mitral leaflet tissue attaches to the left atrial endocardium on the atrial surface and to the left ventricular endocardium on the ventricular surface. A true anatomic annulus cannot be demonstrated.[6,7]

How important is the presystolic annular narrowing in the prevention of mitral valve regurgitation? Our observations so far indicate that during normal hemodynamic conditions and during increased heart rates, atrial-ring narrowing is probably not important because: 1) The valve orifice is relatively small at the onset of ventricular contraction, and 2) it is further reduced in size by the ventricular systole. In contrast, when left ventricular end-diastolic volume was increased and the ejection fraction was reduced, as during acute elevation of aortic pressure, the presystolic narrowing of the annulus associated with atrial contraction was not followed by further reduction in size during ventricular systole.[4] On the contrary, the size of the

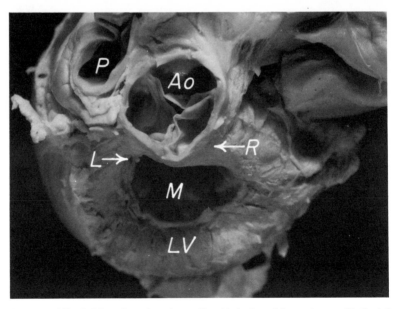

Figure 4. Mitral (M) and aortic valve orifice (Ao) viewed from above with the left atrium removed. R and L indicate the positions of the only two major collagenous structures of the mitral annulus, the right and left fibrous trigones.

26

annulus increased during ventricular ejection, possibly because the basal parts of the left ventricle contracted less than they did during more normal ventricular ejection and therefore could not reduce the size of the annulus. It was during such conditions, when, in addition, atrial annular narrowing was either abolished (by the production of atrial fibrillation) or rendered weak, that mitral regurgitation was observed, presumably caused by a lack of proper leaflet-edge approximation.

REFERENCES

1. Smith, H.L., Essex, H.E., Baldes, E.J.   Study of the movements of heart valves and of heart sounds, *Ann. Intern. Med.* 33:1357, 1950.

2. Hurwitt, E.   Combined Staff Clinic: Mitral stenosis. *Am. J. Med.* 14:216, 1953.

3. Padula, R.T., Cowan, G.S.M., Jr., Camishion, R.C.   Photographic analysis of the active and passive components of cardiac valvular action. *J. Thoracic Cardiovascular Surg.* 56:790, 1968.

4. Tsakiris, A.G., von Bernuth, G., Rastelli, G.C., Bourgeois, M.J., Titus, J.L., Wood, E.H.   Size and motion of the mitral valve annulus in anesthetized intact dogs. *J. Appl. Physiol.* 30:611, 1971.

5. Tsakiris, A.G., Mair, D.D., Seki, S., Titus, J.L., Wood, E.H.   The motion of the tricuspid valve annulus in anesthetized intact dogs. *Circ. Res.* 36:43, 1975.

6. *Titus, J.L.   Anatomy and pathology of the mitral valve.* Edited by F.H. Ellis, Jr. In *Surgery For Acquired Mitral Valve Disease,* Philadelphia, Pa.: Saunders, 1967, p. 49-77.

7. Zimmerman, J., Bailey, C.P.   The surgical significance of the fibrous skeleton of the heart. *J. Thoracic Cardiovascular Surg.* 44:701, 1962.

4 Time-Motion of Both Mitral Leaflets Early in Diastole*

Anastasios G. Tsakiris, M.D.
Douglas A. Gordon
Yves Mathieu, M.D.
Irving Lipton, M.D.

Studies of mitral-valve leaflet motion and position throughout the cardiac cycle, in the intact animal or man, are necessary for the understanding of the closing mechanism of the valve during normal and pathologic conditions.

The following technique has been developed in our laboratory that permits the gathering of precise information concerning the movements and the spatial positions of both mitral cusps in the intact dog: Under normothermic cardiopulmonary bypass, seven small perforated lead beads are sutured on the valve cusps and on the endocardial surface of the apparent annulus in normal dogs (17.3-25 kg bodyweight). One marker is sutured to each commissure at the annular level. One bead is used to mark the middle of the atrial basilar attachment of each cusp. One marker is placed in the middle of the

* Supported in part by Research Grant MA-4159 from the Medical Research Council of Canada, by a grant from the Joseph C. Edwards Foundation and by a grant from the Quebec Heart Foundation.

27

free margin of each leaflet in line with the corresponding annular bead, and the last marker is placed on the atrial surface of the anterior leaflet, midway between the annulus and the free margin.[1,2]

Several weeks or months after the operation the dogs are anesthetized and, after catheter insertion, they are placed in the right decubitus position in a half-body Plexiglas cast. They are then positioned in a single-plane 6-inch image-intensifier system in such a way that the plane of the mitral valve ring is in a vertical position and parallel to the central axis of the roentgen beam with the two commissural beads superimposed. In this position the maximal excursions of the leaflet markers are observed and recorded on cinefilm at speeds ranging from 100 to 120 frames per second, representing sampling intervals of 8 to 10 msec. The cine-camera is synchronized with the oscillographic record by means of an electronic pulse that marks the exposure of each frame. Data analysis consists of determining from the projected cinefilms the spatial coordinates of each marker relative to a fixed image reference throughout the cardiac cycle, and correcting the calculated distances for geometric distortion and for the motion of the mitral annulus. Injections of small amounts of contrast medium (7ml) into the left atrium and left ventricle allow determination of the position of the mitral cusps relative to the ventricular wall and visualization of flow patterns in the left ventricle.

The time-motion of both mitral cusps during diastole was studied in detail, in a series of experiments,[1] during normal sinus rhythm over a wide range of heart rates (42-184 beats/min). Leaflet motion observed during heart rates of 51 and 80 beats/min in the same dog with the atria and ventricles beating in normal sequence is demonstrated in Figures 1 and 2. It can be seen that the time-motion of both cusps was similar throughout diastole except for the delayed opening of the posterior cusp. This delay varied, in the beats analyzed, between 8 and 40 msecs and was not related to heart rate. It is interesting to note that the cusps were never seen to pause at their fully open positions but, following their rapid opening, began to reclose immediately. The diastolic closure was not continuous but showed three distinct time periods, namely a rapid movement, followed by a short pause and by a resumption of the motion towards the atrium at a slower speed (Fig. 1). Cusp motion early in diastole during slow and moderate heart rates was similar (Figs. 1 and 2), whereas at fast heart rates the diastolic leaflet approximation could not be recorded, since it was interrupted by atrial opening.

The fact that diastolic closure was observed to begin immediately after leaflet opening would suggest early vortex formation in the left ventricle. In effect, careful analysis of left atrial angiograms did suggest that contrast medium entering the ventricle spread behind the leaflets early in the filling period, while the ventricular cavity was still

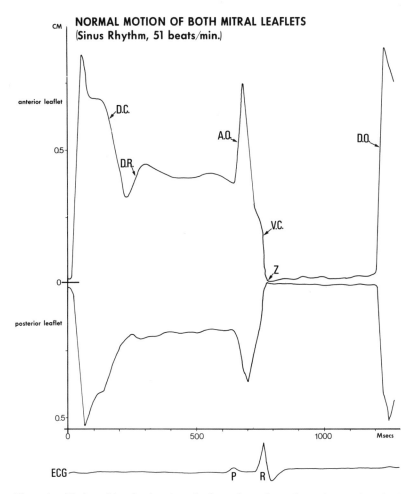

Figure 1. Motion of beads placed on the free edges of anterior and posterior mitral cusps recorded during slow sinus rhythm (51 beats/min). Vertical axis represents the instantaneous linear distance between the leaflet markers and their own reference position (position Z; for explanation see reference No. 1). Time-motion during diastolic closure of both cusps is characterized by immediate reclosure following opening, a short pause, and a resumption of closure at slower speed. Following a small rebound the cusps remain motionless at their semiclosed positions until atrial opening. At end of diastole the valve is closed by the combined effect of atrial and ventricular contractions. DO–diastolic opening, DC–diastolic closure, DR–diastolic rebound, AO–atrial opening, VC–ventricular closure.

30

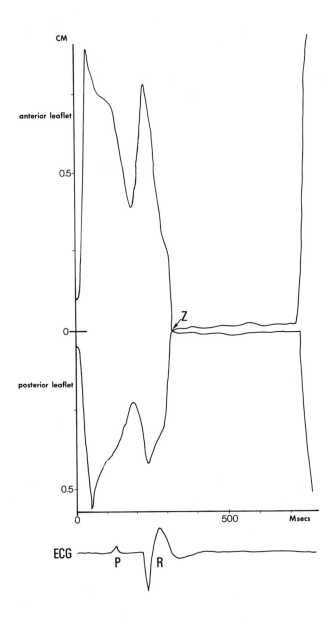

Figure 2. Motion of cusps during atrioventricular pacing at 80 beats/min. Time-motion of both leaflets during diastolic closure is similar to that presented in Fig. 1; diastolic closure and atrial opening are continuous.

small. This appeared to be concomitant with the onset of leaflet movement towards the atrium. Then the ventricle gained volume rapidly and flow appeared to travel mainly toward the apex. This period corresponded to the observed short pause or slowing of leaflet closure. Finally, as the blood stream diverged and ran parallel to the ventricular walls toward the atrioventricular annulus, leaflet closure resumed and continued until blood flow into the ventricle appeared to diminish.

In these experiments the diastolic closing rate of the anterior leaflet averaged 10 ± 3 cm/sec and was higher than values obtained by echocardiography in the open-chest dog.[3]

During slow heart rates after diastolic closure, the cusps remained practically motionless in their semiclosed positions until subsequent atrial or ventricular contraction (Fig. 1). Continuation of closure or leaflet reopening was never observed, and it would appear to us that this floating position (which seemed to be constant in the same animal) is more likely due to a rapid decay of ventricular vortex activity than to tension exerted by the chordae tendineae as has been suggested previously.[4] This latter explanation appears unlikely since, during long diastoles in the presence of a complete atrioventricular block, isolated atrial contractions would invariably produce leaflet reopening.[1]

Since these observations would suggest that the first small quantities of blood entering the ventricle early in diastole do initiate diastolic leaflet closure, it would be unreasonable to expect in the intact heart, during normal ranges of transmitral flow, that the size of the valve orifice would be proportional to volume flow. Indeed, in the individual dog, remarkably little variation was observed both in the maximal excursions of the leaflets and in the distances between them early in diastole.[1]

These observations are probably true only for normal conditions of ventricular diastolic volume, transmitral flow, and degree of ventricular emptying. Delayed valve opening, and diminished and asymmetric diastolic closure, might be expected to occur under pathologic conditions; these possibilities are currently under study.

REFERENCES

1. Tsakiris, A.G., Gordon, D.A., Mathieu, Y., Lipton, I. Motion of both mitral valve leaflets: A cineroentgenographic study in intact dogs. *J. Appl. Physiol.* 39:359, 1975.

2. Tsakiris, A.G., Gordon, D.A., Mathieu, Y., Padiyar, R., Labrosse, C. Sudden interruption of leaflet opening by ventricular contractions: A mechanism of mitral regurgitation. *J. Appl. Physiol.* In press (January 1976).

3. Laniado, S., Yellin, E., Kottler, M., Levy, L., Stadler, J., Terdiman, R. A study of the dynamic relations between the mitral valve echogram and phasic mitral flow. *Circulation* 51:104, 1975.

4. Rushmer, R.F., Finlayson, B.L., Nash, A.A. Movements of the mitral valve. *Circ. Res.* 4:337, 1956.

5 Anatomic-Physiologic Properties of the Mitral Apparatus

Joseph K. Perloff, M.D.

The mitral apparatus is a complex, finely coordinated mechanism that requires for its normal performance the functional integrity of six anatomic elements working in delicate harmony. These elements are: 1) the left atrium, 2) the annulus, 3) the leaflets, 4) the chordae tendineae, 5) the papillary muscles, and 6) the left ventricular wall.[1]

LEFT ATRIUM

Two contributions of the left atrium have been related to competence of the mitral valve: 1) contraction[2] and 2) atrial dilatation.[3] Although it has been affirmed that atrial contraction and relaxation influence mitral valve closure in man[2] (see below), the loss of effective atrial contraction (for example, atrial fibrillation) does not necessarily cause regurgitation.[1] However, left atrial enlargement can contribute to incompetence of the mitral valve (Fig. 1).[3] As that chamber enlarges, its posterior wall is displaced posteriorly and downward.

33

Because of the anatomic continuity of left atrial endocardium and posterior mitral leaflet, displacement exerts tension on this leaflet that may prevent the cusp from contacting its mate, aggravating leaflet malapposition.[1]

MITRAL ANNULUS

The mitral annulus serves two important functions. First, the true annulus is an essential part of the basal attachment or fulcrum of the posterior leaflet.[3] The anterior leaflet is anatomically continuous with the aortic wall and not with the true annulus (Fig. 2). Secondly, the size of the annulus plays a role in preserving competence of the mitral orifice, albeit a role that relates less to dilatation than to a lack of systolic decrease in circumference.[1,2] Annular tissue is pliable, permitting sphincteric contraction during left atrial and left ventricular systole.[2] This contraction diminishes the area that the leaflets must bridge by an estimated 20 to 40%.[1,2,4] Abnormalities causing a decrease in basal left-ventricular circumferential fiber shortening oppose systolic annular contraction. Similarly, with calcification of the

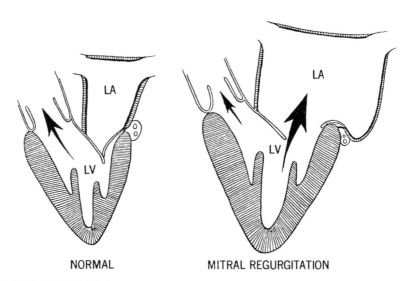

NORMAL   MITRAL REGURGITATION

Figure 1. As the left atrium dilates, its posterior wall tends to exert tension on the posterior mitral leaflet, since this leaflet is continuous with the left atrial endocardium. Note the position of the papillary muscles in the normal left ventricle.

annulus, the mechanism of regurgitation is believed to stem from a loss of sphincteric action.[1]

LEAFLETS

Proper closure of the leaflets represents an important goal of the mitral mechanism. The areas of the two leaflets are nearly identical, but their shapes differ considerably and conform to their functions[1,4] (Fig. 2). The basal attachment of the anterior leaflet is comparatively short, since it is in direct continuity with the aortic wall, which serves as its fulcrum. The basal attachment of the posterior leaflet is comparatively long, since it attaches to the entire length of the true

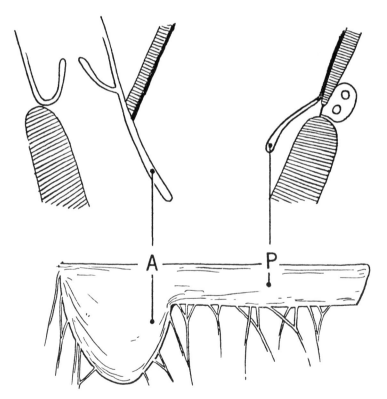

Figure 2. The anterior mitral leaflet (A) is continuous with the aortic wall; the posterior leaflet attaches to the annulus and is primarily a continuation of the mural endocardium of the left atrium. The two leaflets differ in shape but are approximately equal in area.

annulus. However, the basal to free-edge length of the anterior leaflet is two or more times that of the posterior. Consequently, the anterior leaflet is intrinsically more mobile, while the posterior leaflet moves toward its anterior mate chiefly because of movement imparted by the contracting annulus.[1,2] It is not yet clear whether systolic motion of the wall of the aortic root (well seen in echocardiograms) plays a role in the closing movement of the anterior mitral leaflet.

Leaflet abnormalities can be acquired or congenital, with functional derangement resulting from deficient leaflet tissue, excessive leaflet tissue, or restricted leaflet mobility.[1,4] Deficient leaflet tissue has a number of causes; the best known is rheumatic endocarditis, which provokes scarring and contracture. Excessive leaflet tissue results in hoodlike deformities in which the unsupported segment (ruptured chordae tendineae or abnormally long chordae) balloons upward as ventricular systole exerts pressure against its undersurface. Hooding or ballooning of leaflets is seen in the disorder known as the billowing or floppy mitral valve or the systolic click–late systolic murmur syndrome.[1,4] After clicks and late systolic murmurs were initially considered "extracardiac," attention was focused first on prolapse of the posterior leaflet, then on prolapse of both anterior and posterior leaflets; responsible mechanisms now include not only redundant leaflets, but also elongated chordae tendineae and abnormalities of left ventricular wall[1,4,5] (see below). A late systolic murmur and occasionally bizarre musical late systolic whoops or honks may accompany the late systolic regurgitation.[1,4]

Restricted leaflet mobility has a variety of causes. One of the most interesting is the type of leaflet restriction that accompanies congenitally corrected transposition, or l-transposition, of the great arteries (ventricular inversion).[6] In this anomaly, the mitral orifice is equipped with a tricuspid valve (right-to-left inversion of the atrioventricular valves). This left sided A-V valve is often the site of an Ebstein-like anomaly in which the leaflets are attached to the ventricular endocardium by abnormally short chordae, restricting cusp mobility and causing incompetence.[6]

CHORDAE TENDINEAE

Chordal abnormalities that disturb the function of the mitral apparatus include abnormally long chordae, abnormally short chordae, ectopically inserted chordae, fusion of chordae (decreased interchordal slits), and ruptured chordae. Chordae tendineae must be considered in terms of their leaflet attachments, their ventricular attachments, and their individual thicknesses, lengths, and arborization patterns.[1,4] Several different orders of chordae are recognized. Each of the four to six individual heads of the anterior and posterior papillary muscles generally give rise to two primary chordae tendineae. These primary chordae branch and ultimately attach to the edges of the ventricular surfaces of the leaflets as fine, delicate threads—five tertiary chordae for each primary chord. Some chords run as single nonbranching bundles of collagen from their papillary muscle origin to their leaflet insertion. Each of the two papillary muscles, anterior and posterior, give rise to chordae tendineae that cross to and support both anterior and posterior leaflets.

Abnormally long and abnormally short chordae have been commented upon above in the context of leaflet prolapse and ventricular inversion respectively. Ectopically inserted chordae are features of the endocardial-cushion defect and may be prime causes of leaflet incompetence.[6] These chordae spring from the margins of the cleft in the anterior leaflet, not merely from its free edge; they insert directly into septal endocardium, rather than into heads of papillary muscles. Such chordae have no counterpart in the normal heart, and they disturb the vertical axis of tension that contributes to the normal closing motion of the anterior leaflet.[6] Fusion of chordae represents a fault that fundamentally disturbs diastolic flow through the mitral orifice. Flow from left atrium to left ventricle is both central (between the two open leaflets) and peripheral (through interchordal slits). Flow through interchordal slits reciprocally decreases in proportion to the degree of chordal fusion. Chordal rupture (anatomic discontinuity) is functionally important depending upon where in the arborization pattern the discontinuity occurs.[1,4] Rupture of a primary chord results in acute loss of leaflet support and severe regurgitation, while rupture of a tertiary chord may pass unnoticed. In this context, it should be emphasized that the physiologic consequences of acute severe mitral regurgitation stand in contrast to chronic severe mitral regurgitation.[1,4]

PAPILLARY MUSCLES AND LEFT VENTRICULAR WALL

The papillary muscles and left ventricular wall represent the muscular components of the mitral apparatus.[1,4] Papillary muscle dysfunction (Table 1) can occur either with loss in continuity (rupture) or without loss in continuity (fibrosis, ischemia, replacement).

The papillary muscles emerge as single bodies from the left ventricular wall and divide into four to six heads, each serving as an anchor for two primary chordae tendineae.[1] Rupture of a papillary muscle typically results from myocardial infarction, especially of the posteromedial muscle. Sudden loss in continuity causes acute severe mitral regurgitation. The anatomic site at which papillary-muscle rupture occurs is the important determinant of the magnitude of regurgitation and the subsequent clinical course.[1] If rupture is confined to one papillary muscle head, the physiologic derangement is quantitatively similar to rupture of major chordae.[1] If rupture involves the entire papillary muscle, i.e., its central body, approximately half of the support of each leaflet is lost, so that regurgitation is overwhelming and rapidly fatal. In either case, mitral incompetence of papillary-muscle rupture is superimposed upon an acutely infarcted left ventricle, whereas acute regurgitation from chordal rupture usually occurs in an otherwise normal or nearly normal heart.

The anatomic basis of papillary-muscle dysfunction without loss in continuity is still incompletely understood. However, current experimental and clinical evidence indicates that damage confined to a papillary muscle does not necessarily render the mitral valve incompetent unless that damage extends to the adjacent left ventricle.[1] Accordingly, the papillary muscle as a functional unit includes its muscular foundation in the contiguous left ventricular wall.[1] Papillary-muscle dysfunction without loss in continuity can result in either persistent or intermittent mitral regurgitation of varying severity during episodes of ischemia (angina) without infarction.[1,4] See Table 1.

Those aspects of the left ventricular free wall related to the shape of the ventricle per se will now be considered. How might left ventricular enlargement alter the functional integrity of the mitral apparatus? The answer lies chiefly in the effects of altered left-ventricular shape on the position of papillary muscles and the direc-

Table 1.
Papillary Muscle Dysfunction

With Loss in Continuity (Rupture)	Without Loss in Continuity
Infarction	Infarction—Persistent Mitral Incompetence
Trauma (rarely)	Ischemia without Infarction (Angina)—Transient Mitral Incompetence, Mild to Severe

tion of their axes of tension, and on the role of dilatation in preventing the annulus from decreasing its circumferential size during systole[1,4] (see above). The papillary muscles normally arise from the left ventricular wall at its apical and middle thirds (Fig. 1), permitting desirable vertical tension on the chordae tendineae and leaflets during systole, effectively moving the cusps together, and restraining them during ventricular ejection. In contrast, when the papillary muscles are not vertically aligned with the annulus (lateral migration due to spherical dilatation of the left ventricle), the systolic forces exerted on the leaflets via the chordae are in a lateral as opposed to a vertical direction.[3] This lateral tension, especially on the anterior leaflet, interferes with leaflet apposition and contributes to valve incompetence.[1,4] In addition, left ventricular dilatation exerts an unfavorable effect on the annulus by applying a distending pressure that opposes systolic annular contraction, widening the systolic orifice.[1]

Alterations in the shape of the left ventricle have also been held responsible for other varieties of mitral regurgitation. Abnormalities of contraction of the left ventricular wall (segmental changes in left ventricular shape) have been emphasized as contributing causes of mitral valve prolapse.[5] A number of abnormal left ventricular systolic contraction patterns have been observed in this context and may contribute to the inadequate leaflet support that results in or aggravates chordal elongation, leaflet redundancy, and mitral leaflet prolapse.[5]

The change in left ventricular shape associated with aging exerts an unknown effect on the functional integrity of the mitral apparatus. As we grow older, the left ventricular cavity, together with the mitral annulus, normally gets smaller.[4] As cavity and annular sizes decrease, the leaflets and chordae become relatively redundant. Although leaflet and chordal thickening are known to occur in this context,[4] it is not yet clear whether the competence of the mitral valve is affected.

REFERENCES

1. Perloff, J.K., Roberts, W.C. The mitral apparatus. *Circulation* 46:227, 1972.

2. Tsakiris, A.G., von Bernuth, G., Rastelli, G.C., Bourgeois, M.J., Titus, J.L., Wood, E.H. Size and motion of the mitral valve annulus in anesthetized intact dogs. *J. Appl. Physiol.* 30:611, 1971.

3. Levy, M.J., Edwards, J.E. Anatomy of mitral insufficiency. *Prog. in Cardiovasc. Dis.* 5:119, 1962.

4. Roberts, W.C., Perloff, J.K. Mitral valvular disease. *Ann. Int. Med.* 77:939, 1972.

5. Scampardonis, G., Yang, S.S., Maranhao, V., Goldberg, H., Gooch, A.S. Left ventricular abnormalities in prolapsed mitral leaflet syndrome. *Circulation* 48:287, 1973.

6. Perloff, J.K. *The Clinical Recognition of Congenital Heart Disease.* Philadelphia: W.B. Saunders Co., 1970.

7. Edwards, J.E. Mitral insufficiency resulting from "overshooting" of leaflets. *Circulation* 43:606, 1971.

DISCUSSION: PART I

Dr. Frater: I would like to try to get some simplicity back into our discussion of the mitral valve's anatomy. Indeed the anatomy was well described by the old German anatomists. In Figure 1 showing a human mitral valve, there is a large anterior cusp hanging below the root of the aorta. The posterior cusp is smaller but identical in shape and chordal attachments in all mammalian species, and should therefore be regarded as an entity. These two cusps are separated from each other by significant lengths of much shallower tissue, which may be called commissural cusps or commissural tissue, but which are in any case distinct from the anterior and posterior cusps. The description of the chordae may be complicated to almost any degree. The critical part of their description should be related to what they do: namely, support the valve. Except for the short lengths of bare edge in the middle of both anterior and posterior cusps, the whole free edge of the valve is supported by first-order chordae. It does not matter whether these first-order chordae come directly from a papillary muscle or are branches of one sort of arborization or another; cutting any one will result in some insufficiency. The other forms of chordae are the second-order chordae, which are inserted into the body of the anterior cusp away from the edge—the so-called rough-area chordae—and the third order chordae found only on the posterior cusp joining it directly to the wall. There is no need to complicate the description of chordae more than this.

Dr. Bassett: I also want to simplify the anatomy of the chordae. I follow Dr. Ranganathan, but as one first looks at the mitral chordae, one does get confused. First, the point I wish to make is that it becomes simpler if one takes the primary insertions, those attached to the edge of the cusp, as a separate system. They show many variations—they may be single, double, or even triple. They may arborize before their attachment to the cusp. Also they frequently have origin from another group of chordae, usually the one next removed towards the commissures, and the extreme example of this is when they all arise with the commissural chordae and fan out from there.

I regard separately the secondary and tertiary insertions, the "muscle men" of the chordal mechanism. Like others, I recognize three groups to each half of the anterior cusp. In my experience, in 95% of normal valves, these three groups are recognizable. However, it is of interest that less than 50% of abnormal, diseased valves have

41

these groups, the majority having only two, and sometimes one, to one or both halves of the cusp. To illustrate the possible significance of this, consider the case of the valve of a fit lad killed in a motor accident: there was a deformity of the anterior cusp. On turning it over, we found that he had one absent group with hyperplasia of the one next door—what would have happened had he lived?

Dr. Ranganathan: The classification of the chordae presented by the previous speakers here is actually the old classification originally given by Tandler and later by Quain. It is inadequate, in our opinion, if you consider the anatomy of the chordae inserted into the leaflets. I agree entirely with the previous speakers that the location of the leaflet that becomes deficient of chordal support is more important. Implied here is the actual type of chordae that is involved. The "primary chordae," according to the previous definition, would be those that insert into the free edge of the leaflet, and this would correspond to the free-edge branches of the rough-zone chordae. The latter often trifurcate; the free-edge branch would be considered primary while the branch that inserts up into the rough zone along the line of closure would be called "secondary," because it inserts beyond the free edge. So you are actually calling the same chorda by two different names, "primary" and "secondary"; this is incomplete and confusing in itself.

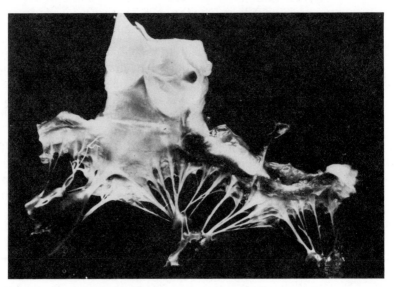

Figure 1. Human mitral valve

Secondly, the commissural chordae would be called "primary" while the basal chordae would be termed "tertiary," and we know the basal chordae may have some function in terms of preventing eversion of the leaflet. Just because the basal chordae are present only in the posterior leaflet does not imply that they are the most important for the integrity of this leaflet. The middle scallop, which is often the largest scallop, has been mistaken for the entire posterior leaflet, and the commissural scallops and their chordae ignored. The unison with which these three scallops move, especially when they are abnormal and prolapsed, shows that they act as a functional unit, as seen in time-motion study of the angiograms. They work together when observed on a pulse duplicator as well. Now if you look at the posteromedial commissural area, we note that it is larger than its anterolateral counterpart. Although it has only a free-edge "primary" chorda, rupture of this chorda can in fact give rise to severe mitral regurgitation because of the wide area of this commissural region. Finally, if you do chordal rupture experiments and if you go step by step, cutting the different types of chordae tendineae, you could demonstrate a variation in the clinical spectrum and hemodynamic degree of mitral regurgitation. So we believe that there is a strong argument in retaining the new classification of chordae, which takes into account the morphologic characteristics of each chorda and its site of insertion rather than lumping them all together.

Dr. Kalmanson: I'd like to put one question to Dr. Tsakiris and to Dr. Perloff. Dr. Tsakiris demonstrated two types of motion of the mitral valve, first that of a sphincter during end-diastole, and second, a downward displacement of the closed mitral floor during systole. On the right side of the heart, i.e., at the site of the tricuspid valve, Dr. C. Veyrat and I have shown that in particular hemodynamic conditions due to right heart disease such as pulmonary stenosis or ventricular septal defect, the physiological downward systolic displacement of the closed tricuspid floor is impeded. Did Dr. Tsakiris or Dr. Perloff meet situations where the downward displacement of the mitral valve—otherwise anatomically normal—was also impeded, for instance in situations such as aortic stenosis?

Dr. Tsakiris: In our experiments, the average magnitude of the excursion of the beads placed on the annulus towards the ventricular apex varied between 3 and 12 mm, under different hemodynamic conditions, and was related to the degree of emptying of the ventricle. In rare occasions, when the ventricular cavity was large and the ejection fraction low, the annulus appeared to remain stationary during ventricular contraction. A motion towards the atrium during sytole was never observed.

Dr. Perloff: In the normal contracting left ventricle, as shown by some of Dr. Tsakiris' slides, and in accord with information from our laboratory in human subjects, the floor of the left atrium moves towards the apex as the long axis of the left ventricle decreases in systole. In a number of conditions there is faulty shortening of the long axis so that the floor of the left atrium may move imperfectly towards the left ventricular apex. One such condition is mitral prolapse with ventricular-wall contractile abnormality. Occasionally in this setting there is virtually no shortening of the long axis of the left ventricle. Similarly in a number of apparently normal elderly people the leaflets tend to move toward the left atrium as the vertical axis or the long axis of the left ventricle diminishes with age. The idea of the floor of the left atrium moving toward the apex, in a fashion analogous to Dr. Kalmanson's observations on the tricuspid valve, certainly does hold in the mitral location, and Dr. Tsakiris's slides of the dog confirm this beautifully. I think he also indicated that the plane of the leaflets remains relatively perpendicular to the long axis as the floor moves toward the apex.

SUMMARY: PART I

Joseph K. Perloff, M.D.

An understanding of the anatomy and physiology of the normal mitral apparatus is a sine qua non for further study. In this context, sophisticated investigation of normal and abnormal structure and function, as well as the design and results of therapeutic interventions, can best be understood. Accordingly, the opening session of the symposium provided a necessary overview and framework within which the topics that followed could be most appropriately considered.

The mitral apparatus is a complex, finely coordinated mechanism that requires for its functional integrity six anatomic elements working in delicate harmony. These elements are: 1) the left atrium, 2) the annulus, 3) the leaflets, 4) the chordae tendineae, 5) the papillary muscles, and 6) the left ventricular wall. Each component must be considered individually, in the context of the apparatus as a whole, in relation to the mode of closure of the normal mitral valve, and in the light of the many acquired and congenital disorders that disturb the harmony of the mechanism, rendering it abnormal. Drs. Ranganathan, Tsakiris, Yacoub, and Perloff all addressed themselves to this topic.

The left atrium affects the function of the mitral apparatus in two ways: contraction and dilatation. It has been affirmed that left atrial contraction and relaxation result in mitral valve closure in humans, but loss of effective atrial contraction does not necessarily result in mitral regurgitation. Experimental observations described by Tsakiris suggest that one of the functions of left atrial contraction is the reduction in size of the mitral annulus before the onset of left ventricular systole. The second way that the left atrium affects mitral apparatus function is dilatation (Perloff). As the left atrium enlarges, it exerts tension on the posterior leaflet because of anatomic continuity of atrial endocardium and posterior mitral cusp, shortening the effective size of the cusp, which intrinsically has a relatively short basal to free-edge length.

The mitral annulus serves two important functions (Perloff). First, it is an essential part of the basal attachment or fulcrum of the posterior leaflet, and second, the annulus acts as a sphincter, decreasing its circumference by as much as 40% from diastole to end systole. Phasic variations in the size, shape, and position of the mitral annulus during the cardiac cycle were experimentally studied by Tsakiris

45

during changes in rate with sinus rhythm, with atrial fibrillation, and with complete AV block, demonstrating eccentric narrowing of the annulus with both left atrial and left ventricular systole.

The areas of the two mitral leaflets are nearly identical, but their anatomy differs and conforms to their functions. Chordae tendineae were considered according to their leaflet and ventricular attachments, thicknesses, lengths, and arborization patterns. Drs. Ranganathan, Yacoub, and Perloff discussed leaflet-chordal anatomy and function. The basal attachment of the anterior leaflet is relatively short because of direct continuity with the aortic wall, which serves as a fulcrum. The basal attachment of the posterior leaflet is comparatively long, because it attaches to the entire length of the true annulus. However, the basal to free-edge length of the anterior leaflet is two or more times that of the posterior, rendering the former more mobile and the latter more supportive. Yacoub described the configuration and measurements of the mitral cusps in 40 calf and 20 human hearts, concluding that the anatomy of the leaflets and chordae is fairly constant and closely related to function. A new classification and nomenclature were proposed, permitting accurate identification of individual chordae. Ranganathan also addressed himself to classification of chordae, especially according to sites of leaflet insertion. Specific fan-shaped chordae defined the commissures between anterior and posterior leaflets. The posterior leaflet was found to be triscalloped (large middle scallop and two smaller commissural scallops), with fan-shaped chordae defining the clefts between the individual scallops.

The papillary muscles and left ventricular wall represent the muscular components of the mitral apparatus. Three morphologic types of left ventricular papillary muscles were defined by Ranganathan, namely, free and fingerlike, completely tethered to the ventricular wall, or intermediate. Arterial supply to papillary muscle was studied by stereoscopic angiography. The papillary muscle as a functional unit includes the contiguous portion of the left ventricular wall; papillary muscle dysfunction with and without loss of continuity was discussed in the light of anatomic and physiologic considerations (Perloff). Finally, left ventricular shape and contraction patterns were assigned roles in the anatomy and function of the mitral apparatus (Perloff). The effects of overall geometric alteration as well as generalized and segmental abnormalities of contraction were identified. Spherical dilatation results in lateral migration of papillary muscles, which then exert an undesirable lateral axis of tension on the leaflets. Spherical dilatation, decreased contractility, and increased wall tension combine to oppose the expected decrease in annular circumferential size during atrial and ventricular systole. The long axis of the left ventricle and the left ventricular cavity get smaller with age, rendering leaflet-chordal length relatively redundant.

In summary, this session dealt with the anatomy and physiology of the six components of the mitral apparatus, setting the stage for the remarks that followed.

PART TWO

PATHOLOGY
OF NATURAL
AND ARTIFICIAL
MITRAL VALVES

6 Recent Advances in the Knowledge of Pathology of Natural and Artificial Valves*

Malcolm D. Silver, M.D.

This is an exciting era for anyone interested in the mitral valve. Recent years have seen a gradual diminution in the frequency of rheumatic valvular disease in developed countries. Because of this and the introduction of new and different methods of clinical investigation, a number of nonrheumatic mitral valve conditions have been defined recently. They are probably not new but were unrecognized in the past because of our tendency to equate mitral and rheumatic disease. Rheumatic disease frequently causes mitral valve dysfunction, but we now appreciate that other pathological entities must be excluded. In this presentation, I will concentrate on a few aspects of the pathology of mitral disease in adults.

MITRAL VALVE STENOSIS

Stenosis of a natural mitral valve may result from an extracardiac object compressing the annular area or from an intracavitary object in

*Supported by grants from the Ontario Heart Foundation.

51

the left atrium impinging on the valve lumen, e.g., an atrial myxoma. Far more often, however, stenosis is the consequence of changes in the valve structures themselves, producing either leaflet stiffening or fusion of adjacent sides of the leaflets in the commissural area (commissural fusion), or a combination of these.[1]

Antecedent and probably recurrent attacks of rheumatic fever are the most common cause of these changes, with the repeated episodes damaging the valve and preparing it for secondary changes induced by altered hemodynamics. These attacks cause the formation, on the valve surfaces, of minute thrombi that subsequently organize to produce leaflet thickening and/or chordal shortening.[2] The clinical outcome may be valvular stenosis, or incompetence, or a combination of these. If stenosis results, the gross lesion presents as a funnel-shaped orifice caused by commissural fusion; chordal changes, involving thickening and fusion, may or may not be marked. In most instances a pathologist can safely make a diagnosis of rheumatic disease on gross findings alone. However, mitral stenosis has been reported in patients with familial pseudoxanthoma elasticum,[3] and if this condition is suspected, histological sections must be made. Elastic fibrillae that are abnormally coarse, curled, and fragmented, and appear like those found in skin lesions, are obvious in the leaflet tissue (Fig. 1). Whether this condition may be differentiated from rheumatic mitral stenosis by echocardiography or other clinical methods remains to be determined.

MITRAL VALVE INCOMPETENCE

Closure of a natural mitral valve involves the coordinated action of components of the valve complex.[4] Any pathological process that interferes with their function, either singly or in combination, may cause insufficiency. Let us discuss some of these processes.

Prolapse of the Mitral Valve

This condition is presently the subject of intense interest with regard to its auscultatory, electrocardiographic, echocardiographic, and angiographic findings.[5-16] Clinically, it is associated with several congenital and acquired conditions. Pathological correlations have developed slowly, because few patients have disease severe enough to warrant sugical intervention or to cause death.[17-25]

Myxomatous degeneration of the mitral valve is one common cause.[5-24] It occurs in families,[26] especially in those with Marfan's syndrome,[27,28] or as an isolated phenomenon. Usually, more females are affected than males.

Part or all of the anterior and/or posterior leaflet, but particularly the latter, is abnormal in the gross; other heart valves or the aorta may be affected in the same individual. The involved mitral leaflet is voluminous, soft, thickened, and grey-white. It has a shiny surface, a moist, gelatinous appearance when sectioned, and is deformed (prolapsed) towards the left atrium. If the deformity is not marked it is dome-shaped, and the rough zone, where chordae insert, is principally affected. Coaptation may be normal at this stage, but an abnormal movement of leaflets or chordae produces a midsystolic click. If severe, the leaflet deformity is hoodlike; both rough zone and more of the leaflet's base are involved (Fig. 2). Then, due to the prolapse, normal coaptation is impossible, and a midsystolic murmur is heard. A variation in extent of the leaflet involvement probably explains the variable echocardiographic findings. Possibly, the severity

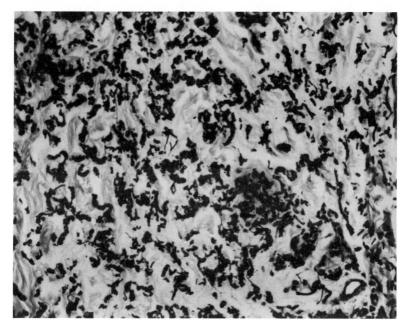

Figure 1. Coarse, fragmented, and curled elastic fibers found in the mitral valve in familial pseudoxanthoma elasticum, here demonstrated in a skin lesion. Combined Verhoeff Elastic-Masson trichrome stain X50.

54

of the deformity mirrors chronicity. If marked, thrombus forms at the base of the leaflet in the angle between it and the adjacent left ventricular wall. Yet thromboembolic phenomena have not been emphasized clinically. Rarely, myxomatous leaflets are calcified. Near their free margins, severely deformed leaflets may look like a series of arches because of extra indentations in their substance and free edge. The indentations must be differentiated from normal clefts in the posterior leaflet to prevent errors in the angiographic/pathologic correlations now possible.[10,11] Chordae attached to the deformed leaflets are often elongated. They may be attenuated, but are usually thickened and may be fused near their insertion. Also, rough zone chordae inserting into the affected leaflet may show more than their usual complement of cords.

The hearts examined at autopsy showed a variable amount of coronary artery disease, usually not severe. Focal areas of fibrosis are found in the subendocardium of the left ventricle. The relationship of these findings both to a patient's chest pain and to the abnormal

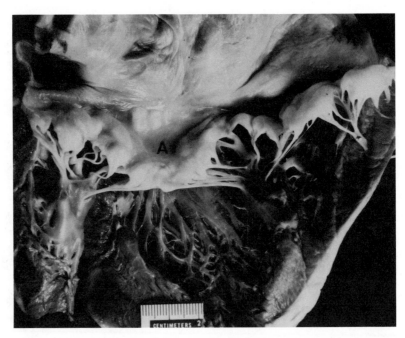

Figure 2. Gross appearance of prolapsed mitral valve due to myxomatous degeneration affecting both anterior (A) and posterior leaflets—here with four scallops. Note hooded appearance of thickened scallops, elongated chordae.

movements of the left ventricular wall noted in the condition[29] is still not clear.

Histologically, the central core of the leaflet (fibrosa and spongiosa) is replaced by loosely arranged myxomatous tissue rich in glycoprotein, with the change becoming more marked as one proceeds distally (Fig. 3). In my view, the change must affect the central plate diffusely to justify a diagnosis of prolapse, since focal myxomatous degeneration may be found in the mitral leaflets in other conditions. Part of the leaflet thickening is caused by this change and part by connective tissue sclerosis on both surfaces, but particularly in the atrial surface. Areas of myxomatous degeneration are often obvious in the mitral annulus and adjacent chordae. These changes

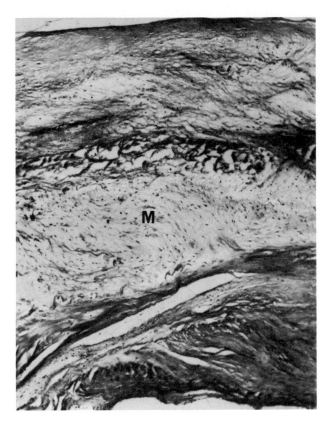

Figure 3. Myxomatous change (M) affecting spongiosa and to a lesser extent fibrosa of posterior mitral valve leaflet. Atrial (upper) and ventricular surfaces are thickened by connective tissue. Hematoxylin & eosin X16.

make the patients prone both to chordal rupture, usually manifested by a sudden worsening of their clinical state (7 in this series of 26 cases), and to prosthesis dehiscence if the valve is replaced. Infective endocarditis, aneurysm formation in the leaflets, and a patient's liability to sudden death are other complications.

Some cases of myxomatous degeneration are due to a congenital abnormality of the connective tissue.[27,28] The cause in others is unknown. Possibly the lesion represents a bizarre reparative response, induced by abnormal stress or strains placed on chordae or leaflets by a dyssynchronous contraction of the left ventricle, mirrored by electrocardiographic findings.[30]

Myxomatous degeneration, with or without chordal rupture, is not the only cause of mitral valve prolapse. Five other patients had anomalous arrangements of their chordae tendineae.[31] The leaflet tissue was myxomatous and thrown into folds. Another young female had a prolapsed mitral valve with morphological features of incomplete differentiation.[32] Two others had an accentuated form of nodular sclerosis affecting most of the leaflets, with only focal myxomatous degeneration histologically. Possibly this latter condition is like that which causes mitral insufficiency and heart failure in elderly dogs. Thus, the pathologist sees a variety of lesions producing mitral valve prolapse. Defining clinical/pathological correlations will keep us all intrigued and busy in the future.

Patients with ruptured chordae tendineae or papillary muscles usually have a sudden onset of symptoms and distinct clinical findings,[33,34] but differentiation from prolapse due to myxomatous change may be difficult. Pathological differentiation depends upon microscopic findings. Such valves do not show diffuse myxomatous changes in their leaflets, but may have myxomatous foci in the affected chordae.

Whipple's Disease

McAllister and Fenoglio[35] have redrawn attention to the cardiac involvement in Whipple's disease. In particular, some of their patients had soft, apical systolic murmurs and, in the gross, marked thickening of leaflets and chordae comparable to that produced by rheumatic valvular disease. Histologically, macrophages filled with periodic acid–Schiff positive granules were found in the sclerosed mitral valve leaflets. Rod-shaped bodies that resemble bacteria and are observed in jejunal biopsies of patients with the disease were demonstrable in the macrophages by electron microscopy (Fig. 4). The findings provide the first morphological demonstration that a mitral valvular deformity may be caused by a persistent, intrinsic, infectious agent.

Systemic Lupus Erythematosus

Bulkley and Roberts[36] described three patients in whom the use of steroids prolonged life and permitted, in their opinion, the healing of Libman-Sacks endocarditis. As a result, the posterior leaflets and their chordae were firmly bound to the underlying mural endocardium by dense fibrous tissue containing plasma cells and calcium deposits, while the anterior leaflets were diffusely scarred. The changes caused severe mitral regurgitation, fatal in two patients, and heart failure requiring valve replacement in a third.

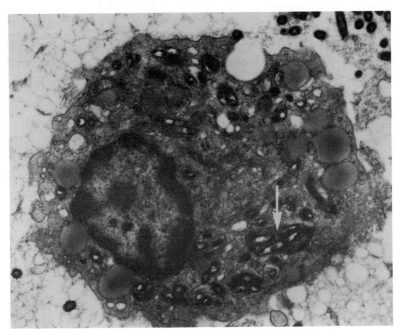

Figure 4. Electron micrographs of P.A.S. positive macrophage from case of Whipple's disease. Arrow defines rod-like bacteria in cytoplasm. Similar macrophages are found in pericardium, myocardium, and endocardium.

STENOSIS AND INCOMPETENCE OF MITRAL
PROSTHETIC VALVES

Certain complications that cause stenosis or incompetence and induce prosthetic malfunction are common to all types; others are uniquely associated with particular prostheses because of their design or structure.[37-39] The clinical manifestations they produce depend upon the severity of the resultant malfunction.

Stenosis of Prostheses

The resting pressure gradient found across each prosthesis after insertion means that each produces a minimal degree of stenosis. Bland thrombus formation and thrombotic vegetations associated with infective endocarditis are the major causes of acquired prosthetic stenosis (Fig. 5). These thrombi, or a tough pannus formed by their organization, extend into or across the orifice. Such bland thrombi form rapidly if a patient develops heart failure or stops taking an-

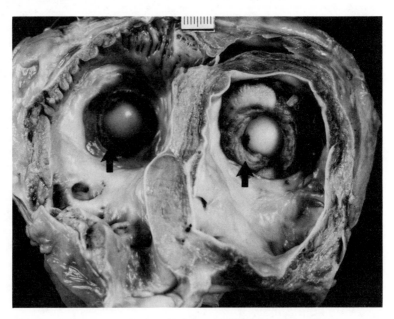

Figure 5.   Atrial aspects of tricuspid (left) and mitral Starr-Edwards prostheses inserted three years before death. Thrombus (arrows) deposited at the interface between cloth sewing ring and metal inner ring constricts the lumen of both prostheses. (Scale = 1 cm)

ticoagulants. They are more troublesome in disc than ball-valve prostheses.

Incompetence of Prostheses

Prosthetic incompetence is caused by pathological processes that act beyond the prosthesis or directly affect its function.

Complications Common to All Prostheses Small paravalvular leaks occur when sutures or tissue separate at the perimeter of a prosthesis. They are uncommon and diminish in frequency as the technical expertise of a surgical team increases. Pre-existing changes in the annular tissue increase the risk of suture separation. For example, sutures may be difficult to set in a heavily calcified annulus, or diseases, such as infective endocarditis or myxomatous change, may weaken the tissue. Large dehiscences are often caused by infective endocarditis. They may tilt the valve and cause abnormal rocking or tilting during the cardiac cycle which is obvious on fluoroscopy. All dehiscences increase the risk of red cell destruction.

Thrombus (bland or vegetations of infective endocarditis), or tissue projecting into a prosthetic cage as a result of ingrowth, or disproportion between a prosthesis and the chamber into which it projects may interfere with the normal movement or seating of an occluder (Fig. 6).

Complications Unique to Certain Prostheses Wearing at the edge of a disc poppet may make it incompetent or cause it to catch in a tilted position. The cloth covering of ball or disc valves may also wear and interfere with poppet movement. Alternatively, thrombus may accumulate on the cloth at the apex of the cage, and a poppet will stick fast to it. Fracture of the struts of cages has occurred in some prostheses, with sudden incompetence.

The cusps of allograft and heterograft prostheses may perforate following infection, or they may disintegrate as a result of degenerative processes or heavy calcification. Fascia lata valves, particularly those in mitral and tricuspid areas, become incompetent as a result of cusp shrinkage.

I have briefly reviewed some of the pathology of the mitral valve revealed as the incidence of rheumatic valvular disease diminishes and new methods of diagnosing and treating valvular heart disease are introduced. I hope an epidemiologist will challenge my assumption of a cause/effect relationship here, so that the effect of some presently unsuspected noxious agents that might induce mitral disease will not be missed.

60

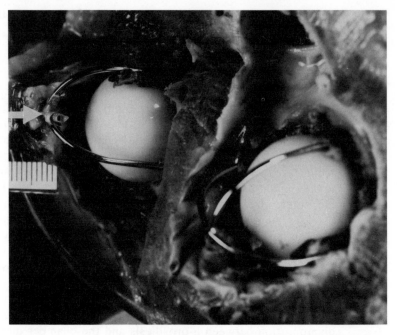

Figure 6. Ventricular aspect of prostheses illustrated in Figure 5 (tricuspid valve to left). Note thrombus formation along struts of cage. Disproportion between the tricuspid prosthesis and right ventricular cavity has caused one strut and the apex of the cage (arrow) to become incorporated into the ventricular wall, interfering with poppet movement and causing prosthesis dysfunction. (Scale = 1 cm)

REFERENCES

1. Rusted, I.E., Scheifley, C.H., Edwards, J.E. Studies of mitral valve; certain anatomic features of the mitral valve and associated structures in mitral stenosis. *Circulation.* 14:398, 1956.

2. Magarey, F.R. Pathogenesis of mitral stenosis. *Brit. Med. J.* 1:856, 1951.

3. Coffman, J.D., Sommers, S.C. Familial pseudoxanthoma elasticum and valvular heart disease. *Circulation* 19:242, 1959.

4. Silverman, M.E., Hurst, J.W. The mitral complex; interaction of the anatomy, physiology, and pathology of the mitral annulus, mitral valve leaflets, chordae tendineae, and papillary muscles. *Am. Heart J.* 76:399, 1968.

5. Barlow, J.B., Bosman, C.K. Aneurysmal protrusion of

the posterior leaflet of the mitral valve. An auscultatory-electrocardiographic syndrome. *Am. Heart J.* 71:166, 1966.

6. Criley, J.M., Lewis, K.B., Humphries, J.O., Ross, R.S. Prolapse of the mitral valve: clinical and cine-angiographic findings. *Br. Heart J.* 28:488, 1966.

7. Hancock, E.W., Cohn, K. The syndrome associated with midsystolic click and late systolic murmur. *Am. J. Med.* 41:183, 1966.

8. Barlow, J.B., Bosman, C.K., Pocock, W.A., Marchand, P. Late systolic murmurs and non-ejection ("mid-late") systolic clicks. An analysis of 90 patients. *Br. Heart J.* 30:203, 1968.

9. Engle, M.A. The syndrome of apical systolic click, late systolic murmur, and abnormal T waves. *Circulation* 39:1-2, 1969.

10. Jeresaty, R.M. Mitral valve prolapse-click syndrome. *Prog. Cardiovasc. Dis.* 15:623, 1973.

11. Ranganathan, N., Silver, M.D., Robinson, T.I., Kostuk, W.J., Felderhof, C.H., Patt, N.L., Wilson, J.K., Wigle, E.D. Angiographic-morphologic correlation in patients with severe mitral regurgitation due to prolapse of the posterior mitral valve leaflet. *Circulation* 48:514, 1973.

12. Ranganathan, N., Silver, M.D., Wigle, E.D. Mitral valve prolapse (letter to the editor). *Circulation* 49:1268, 1974.

13. Dillow, J.C., Haine, C.L., Chang, S., Feigenbaum, H. Use of echocardiography in patients with prolapsed mitral valve. *Circulation* 43:503, 1971.

14. Popp, R.L., Brown, O.R., Silverman, J.F., Harrison, D.C. Echocardiographic abnormalities in the mitral valve prolapse syndrome. *Circulation* 44:428, 1974.

15. DeMaria, A.M., King, J.F., Bogren, H.G., Lies, J.E., Mason, D.T. The variable spectrum of echocardiographic manifestations of the mitral valve prolapse syndrome. *Circulation* 50:33, 1974.

16. Betriu, A., Wigle, E.D., Felderhof, C.H., McLoughlin, M.J. Prolapse of the posterior leaflet of the mitral valve associated with secundum atrial septal defect. *Am. J. Cardiol.* 35:363, 1975.

17. Fernex, M., Fernex, C. La dégénérescence mucoide des valvules mitrales his repercussions functionelles. *Helv. Med. Acta.* 25:694, 1958.

18. Read, R.C., Thal, A.P., Wendt, V.E. Symptomatic valvular myxomatous transformation (the floppy valve syndrome). A possible forme fruste of the Marfan Syndrome. *Circulation* 32:897, 1965.

19. Bittar, N., Sosa, J.A. The billowing mitral valve leaflet. Report on fourteen patients. *Circulation* 38:763, 1968.

20. Pomerance, A. Ballooning deformity (mucoid degeneration) of atrioventricular valves. *Br. Heart J.* 31:343, 1969.

21. Frable, W.J. Mucinous degeneration of the cardiac valves: the "floppy valve" syndrome. *J. Thorac. and Cardiovasc. Surg.* 58:62, 1969.

22. Trent, J.K., Adelman, A.G., Wigle, E.D., Silver, M.D. Morphology of a prolapsed posterior mitral valve leaflet. *Am. Heart J.* 79:539, 1970.

23. Davis, R.H., Schuster, B., Knoebel, S.B., Fisch, C. Myxomatous degeneration of the mitral valve. *Am. J. Cardiol.* 28:449, 1971.

24. Kern, W.H., Tucker, B.L. Myxoid changes in cardiac valves: pathologic, clinical, and ultrastructural studies. *Am. Heart J.* 84: No. 3, 294, 1972.

25. McKay, R., Yacoub, M.H. Clinical and pathological findings in patients with "floppy" valves treated surgically. *Circulation,* Suppl. III to Vols. 47 and 48, 63, 1973.

26. Hunt, D., Sloman, G. Prolapse of the posterior leaflet of the mitral valve occurring in eleven members of a family. *Am. Heart J.* 78:149, 1969.

27. Anderson, R.E., Grondin, C., Amplatz, K. The mitral valve in the Marfan's Syndrome. *Radiology* 91:910, 1968.

28. Bowers, D. Pathogenesis of primary abnormalities of the mitral valve in Marfan's Syndrome. *Br. Heart J.* 6:679, 1969.

29. Scampardonis, G., Yang, S.S., Maranháo, V., Goldberg, H., Gooch, A.S. Left ventricular abnormalities in prolapsed mitral leaflet syndrome. *Circulation* 48:287, 1973.

30. Ranganathan, N. Personal communication, 1975.

31. Edwards, J.E. Mitral insufficiency resulting from 'overshooting' of leaflets. *Circulation* 43:606, 1971.

32. Bharati, S., Lev, M. Congenital polyvalvular disease. *Circulation* 47:575, 1973.

33. Auger, P., Wigle, E.D. Sudden, severe mitral insufficiency. *Canad. Med. Assoc. J.* 96:1493, 1967.

34. Selzer, A., Kelly, J.J. Jr., Vannitamby, M., Walker, P., Gerbode, F., Kerth, W.J. The syndrome of mitral insufficiency due to isolated rupture of the chordae tendineae. *Am. J. Med.* 43:822, 1967.

35. McAllister, H.A. Jr., Fenoglio, J.J. Cardiac involvement in Whipple's disease. *Circulation.* 52:152, 1975.

36. Bulkley, B.H., Roberts, W.C. Systemic lupus erythem-

atosus as a cause of severe mitral regurgitation. *Am. J. Cardiol.* 35:305, 1975.

37. Hudson, R.E.B. *Cardiovascular Pathology.* Vol. 1-3. London: Edward Arnold, 1965.

38. Roberts, W.C., Bulkley, B.H., Morrow, A.G. Pathologic anatomy of cardiac valve replacement. A study of 224 necropsy patients. *Prog. Cardiovasc. Dis.* 15:539, 1973.

39. Silver, M.D. Cardiac Pathology—A look at the last five years: II. The pathology of cardiovascular prostheses. *Hum. Pathol.* 1:127, 1974.

7 Pathology of the Mitral Valve

Introduction to Plastic and
Reconstructive Valve Surgery

A. Carpentier, M.D., Ph.D.
J. Guerinon, M.D.
A. Deloche, M.D.
J.N. Fabiani, M.D.
J. Relland, M.D.

The development of techniques for mitral valve reconstruction presupposes a precise knowledge of the lesions encountered. The present study analyzes the anatomic findings at autopsy of 100 human hearts with either rheumatic or dystrophic noncalcified valvular disease, and those observed at the time of operation in a series of 400 mitral valve repairs. Anatomic study consisted of a precise measurement of the various valve structures; intra-operative observations allowed us to analyze accurately the shape of the annulus and the physiology of the leaflets of the living, beating heart.

TERMINOLOGY

Since several terms are used in the literature to define the same structure of the mitral valve, it is necessary to begin by reviewing the terminology used in the present study. Aortic (anterior) and the mural (posterior) leaflets are separated by anteroseptal and postero-medial

65

commissures, which can be identified by the tips of the corresponding papillary muscles,[9,10] and by the commissural chordae.[7] The commissural chordae arise from the tip of the papillary muscle as a single stem that branches radially in a fan-like fashion to insert into the free margin of the commissural regions[6] (Fig. 1).

The anterior and posterior leaflets present a rough zone which is the area of contact of both leaflets during systole. In this study, this zone is called the "closure area." The margin of the mural leaflet generally presents two indentations, giving rise to a scalloped appear-

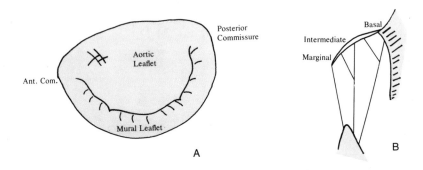

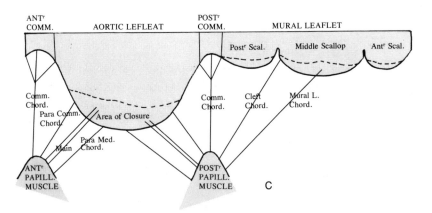

Figure 1. Schematic representation of the normal anatomy of the mitral valve apparatus. A—View from left atrium. B—Cross sectional view showing site of insertion of the chordae on the leaflet. C—Mitral apparatus opened showing the various components.

ance. A middle scallop, a postero-medial scallop, and an antero-lateral scallop may be identified.[7]

The chordae are categorized according to the site of their insertion on the leaflets: marginal, basal, and intermediate. This classification is the most reliable and useful for surgical application (Fig. 1 B).

Marginal chordae insert into the free margin of the leaflet, whether or not they have a prolongation of their insertion on the ventricular surface of the leaflet.

Basal chordae insert at the point of attachment of the leaflet to the annulus.

Intermediate chordae insert in the middle area between the free margin and the base of the leaflet.

Chordae are also defined as belonging to their corresponding leaflets (Fig. 1 C).

Aortic leaflet chordae arising from the anterior papillary muscle consist of three types: Main chordae anterior—large chordae of the intermediate type inserted on the rough zone of the leaflet. Paramedial anterior—thin chordae of the marginal type inserted near the middle of the edge. Paracommissural anterior—thin chordae of the marginal type inserted between the main chordae and the commissural chordae.

Aortic chordae arising from the posterior papillary muscle include: Main chordae posterior—large chordae of the intermediate type inserted on the rough zone of the leaflet. Paramedial posterior—thin chordae of the marginal type inserted near the middle of the edge. Paracommissural posterior—thin chordae of the marginal type inserted between the main chordae and the commissural chordae.

Commissural chordae arising from the anterior papillary muscle: Anterior commissural chordae—thin chordae of the marginal type arising as a single stem and inserting into valves at the anterior commissure.[6]

Commissural chordae arising from the posterior papillary muscle: Posterior commissural chordae—thin chordae of the marginal type arising as a single stem and inserting into valves at the posterior commissures.

Mural leaflet chordae: Chordae of the middle scallops—thin chordae of the marginal intermediate or basal type. Cleft chordae corresponding to the indentations of the leaflet— thin chordae of the marginal type.[6]

MATERIAL AND METHODS

The 100 human hearts with rheumatic or dystrophic valvular disease were compared with 50 normal hearts which served as reference. The average weight of the normal hearts was 340 gm. The 100 pathological hearts were divided into four groups.

Rheumatic valvular insufficiency: 30 specimens—average weight: 620 gm. This group was characterized by major insufficiency with a commissural fusion of less than 5 mm and without ruptured chordae.

Rheumatic combined valvular insufficiency and stenosis: 30 specimens—average weight: 580 gm. This group consisted of cases of non calcified mitral valve disease with associated insufficiency and mild stenosis (1 to 2 finger breadths).

Dystrophic mitral insufficiency: 20 specimens—average weight: 630 gm. This group included cases of mitral valve insufficiency with no previous history of rheumatic fever, and without typical rheumatic lesions, i.e., fusion of the commissures, shortening and fusion of the chordae, thickening and shrinkage of the leaflets.

Dystrophic mitral insufficiency with ruptured chordae: 20 specimens—average weight: 560 gm. Ruptured chordae of rheumatic origin or due to bacterial endocarditis were excluded from this group. The ruptured chordae belonged to the mural leaflet in 11 cases, to the aortic leaflet in 5 cases, and to both leaflets in 4 cases.

The hearts used in the anatomic study were obtained at autopsy. In contrast to most studies, no distinction was made between the measurements on the basis of sex, because it was felt that the differences were related more to body size than to sex. The average height of the subjects studied measured 1.66 m, with a range of 1.50 m to 1.82 m ($\pm$ 10%). All measurements represent averages which have been rounded off to the nearest millimeter.

Intra-operative observations were made on a series of 400 mitral valve repairs carried out under extra-corporeal circulation. The mitral valve was approached through a median sternotomy and a left atriotomy. The heart was kept beating. The shape of the annulus was analyzed while the aorta was unclamped. The motion of the leaflets was observed, with the aorta crossclamped to avoid air embolism.

RESULTS

Table 1
Normal Heart

Circumference: 116 mm ± 3.5	
Aortic leaflet	
Attachment	32 mm ± 1.3
Height	23 mm ± 0.9
Closure area	14 mm ± 1.1
Main chordae anterior	19 mm ± 0.4
posterior	17 mm ± 0.2
Para-commissural anterior	17 mm ± 0.3
Para-medial anterior	15 mm ± 0.5
Mural leaflet	
Attachment	55 mm ± 2.2
Height middle scallop	14 mm ± 0.9
anterior scallop	9 mm ± 1
posterior scallop	10 mm ± 1.2
Closure area middle scallop	8 mm ± 0.9
Middle scallop chordae marginal	14 mm ± 2.9
basal	8 mm ± 1.7
Cleft chordae	13 mm ± 3.7
Anterior commissural leaflet	
Attachment	12 mm ± 3.3
Height	8 mm ± 1
Commissural chordae	13 mm ± 0.2
Posterior commissural leaflet	
Attachment	17 mm ± 0.8
Height	8 mm
Commissural chordae	15 mm ± 0.05

Table 1 shows the measurements of the **normal heart.** The shape of the normal orifice is ovoid, the main axis being transverse from one commissure to the other. However, the orifice becomes kidney-shaped when the aorta is filled, due to the redundance of the aortic root. With the heart beating, the orifice area is reduced during systole by the advancement of the base of the aortic leaflet and the contraction of the annulus at the mural leaflet. This reduces the orifice area by approximately 25%.

Table 2 presents the measurements of hearts with **rheumatic valvular insufficiency.** Comparison of these measurements with those of normal valve (N =. . .) and operative findings suggested the following (Fig. 2):

Dilatation of the annulus was significant, being approximately 25% more than normal, and affected mainly the posterior commissure. Dilatation of the aortic leaflet was not significant.

Table 2
Rheumatic Valvular Insufficiency

Circumference: 147 mm ± 4.9 (normal 116 mm) p < 0.05

Aortic leaflet

Attachment	35 mm ± 1.9 (N = 32 mm)†
Height	24 mm ± 1.9 (N = 23 mm)†
Closure area	17 mm ± 1.6 (N = 14 mm)*
Main chordae anterior	22 mm ± 0.7 (N = 19 mm)*
posterior	15 mm ± 0.6 (N = 17 mm)*
Para-commissural anterior	23 mm ± 1.2 (N = 17 mm)*
Para-medial anterior	23 mm ± 1.5 (N = 15 mm)*

Mural leaflet

Attachment	71 mm ± 3.6 (N = 55 mm)*
Height middle scallop	15 mm ± 1.1 (N = 14 mm)†
Closure area middle scallop	7 mm ± 1 (N = 8 mm)†
Middle scallop chordae marginal	10 mm ± 0.3 (N = 14 mm)*
basal	6 mm ± 0.6 (N = 8 mm)†
Cleft chordae	11 mm ± 0.8 (N = 13 mm)†

Anterior commissural leaflet

Attachment	15 mm ± 1 (N = 12 mm)*
Commissural chordae	14 mm ± 1.2 (N = 13 mm)†

Posterior commissural leaflet

Attachment	25 mm ± 2.3 (N = 17 mm)*
Commissural chordae	19 mm ± 0.2 (N = 15 mm)*

* Statistically significant (Student's test)
† Not statistically significant.

The chordae of the anterior leaflet were elongated, particularly the paramedial and the paracommissural chordae.

The posterior commissural chordae were also elongated, whereas the anterior commissural chordae were not.

In contrast with these, the chordae of the mural leaflet were shortened and often thickened, which seems to be characteristic of rheumatic mitral valve insufficiency.

The height of the leaflets was not significantly changed.

It should be pointed out that all of the structures were altered, but not necessarily in the same manner. In spite of the fact that the average length of the chordae was increased, some chordae were shortened, particularly the intermediate chordae of the mural leaflet.

The valvular tissue displayed marked changes: the mural leaflet was thickened and the clefts were no longer visible. The anterior leaflet was less altered, with the exception of the closure area, which was thickened and sometimes calcified. Commissural areas were thickened, making it difficult to recognize the exact site of the commissures. The shape of the annulus was changed: the main axis became vertical instead of horizontal, and in most cases the deformation was asymmetrical, the dilatation being more marked at the posterior commissure. With the heart beating, there was no change in the shape of the orifice and no reduction in its size during systole.

Table 3 shows that, in the case of **combined mitral valve disease and insufficiency,** the size of the annulus was significantly reduced due to the retraction of the commissures and the mural leaflet. The aortic valve attachment was normal or even slightly dilated. The valvular tissue was thickened and retracted, particularly at the mural leaflet and the commissure (Fig. 3).

All of the chordae were shortened, thickened, or fused. Some were selectively elongated. It is of some practical importance to point out that thickening and rigidity of the mural leaflet were often due

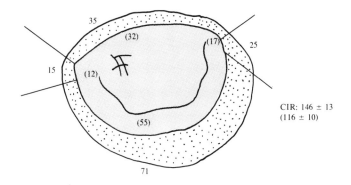

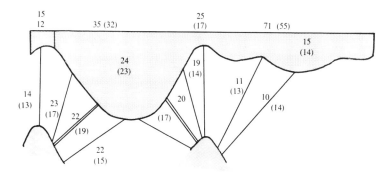

Figure 2. Rheumatic valvular insufficiency. Measurements of the various structures in comparison with normal measurements shown in parentheses.

Table 3
Combined Mitral Valve Disease and Insufficiency

Circumference: 106 mm ± 1.7 (N = 116 mm) p < 0.005*
Aortic leaflet

Attachment	34 mm ± 2 (N = 32 mm)†
Height	24 mm ± 1.7 (N = 23 mm)†
Closure area	9 mm ± 0.8 (N = 14 mm)*
Main chordae anterior	12 mm ± 1.9 (N = 19 mm)*
posterior	11 mm ± 1.7 (N = 17 mm)*

Para-commissural and para-medial chordae were most often fused with the main chordae. In some cases, however, they were well individualized and elongated.
Mural leaflet and fused anterior and posterior commissural leaflets:

Attachment	72 mm ± 2.05 (N = 84 mm)*
Height middle scallop	12 mm ± 1.4 (N = 14 mm)†
Closure area	5 mm ± 0.7 (N = 8 mm)*
Middle scallop chordae marginal	9 mm ± 0.8 (N = 14 mm)*

* Statistically significant (Student's test)
† Not statistically significant.

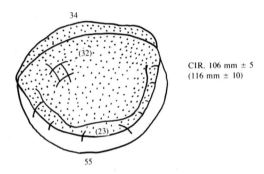

CIR. 106 mm ± 5
(116 mm ± 10)

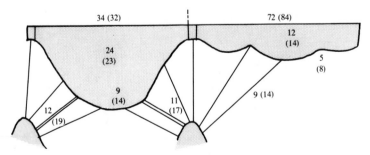

Figure 3. Combined mitral valve disease and insufficiency. Measurements of the various structures in comparison with normal measurements shown in parentheses.

more to retracted and hypertrophied intermediate chordae than to the thickening of the leaflet tissue itself. After resection of intermediate chordae, the leaflet became more pliable. The ventricular cavity was much smaller than in mitral insufficiency. With the heart beating, little change was observed in the annulus size area.

Table 4
Dystrophic Mitral Insufficiency

Circumference: 148 mm ± 5.5 (N = 116 mm) p < 0.005*

Aortic leaflet	
Attachment	35 mm ± 2 (N = 32 mm)†
Height	30 mm ± 1.4 (N = 23 mm)*
Closure area	18 mm ± 1 (N = 14 mm)*
Main chordae anterior	21 mm ± 0.9 (N = 19 mm)†
posterior	19 mm ± 0.5 (N = 17 mm)*
Paracommissural anterior	24 mm ± 1.8 (N = 17 mm)*
Paramedial anterior	28 mm ± 2.1 (N = 15 mm)*
Mural leaflet	
Attachment	85 mm ± 3.7 (N = 55 mm)*
Height middle scallop	17 mm ± 2.9 (N = 14 mm)*
Closure area middle scallop	8 mm ± 0.5 (N = 8 mm)†
Middle scallop chordae marginal	23 mm ± 1.9 (N = 14 mm)*
basal	17 mm ± 3 (N = 8 mm)*
Cleft chordae	18 mm ± 1.6 (N = 13 mm)*
Anterior commissural leaflet	
Attachment	13 mm ± 1.4 (N = 12 mm)†
Commissural chordae	17 mm ± 1.1 (N = 13 mm)*
Posterior commissural leaflet	
Attachment	18 mm ± 1.1 (N = 17 mm)†
Commissural chordae	17 mm ± 0.8 (N = 14 mm)*

* Statistically significant (Student's test)
† Not statistically significant.

The typical features which can be drawn from the measurements of **dystrophic mitral insufficiency** (Table 4) are the following: There was an approximately 20% increase in annulus size, due mainly to the dilatation of the annulus at the mural leaflet. It is interesting to note that the commissural areas were only slightly dilated in contrast to rheumatic mitral valve insufficiency. The annulus was deformed, with the longer axis being vertical, and the deformation was symmetrical, as opposed to rheumatic valve disease, in which it was most often asymmetrical (Fig. 4).

All of the chordae were elongated, including the commissural chordae of the anterior commissure and the chordae of the mural leaflet. Another point of contrast with rheumatic valve disease was that the chordae were thinner than normal.

The leaflet tissue was abnormal in certain areas. The height of the leaflet was significantly increased in contrast to rheumatic valve disease. In some areas, it appeared to have an excess of tissue, resulting in a ballooning effect of the leaflets. Unlike rheumatic valve disease, certain areas appeared absolutely normal. This heterogeneity in the distribution of the lesions may be considered as a significant difference from the homogeneous lesions of rheumatic valvular disease. With the heart beating, the annulus was completely immobile.

These measurements for **dystrophic mitral insufficiency with ruptured chordae** (Table 5, p. 76) are similar to those obtained in the

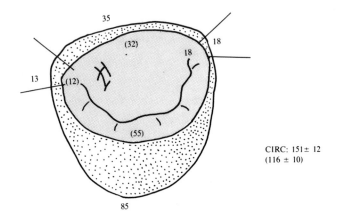

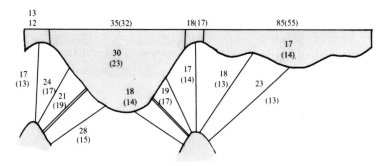

Figure 4. Dystrophic mitral insufficiency. Measurements of the various structures in comparison with normal measurements shown in parentheses.

preceding group. They show that both groups represent different evolutions of the same pathological process (Fig. 5).

CONCLUSION

This study is, to our knowledge, the first to present detailed, numerical data on the pathological findings of usual causes of mitral valve insufficiency. The differentiation of these heterogeneous lesions into their components provides a rational basis for the development of a variety of new mitral-valve reconstructive techniques and for the specific indications governing their use in each of the disease groups.

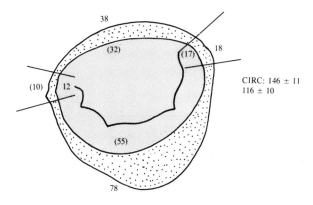

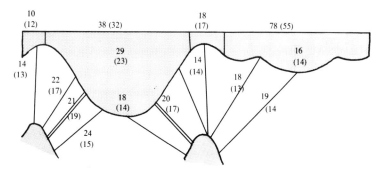

Figure 5. Dystrophic mitral insufficiency with ruptured chordae. Measurements of the various structures in comparison with normal measurements shown in parentheses.

Table 5
Dystrophic Mitral Insufficiency with Ruptured Chordae

Circumference: 144 mm ± 5.1 (N = 116 mm) p 0.005
Aortic leaflet

Attachment	38 mm ± 2.2 (N = 32 mm)*
Height	29 mm ± 1.5 (N = 23 mm)*
Closure area	18 mm ± 1.2 (N = 14 mm)†
Main chordae anterior	21 mm ± 0.3 (N = 19 mm)*
posterior	20 mm ± 1.9 (N = 17 mm)†
Paracommissural anterior	22 mm ± 1 (N = 17 mm)*
Paramedial anterior	24 mm ± 0.9 (N = 15 mm)*

Mural leaflet

Attachment	78 mm ± 3.6 (N = 55 mm)*
Height middle scallop	16 mm ± 1.5 (N = 14 mm)†
Closure area middle scallop	9 mm ± 0.9 (N = 8 mm)†
Middle scallop chordae marginal	19 mm ± 1.4 (N = 14 mm)*
basal	14 mm ± 0.8 (N = 8 mm)*
Cleft chordae	18 mm ± 2.8 (N = 13 mm)*

Anterior commissural leaflet

Attachment	10 mm ± 2 (N = 12 mm)†
Commissural chordae	14 mm ± 0.9 (N = 13 mm)†

Posterior commissural leaflet

Attachment	18 mm ± 2.8 (N = 17 mm)†
Commissural chordae	14 mm ± 0.9 (N = 14 mm)†

* Statistically significant (Student's test)
† Not statistically significant.

REFERENCES

1. Brock, R.C. The surgical and pathological anatomy of the mitral valve. *Brit. Heart J*. 14:489, 1952.

2. Carpentier, A. La valvuloplastie reconstitutive. *Presse Méd*. 77:7, 1969.

3. Carpentier, A., Deloche, A., Dauptain, J., Soyer, R., Prigent, Cl., Blondeau, P., Piwnica, A., Dubost, C. A new reconstructive operation for correction of mitral insufficiency. *J. Thor. Cardiovasc. Surg*. 61:1, 1970.

4. Chiechi, M.A., Less, W.M., Thompson, R. Functional anatomy of the normal mitral valve. *J. Thor. Surg*. 32:378, 1956.

5. Edwards, J.E., Burchell, H.B. Pathologic anatomy of mitral insufficiency. *Proc. Staff Mayo Clinic* 33:497, 1958.

6. Lam, J.H.C., Ranganathan, N., Wigle, E.D., Silver, M.D. Morphology of human mitral valve: I-Chordae tendineae: A new classification. *Circulation* 41:449, 1970.

7. Ranganathan, N., Lam, J.H.C., Wigle, E.D., Silver,

M.D.   Morphology of the human mitral valve: II The valve leaflets. *Circulation* 41:459, 1970.

8.   Roberts, W.C., Perloff, J.K.   Mitral valvular disease. A clinicopathologic study of the conditions causing the mitral valve to function abnormality. *Ann. Int. Med.* 77:939-975, 1972.

9.   Rusted, I.E., Schiefley, C.H., Edwards, J.E.   Studies of the mitral valve: I Anatomic features of the normal mitral valve and associated structures. *Circulation* 6:825, 1952.

10.   Rusted, I.E., Schiefley, C.H., Edwards, J.E. et al.   Guides to the commissures in operations upon the mitral valve. *Proc. Staff Meet Mayo Clin.* 26:297, 1951.

11.   Silverman, M.E., Hurst, J.W.   The mitral complex. *Am. Heart. J.* 73:399, 1968.

12.   Sokoloff, L., Elster, S.K., Righthand, H.   Sclerosis of the chordae tendineae of mitral valve. *Circulation* 1:782, 1950.

13.   Tandler, J.   Anatomie des Herzens: Handbuch des anatomies des Menschen. Bandelben. Gustav Fischer, Vol. 3, Abt i. Jena, Verlagsbuchandlung. 1913, p.84.

14.   Tsakiris, A.G., Von Bernuth, G., Rastelli, G.C., Bourgeois, M.G., Titus, J.L., Wood, E.H.   Size and notion of the mitral valve annulus in dogs. *Appl Physiol.* 30:5, 1971.

15.   Walmsley, Thomas (ed.)   *Quain's Anatomy*. The Heart. Part III, Vol V. London: Longman, Green & Co, 1929 p.81.

8 Pathology of Congenital Mitral Valve Disease

Henry N. Neufeld, M.D.
Leonard C. Blieden, M.B.B.Ch.

Exclusive of rheumatic heart disease, the causes of mitral valve disease in children are numerous and are related to local cardiac abnormalities as well as generalized disease processes. The pathological changes in the mitral valve may be confined to that structure or may be part of a more generalized anomaly involving several other cardiac structures. Of note in this group is papillary muscle dysfunction which is secondary to conditions such as aortic stenosis or endocardial fibroelastosis. When the heart is part of a generalized disease process involving other organs of the body, such as in the inherited disorders of metabolism, the mitral valve is commonly the predominant cardiac structure involved. In these generalized conditions, the mitral valve involvement in some cases may be an incidental finding at autopsy; in other cases, the incompetent valve may be the cause of congestive cardiac failure and death.

Irrespective of whether the mitral pathology is isolated or part of a cardiac syndrome or some generalized condition, the pathological features are best understood by classifying the lesions according to involvement (either singly or collectively) of the four anatomic components of the mitral valve apparatus. To make this classification meaningful, it is necessary to consider briefly the structure of the normal mitral valve.

NORMAL MITRAL VALVE

The normal mitral valve has two leaflets, the anterior (septal) and posterior (parietal). These leaflets are connected by two bridges of tissue called commissures. The commissures are named by the position they occupy—either anterolateral or posteromedial. Chordae tendineae run between each leaflet to the anterolateral and posteromedial papillary muscles of the left ventricle. Conversely, a set of chordae runs from each papillary muscle to the corresponding aspect of each leaflet.

CLASSIFICATION OF MITRAL VALVE LESIONS

Congenital abnormalities of the mitral valve may involve the leaflets, the commissures, the chordae tendineae, or the papillary muscles[1] (or varying combinations of these structures).

Abnormalities Involving the Leaflets

Cleft Mitral Leaflet   This may rarely occur as an isolated anomaly. Usually it is part of the complex lesion—persistent common atrioventricular (AV) canal; it may also occur with a ventricular septal defect of the AV canal type. The crucial problem in these associated conditions is the abnormal attachment of chordae tendineae between the edges of the valve cleft and the rim of the ventricular septal defect.

Supravalvular ring of the left atrium   This consists of a circumferential ridge of connective tissue attached to the base of the atrial surfaces of the mitral leaflets and protruding into the orifice of the mitral valve.[2] Depending upon the diameter of the ring, there are differing degrees of obstruction to flow across the mitral valve. In most cases, no significant obstruction occurs, but in the relatively few cases with the fully developed deformity, the supravalvular ring acts as a significantly stenosing diaphragm. Supravalvular ring is frequently a part of the Parachute Mitral Complex (see below). Only very rarely is surgical relief of this obstruction necessary.

Accessory orifice of the mitral valve This is characterized by a circular deficiency of varying size in the substance of the valve leaflet. From the circumference of the accessory orifice, chordae tendineae pass to be inserted into an independent papillary muscle. The valve may be incompetent (Fig. 1). This condition is very rare.[3]

Ebstein's Malformation of Inverted Tricuspid Valve In congenitally corrected transposition of the great vessels, the ventricles and atrioventricular valves are inverted, so that the left atrioventricular valve has the structure of the usual tricuspid valve. The inverted tricuspid valve may be subject to Ebstein's malformation, which is an abnormality of the normally situated tricuspid valve. The incidence of this valvular abnormality varies between 50–80% of the cases with "corrected" transposition. In most cases the degree of incompetence of the valve is mild. In some instances severe incompetence is present, and this leads to congestive cardiac failure. Valve replacement

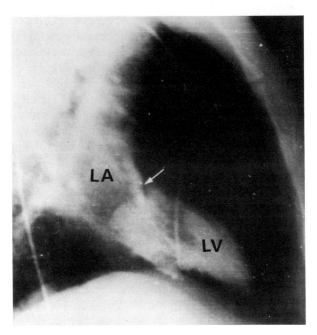

Figure 1. Left ventriculogram, lateral view, showing regurgitant jet (arrow) directed upward toward the atrial septal wall. LV – Left Ventricle, LA – Left Atrium.

may be necessary in these patients, in spite of the fact that the surgical risk is very high.

Accessory Valvular Tissue   This is a rare condition which may cause obstruction at the mitral valve level. It may be associated with other forms of mitral lesions, such as supravalvular ring or parachute mitral valve. In cases associated with complete transposition of the great vessels the presence of additional mitral valve tissue may be responsible for the production of subpulmonic obstruction.

"Billowing" (Prolapsing) Mitral Leaflet   The syndrome characterized by a systolic click, late systolic murmur, a distinctive electrocardiographic pattern, and mitral valve prolapse was defined by Barlow and associates and recently reviewed by them.[4] Numerous facets of this condition are still being reported.

Myxomatous changes of the mitral leaflets constitute the cornerstone of this syndrome. Although the condition has been reported in the pediatric age group, the number of reported cases remains small. This suggests that although the condition may be genetically determined, its manifestations only became evident after childhood. Cases of prolapsed mitral valve have been reported in association with cardiomyopathy or abnormally contracting left ventricle (Fig. 2). This association may be a critical factor in the pathogenesis of the condition. Possibly the abnormal contraction of the ventricle is the initial feature which causes irregular closure of the mitral valve and leads to myxomatous changes (i.e., degeneration). Progression of this condition would then lead to prolapse.

Dysrhythmia and subactue bacterial endocarditis may be associated with this condition. In some cases the degree of mitral regurgitation produced is significant and the valve needs to be replaced. It is noteworthy that this type of mitral abnormality is being described more and more frequently in association with secundum-type atrial septal defects. The clinical significance of this association has yet to be adequately demonstrated.

Mitral Valve Abnormalities and the Cardiomyopathies   It is not possible to discuss mitral valve abnormalities without at least mentioning their role in the cardiomyopathies and specifically in I.H.S.S. (Idiopathic Hypertrophic Subaortic Stenosis). Characteristically, in the obstructive phase of this disease, the anterior leaflet of the mitral valve moves into the left ventricular outflow tract during systole, causing or contributing to the obstruction. This systolic anterior movement of the mitral valve produces a characteristic pattern on echocardiography. The abnormal contraction of the left ventricle in this cardiomyopathy may also be associated with prolapse of the mitral leaflet(s). The exact mechanism for the obstruction related to the mitral leaflet has not been elucidated. It is noteworthy that all of the mitral apparatus, including chordae tendineae and papillary muscles, may be thickened and hypertrophied. One surgical approach recommended for relief of the obstruction in these cases is replacement of the mitral valve.

Anomalies of the Commissures

Congenital fusion of the commissures is a very rare condition which has features similar to those observed in rheumatic mitral stenosis.

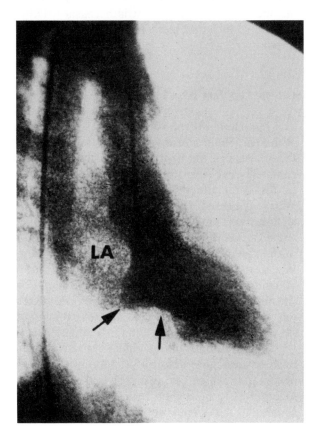

Figure 2. Left ventriculogram, lateral view. Note prolapse of posterior leaflet and irregular contraction of ventricular wall (arrows). LA – Left Atrium.

Anomalies of the Chordae Tendineae

Abnormal insertion or length of the chordae tendineae may interfere with the functional integrity of the mitral valve. Basically two types of involvement are seen:

Short chordae tendineae limit the mobility of the valve leaflets, and fix them along the wall of the left ventricle. This causes mitral obstruction or insufficiency. When short chordae tendineae form part of a more generalized involvement of the valve leaflet and papillary muscle, surgical therapy may be warranted.

Long chordae tendineae This condition may be associated with Marfan's syndrome. If this is the case, redundant ("billowing") leaflets may also be present. Mitral insufficiency results, and in some instances valve replacement is necessary. Other connective tissue disorders, such as Ehlers–Danlos syndrome, may show similar features.

Anomalies of the Papillary Muscles

Parachute Mitral Valve Complex The developmental complex of the parachute mitral valve with associated obstructive lesions on the left side of the heart is now a well-recognized entity. The first comprehensive report of this condition was by Shone and Associates.[5] In the parachute mitral valve, a single left ventricular papillary muscle is present (Fig. 3). The chordae tendineae from both mitral leaflets insert into the papillary muscle. The leaflets and commissures are normal. Mitral stenosis may be associated with the parachute mitral valve because of several anatomic features. The chordae tendineae in this condition are usually short and thickened, thereby allowing only limited movement of the leaflets. The primary orifice of the mitral valve is reduced in size as a result of the convergence of all the chordae tendineae into the solitary papillary muscle, so that blood flow occurs through the secondary orifices between the chordae.

Although only one papillary muscle is present in the classical form of parachute deformity of the mitral valve, cases have been observed in which two papillary muscles were present but so close together as to border on being a single muscle. The obstruction is sometimes sufficiently severe to warrant replacement of the mitral apparatus.

Anomalous Mitral Arcade In this condition the anterolateral and posteromedial papillary muscles form an arcade, together with the anterior mitral leaflet. A bridge of fibrous tissue is continuous with the free aspect of the anterior mitral leaflet and the two papillary muscles. The commissures are not fully developed and the chordae are thickened and short. The papillary muscles themselves may be hypertrophied. This complex may give rise to significant obstruction and may necessitate replacement of the mitral apparatus with a prosthetic valve.[6]

Abnormal size and position of papillary muscles Markedly hypertrophied or abnormally inserted papillary muscles may occur. The former condition causes obstruction. The latter condition is usually associated with endocardial fibroelastosis in which case infarction of the papillary muscles and mitral insufficiency may occur.

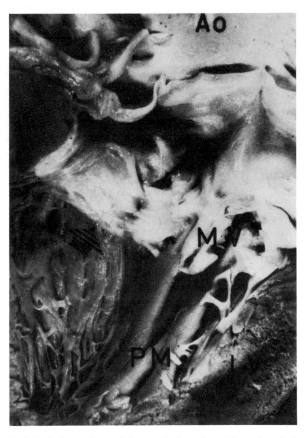

Figure 3. Pathological specimen, left ventricular view. Note the single papillary muscle. MV – Mitral Valve, PM – Papillary Muscle, Ao – Aorta.

ASSOCIATED CONGENITAL HEART DISEASE

Primary

In addition to the conditions mentioned above, complete transposition of the great vessels is quite commonly associated with mitral involvement of varying pathology. Double outlet right ventricle may also have associated mitral involvement, usually obstruction. In addition to cases of the "parachute" complex, coarctation of the aorta may be associated with mitral regurgitation due to varying abnormalities of the mitral apparatus.

Secondary

In this group of cases, myocardial infarction of the papillary muscles and free wall of the left ventricle may lead to mitral regurgitation. The abnormalities involved include anomalous origin of the left coronary artery from the pulmonary artery (Fig. 4), endocardial fibroelastosis, and aortic stenosis.

The mitral valve may quite often be involved in the inherited disorders of metabolism. These are genetically determined abnormalities of enzyme function that lead to the accumulation of a metabolic product as a result of deficiency or low concentration of a specific enzyme. This "stored" substance may be present in the leaflets, chordae, and/or papillary muscles, giving rise to dysfunction—usually mitral regurgitation. The disorders include metabolic abnormalities of a) mucopolysaccharides (Hurler's, Hunter's, and Sanfillipo syndromes), b) protein (aspartylglucosaminurea, c) amino acids (alkaptonurea), and d) lipids (Fabry's disease, Sandhoff's disease, GM I gangliosidosis, hyperlipoproteinemia II and III). Usually the basic metabolic disease dominates the clinical picture; occasionally the mitral disease is dominant, leading to congestive cardiac failure and death.[7]

COMMENT

In this presentation, we have classified the mitral valve anomalies seen in childhood and which are of congenital origin. The classification is dependent on the anatomical component of the mitral apparatus involved. In many cases, more than one component of the mitral valve is involved. In some patients the severity of the lesion

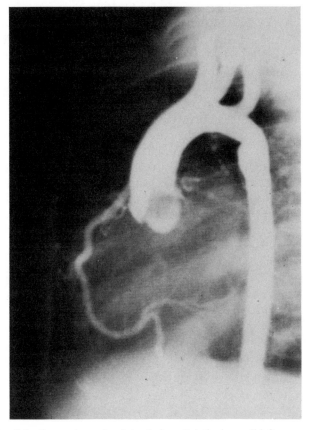

Figure 4. Selective aortography, lateral view. Relatively small left coronary artery arising from pulmonary artery and filling in retrograde fashion from the right coronary artery (via collaterals).

necessitates surgical intervention. Several of these cases may benefit from reconstruction or repair of the abnormality, but a high percentage will require prosthetic valve replacement. When the mitral valve is associated with generalized conditions such as the inborn errors of metabolism, more often than not the cardiac involvement is of secondary importance.

REFERENCES

1. Davachi, F., Moller, J.H., Edwards, J.E. Diseases of the mitral valve in infancy. *Circulation* 43:565, 1971.

2. Johnson, N.J., Dodd, K. Obstruction to left atrial outflow by a supravalvular stenosing ring. *J. Pediat.* 51:190, 1957.

3. Schlesinger, Z., Kraus, Y., Deutsch, V., Yahini, J.H., Neufeld, H.N. An unusual form of mitral valve insufficiency simulating aortic stenosis. *Chest* 58:385, 1970.

4. Pocock, W.A., Barlow, J.B. Etiology and electrocardiographic features of the billowing posterior mitral leaflet syndrome: analysis of a further 130 patients with a late systolic murmur or nonejection systolic click. *Am. J. Med.* 51:731, 1971.

5. Shone, J.D., Sellers, R.D., Anderson, R.C., Adams, P. Jr., Lillehei, C.W., Edwards, J.E. The developmental complex of 'parachute mitral valve,' supravalvular ring of left atrium, subaortic stenosis and coarctation of aorta. *Am. J. Cardiol.* 11:714, 1963.

6. Castaneda, A.R., Anderson, R.C., Edwards, J.E. Congenital mitral stenosis resulting from anomalous arcade and obstructing papillary muscles. Report of correction by use of ball valve prosthesis. *Am. J. Cardiol.* 24:237, 1969.

7. Blieden, L.C., Moller, J.H. Cardiac involvement in the inherited disorder of metabolism. *Progress in Cardiovascular Dis.* 16:615, 1974.

DISCUSSION: PART II

Dr. Oury: I want to discuss the differences in mitral valve pathology noted in two cardiovascular centers on the West Coast as contrasted to that seen during my period of study in Paris, France.

For the purpose of this comparison, we have reviewed the two years experience in mitral valve surgery at the Naval Hospital, San Diego, as well as the University of California Medical School, San Diego. We make the assumption that our experience is similar to that reported from other cardiovascular centers in the United States. Our total experience covering this time period is 80 mitral valve procedures (Fig. 1). As you can see, the procedures involved reconstruction in 34 patients (43%) and replacement of the valve in 46 patients (57%). Recently, mitral valve reconstruction utilizing the Carpentier ring annuloplasty has been used in approximately 20% of these reconstructive procedures, and we will detail this experience later at this conference. The average age of patients in the mitral replacement group was 51 with a range of 32 to 67 years; in the mitral reconstruction group, the average age was 41 with a range of 21 to 66. The male to female ratio was 16 males, 30 females in the mitral replacement group and 3 males, 31 females in the reconstruction group. The great majority of patients in both categories of reconstruction or replacement were classes three to four, New York Heart classification. Previous mitral procedures have been performed in 37% of the replacement group and 20% of the reconstruction group. The presence of calcification, which we regard as an important criterion to determine whether the patient will receive mitral replacement or reconstruction, was noted in 48% of the mitral replacement group and in 16% of the reconstruction group.

The experience at the University of California Medical School, San Diego, reviewed by Drs. Peterson and Daily, revealed that there was roughly the same number of patients over the same time span. The age range was similar and the only important difference between these two series was that the majority of patients in the San Diego series have valve replacement (over 90%) as compared to our series in which almost 50% underwent reconstruction. I think this has a great deal to do with a more advanced spectrum of mitral valve disease seen in the University series and, I also think, with the enthusiasm of the surgeon toward reconstructive procedures.

The point I would like to make (Figs. 2a, 2b) is that a much higher percentage of the patients with mitral valve replacement had calcification of the valve: both in the pure insufficiency category, 2 out of 3 in the pure stenosis category, and 15 out of 21 in the mixed stenosis and insufficiency category. With the recent increased enthusiasm toward reconstruction, we feel that patients in this category who do not have calcified valves will be amenable to reconstructive procedures.

The functional results in these two categories are as expected (Fig. 3). The patients who underwent reconstructive procedures were in general younger, and the longevity of their symptomatology and severity of disease was less in general. The functional result was therefore correspondingly better. The vast majority of patients in both categories, however, improved by at least one New York Heart Association class.

My conclusion is that the majority of patients presenting for mitral valve procedures in the United States will continue to require mitral valve replacement because of the advanced nature of their disease. We have, however, utilized reconstructive procedures with increasing frequency in the past two years, and our approach would appear to be justified in a significant number of patients with mitral valve disease on the basis of low operative mortality (zero mortality in the reconstruction group vs 11% for mitral replacement) and the excellent functional result. We feel the major contraindication to reconstruction is heavy calcification of the valve.

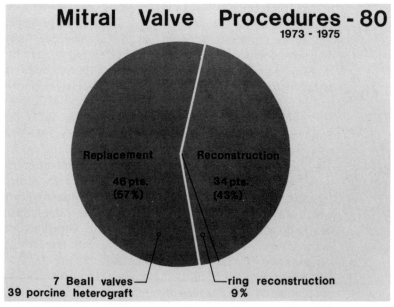

Figure 1. Mitral valve procedures—two-year experience, Naval Hospital, San Diego.

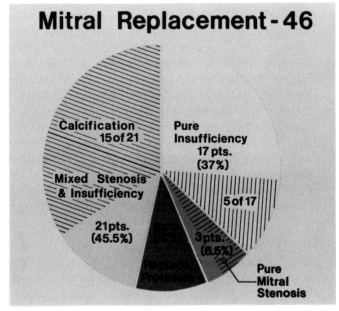

Figure 2a. Diagnostic classification of patients requiring valve replacement—presence of calcification.

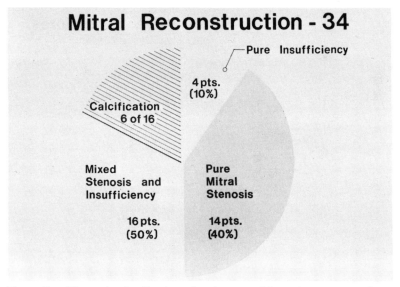

Figure 2b. Diagnostic classification of patients requiring valve reconstruction—presence of calcification.

Dr. Carpentier: I note with interest that changes are occurring not only in France but on the other side of the Atlantic as well. Mitral valve surgery is becoming more eclectic and in treating mitral lesions, surgeons are considering alternative methods to mitral valve replacement. One of the objections frequently voiced in the United States is that the lesions seen there are most often far advanced and calcified, and therefore not amenable to reconstruction. Dr. Oury's and Dr. Angell's experience shows that, at least in certain groups, almost half the cases can be treated by reconstructive surgery.

Next, I have two questions for Dr. Silver: First, what is the average age of the patients with floppy valve syndrome? Second, what is the pathology of the floppy valve syndrome? Is it the result of primarily diseased chordae or is it a combined disease of both leaflets and chordae?

Dr. Silver: Most of the patients who had floppy valves examined after surgery or at autopsy were 45–50 years old, and the majority were women, but I have seen this condition in a 12-year-old child who had incomplete differentiation of the mitral valve. So the majority of the cases seen by the pathologist occur in the older group, while clinicians see cases in younger people.

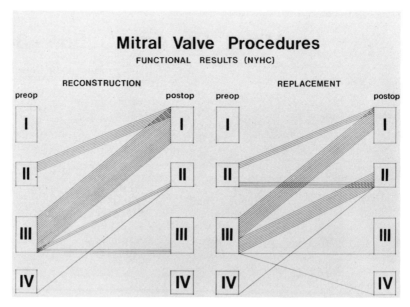

Figure 3. Functional result of mitral valve procedures—comparison of reconstruction vs. replacement.

The second question is both fascinating and important. Here, I think, one must tread warily and not be like the gentleman walking down the boulevard who is fascinated by an attractive young lady and completely misses the fact that her accomplice picks his pockets. One must watch the pretty girl and the accomplice. Equally, one must consider that a floppy valve may be the result of lesions either of the chordae or of the leaflets or indeed of both. As Dr. Perloff explained today, there are many conditions that may lead to mitral insufficiency. I will bet now that there are many different conditions that produce floppy valves. Thus, at this stage I am unwilling to answer the question; in other words, I tend to be a "lumper"—I am putting all examples of floppy valves into one basket and when I have enough I will sort out those which have primary leaflet disease and those which have primary chordal lesions.

Dr. Chiche: Dr. Silver, since the localization of myxomatous degeneration at the site of the aortic valve is usually associated with connective tissue disease, don't you think that the floppy valve is also a primary location of such a syndrome?

Dr. Silver: Yes, the association of myxomatous degeneration and Marfan's syndrome suggests that a congenital abnormality of connective tissue and cusp predisposes the patient to floppy valve and that the lesion may be due to a cusp abnormality. But, in the mitral area, connective tissue is present in both leaflets and chordae, and I do not know which is affected first. Again, as our experience widens, we have encountered a large group of individuals with floppy valves who do not have Marfan's syndrome or a forme fruste. At the moment I must "lump" and cannot define the initiating mechanism of the pathological changes.

Dr. Frater: I want to congratulate Dr. Deloche and Dr. Carpentier for the really superb anatomical studies they have done. At the same time, I believe they must be made more simple to persuade cardiac surgeons to repair rather than replace. There are two essential points I want to make (Fig. 4): the distance C from the papillary muscle to the plane of the atrioventricular ring is always greater than the distance B from the papillary muscle to the free edge of any portion of the valve, and the sum of the lengths of the anterior A and posterior P cusps always exceeds the diameter D of the contracted ring during systole. If the free edge of the valve (Fig. 5a) rises above the plane of the atrioventricular ring, there will inevitably be insufficiency, and this applies to the anterior cusp, the posterior cusp, or the posteromedial commissural tissue. Alternatively, if the length of the anterior and posterior cusps (Fig. 5b) does not match the orifice, and this may be a normal orifice with a contracted posterior cusp or an abnormal orifice with normal anterior and posterior cusps, then there will be insufficiency. Therefore, it is not necessary to know the precise dimensions that Dr. Deloche has so brilliantly described. At the operating table, simple comparative dimensions will define the mechanism of insufficiency that one is dealing with.

Dr. Taylor: In reference to what Dr. Silver was saying about the probability of there being more than one cause for the floppy valve syndrome, and to Dr. Perloff's comments on the papillary muscle

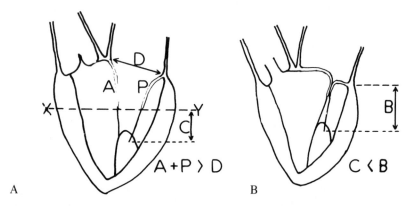

Figure 4. Dimensional relationship between anatomical components of the mitral apparatus in a competent valve. (a) diastole (b) systole. See text.

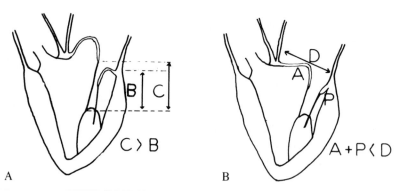

Figure 5. Dimensional relationship between anatomical components of the mitral apparatus leading to mitral incompetence: in both eventualities (a) and (b), mitral regurgitation is inevitable. See text.

syndrome, in our experimental studies on papillary muscle inactivation we have on rare occasion produced similar states in the dog (Taylor et al., *Cardiovascular Research,* 319-326, 1970). The lesions were produced by the injection of ethanol. In a few animals, about one in ten, lesions with "vegetations" which progressed to calcific plaques and chordal shortening occurred. It is certainly possible to produce an experimental analogue of the papillary muscle syndrome and the floppy valve syndrome, but because of the rarity with which persistent dysfunction is produced, I would not recommend it unless one has a large amount of both time and money.

SUMMARY: PART II

M. Silver, M.D.

Dr. Silver presented the pathology of several conditions causing stenosis or insufficiency in natural or artificial heart valves; Dr. Deloche described anatomical studies he and his colleagues had done on valves insufficient as a result of different pathological processes; and Dr. Neufeld discussed the pathology of congenital lesions of the mitral valve.

Dr. Silver emphasized that myxomatous degeneration is the most common cause of a prolapsed mitral valve, but indicated that other conditions may induce prolapse. Dr. Taylor provided evidence from experimental studies to support the latter viewpoint but indicated that only 10% of experimental animals developed myxomatous changes. During the discussion, Dr. Silver was cautious when pressed on a question as to whether the main change affected mitral leaflets or chordae. His caution may be justified, at present, because pathological correlations lag behind clinical findings. The pictorial display of heart valve complications should be remembered by all. Individually, the complications may be uncommon but each caused morbidity or the death of a patient. This is often forgotten when one listens to a cold statistical analysis defining the efficiency of a prosthesis. It should not be, for each complication is a challenge to continue improving valve design and function.

The painstaking work of Dr. Deloche and his colleagues provides a sound anatomic basis for the surgical correction of mitral valve lesions without using a prosthesis to replace them. This is an important alternative in countries where the cost of a prosthesis may be an important consideration. Dr. Frater, in discussing that paper, argued that it was unnecessary to know the precise dimensions described by Dr. Deloche. He provided a simplified method of determining if a valve is insufficient. His point was valid but not germane if a valve is to be reconstructed properly. Then, the measurements provided by Dr. Deloche's continuing studies are vital.

The pathology of mitral valve problems encountered in the pediatric age group was presented most lucidly by Dr. Neufeld. In particular, he emphasized that the relationship between congenital lesions, myxomatous degeneration, and prolapsed mitral leaflets in the adult need further study.

PART THREE

FLOW
DYNAMICS
OF THE
NORMAL
MITRAL
VALVE

9 Fluid Mechanics of a Model Mitral Valve

B.J. Bellhouse, M.A., D. Phil.

INTRODUCTION

The closure mechanism of the mitral valve has been studied by many investigators with widely differing methods and conclusions. The use of ultrasonic techniques to record anterior cusp position[1] has shown that the anterior cusp opens wide early in diastole, moves towards closure during mid-diastole, partially reopens at the onset of atrial systole, and moves again towards closure before the end of diastole. These measurements appear to be inconsistent with the view expressed by Rushmer, Finlayson, and Nash[2] that the mitral valve cusps were drawn towards apposition during diastole by traction exerted through the chordae tendineae by the papillary muscles. The purpose of the present investigation was to see if the diastolic movements of the mitral cusps could be explained by flow patterns within the left ventricle, and by accelerations and decelerations of blood-flow through the mitral valve, rather than by muscular traction by the papillary muscles.

METHODS

A model of the left ventricle was built (Fig. 1), consisting of a rigid base made of Perspex, incorporating a mitral valve (A) and an aortic valve (B), with a transparent rubber bag (C) simulating the remainder of the ventricle. The model ventricle was fixed inside a Perspex tank (D), which was filled with water and connected at (E) to a piston pump to actuate the ventricle.

The aortic valve was connected by a pipe (F) to a header tank which overflowed to a lower tank, which in turn discharged through a viewer (G) to the mitral valve. The aortic valve had three thin (0.1 mm) flexible cusps made of silicone rubber reinforced with fabric, and also had three sinuses.

The mitral valve (Fig. 2) consisted of a sleeve of nylon net coated with silicone rubber, shaped to make two cusps 0.1 mm thick and 28 mm long. The sleeve was shaped on a divergent-cone mold (semi-

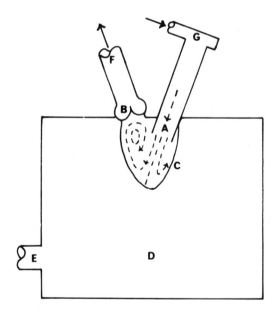

Figure 1. Diagram of the model left ventricle, showing the mitral valve (A), aortic valve (B), and a transparent rubber bag (C) simulating the remainder of the ventricle. Water was pumped in and out of the Perspex tank (D), by a piston pump connected at (E), to actuate the ventricle. The ventricle pumped water round a separate circuit, through the aorta (F) to two header tanks back through a viewer (G) into the ventricle.

angle 14°), with the narrower end attached to the mitral ring. The free margins of the cusps were connected by threads to a fixed support 45 mm from the mitral ring, to prevent prolapse of the valve during systole.

Atrial systole was simulated by connecting a balloon pump, in addition to the piston pump, to the Perspex tank (Fig. 1). The balloon pump was driven by compressed air and was triggered by switches attached to the piston pump. Thus the timing, duration, and stroke volume of atrial systole could be varied.

Through the viewer (G), the positions of the mitral valve cusps could be observed from the atrial side (Fig. 1). A timing light was tripped by the piston pump, and the light and valve were filmed simultaneously at 50 frames s⁻¹. The film was then analyzed frame-by-frame, and the area of the mitral cusp orifice was measured as a function of time.

Velocity was measured at the mitral ring, with a heated-element needle-gauge.[3] The velocity signal and voltage pulse for the timing

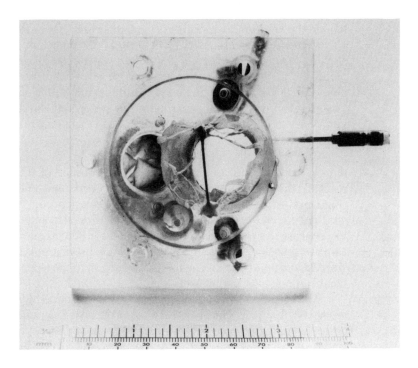

Figure 2. Photograph of the base of the model ventricle showing the mitral valve, the chordae tendineae, and the fixed bar to which they are attached.

light were recorded simultaneously, to permit correlation of fluid velocity with cusp position (recorded on the ciné film).

EXPERIMENTAL RESULTS

Small Ventricle

When the ventricle was actuated by the piston pump (which produced a sinusoidal flow, one half for diastole, the other for systole), the mitral valve opened rapidly at the start of diastole, but it did not open to its fullest extent, and the chordae tendineae were slack. As the valve opened, a small starting vortex was formed at the free margins of the cusps; when the mitral valve had opened, the incoming jet struck the apex of the ventricle and spread out to flow up the walls to the base of the ventricle, then turned back behind the cusps towards the apex again to form a ring vortex. The vortex was asymmetrical, with its main strength concentrated in the outflow tract, behind the anterior cusp. This vortex had swept up the small starting vortex and absorbed it. After peak diastole, the anterior cusp moved steadily towards closure, and just before ventricular filling was complete, the posterior cusp started to close also. Solid particles suspended in the water showed that very little reversed flow was required to seal the valve. In this experiment the end-systolic volume of the ventricle was 107 ml, the stroke volume was 173 ml, and the pulse rate was 24/min.

Ciné film of the mitral valve was taken from the atrial side. The film was projected frame-by-frame and the outline of the cusp free margins, the supporting bar for the chordae tendineae, and the mitral ring were traced onto white paper. The areas between the anterior cusp and the bar (A_1) and between the posterior cusp and the bar (A_2) were measured with a planimeter. In addition, the area of the mitral ring was measured. Since the plane of the cusps' margins and the ring were 28 mm apart during diastole, a correction for perspective (8.1%) has been made to the measurements.

The results for the small ventricle (end-systolic volume 107 ml) are shown in Fig. 3. Time is plotted along the abscissa, with zero time corresponding to the end of diastole. The velocity through the mitral ring is shown in (a), the cusp orifice area divided by the ring area ((A_1 + A_2)/A_0) is shown in (b), and the nondimensional opening areas of

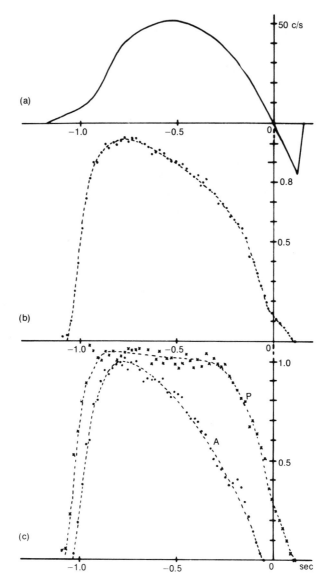

Figure 3. Effect of end-systolic volume on mitral valve closure (small ventricle). (End systolic volume 107 ml, stroke volume 173 ml, frequency 24/min.) Velocity at the mitral ring is shown in (a), the area of the mitral cusp orifice divided by the area of the ring is drawn in (b). The opening-areas of the anterior cusp (A) and posterior cusp (P) are plotted nondimensionally in (c). See text.

anterior cusp $\dfrac{2A_1}{A_0}$ is plotted, and for the posterior cusp $\dfrac{2A_2}{A_0}$ is plotted.)

It is seen that both cusps opened rapidly at the beginning of diastole and that the anterior cusp then started to move towards the closed position, followed by the posterior cusp towards the end of diastole. By the end of diastole the valve was 88% closed, and a small amount of reversed flow at the onset of systole was required to seal the valve.

The difference between the movements of the anterior and posterior cusps appeared to be due to the asymmetry of the ventricular vortex. However, small differences in cusp stiffness could also account for their different closure rates. To examine this possibility, the mitral valve was rotated by 180° so that the cusps changed position, and the experiment was repeated. The new anterior cusp performed exactly as the previous anterior cusp had done, and the same was true of the posterior cusps. Thus different cusp stiffness was not the cause of dissimilar cusp movements in diastole.

Large Ventricle

Flow acceleration and deceleration through the mitral ring would affect both cusps equally. To study this effect in isolation from the ventricular vortex, the end-systolic volume was enlarged to 1216 ml, and the experiment was repeated, keeping the stroke volume fixed at 173 ml and the frequency at 24 min^{-1}. The large end-systolic volume, compared with stroke volume, ensured that the energy in the jet through the mitral valve was dissipated within the ventricle, and only a very weak vortex was formed. The starting vortex was again apparent, but this was propelled across the ventricle like a smoke-ring, and decayed rapidly. In this experiment (Fig. 4), both anterior and posterior cusps remained wide open until, towards the end of diastole, they started to close simultaneously. At the end of diastole the valve was only 28% closed.

Atrial Systole

The effect of atrial systole on the model valve can be seen in Figs. 5 and 6. The velocity through the mitral valve is shown in (a); the cusp orifice area divided by ring area (derived from frame-by-frame analysis of ciné film) is plotted in (b); and each cusp opening-area is

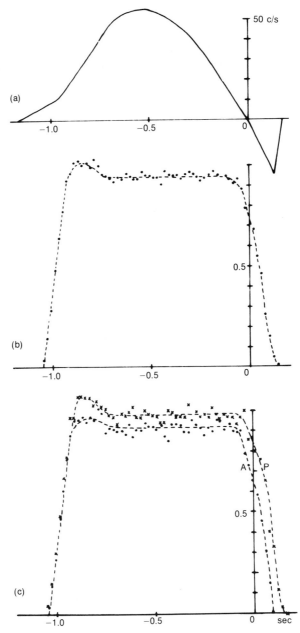

Figure 4. Effect of end-systolic volume on mitral valve closure (large ventricle). (End systolic volume 1216 ml, stroke volume 173 ml, frequency 24/min.) (a), (b), (c) as in Figure 3.

106

shown separately in (c). In both cases the mitral valve opened wide at the beginning of diastole, and then moved steadily towards closure until atrial systole intervened to cause partial reopening, followed by a resumption of closure once the peak of velocity had passed. The posterior cusp responded to atrial systole by opening wide; the anterior cusp also responded in the same way, but to a smaller extent.

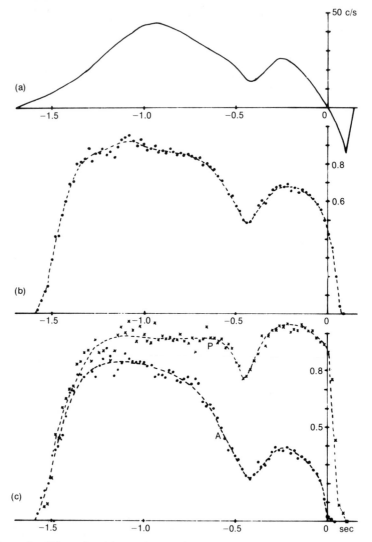

Figure 5. Effect of atrial systole on mitral valve closure (case 1). (End-systolic volume 183 ml, stroke volume 191 ml, frequency 24/min.) (a), (b), and (c) as in Fig. 3.

ANALYSIS OF THE RESULTS

The ventricular vortex can be seen as a mechanism for recovering dynamic head from the jet entering the left ventricle through the mitral valve. If the end-systolic volume of the ventricle is small compared with the stroke-volume of the ventricle, then most of the

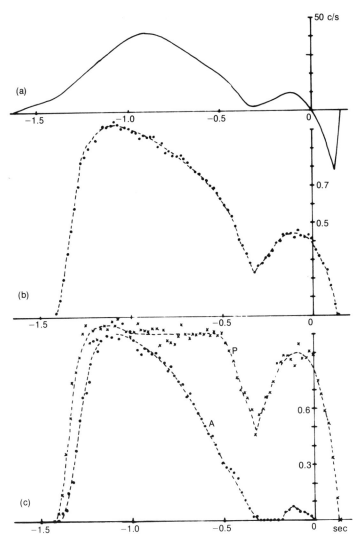

Figure 6. Effect of atrial systole on mitral valve closure (case 2). (End-systolic volume 201 ml, stroke volume 154 ml, frequency 24/min.) (a), (b) and (c) as in Fig. 3.

energy in the jet is transferred to the ventricular vortex, which, because of the shape of the left ventricle and position of the mitral valve, exerts a thrust on the anterior cusp, pushing it towards its closed position. A large end-systolic volume, on the other hand, ensures that the energy of the jet is dissipated when entering that large volume of stagnant fluid. Flow acceleration through the mitral ring tends to open the cusps, because the pressure at the ring is greater than in the ventricle, thus providing a higher pressure on the atrial side of the cusps than on the ventricular side. Flow deceleration through the mitral ring tends to close the cusps, because pressure is greater inside the ventricle than at the mitral ring. In addition, a Venturi effect acts as the cusps move towards apposition, causing the pressure in the plane of the cusp free margins to be lower than at the mitral ring. This counteracts the efforts of flow deceleration and the ventricular vortex to close the valve by trying to keep the cusps parallel.

The same explanations account for the second opening of the mitral valve during atrial systole, and are supported both by pressure measurements and detailed calculations reported elsewhere.[4]

DISCUSSION

The smallest end-systolic volume that could be used without rupturing the rubber ventricle on the mitral valve support-bar was about 107 ml. This is larger than normal in man, so the stroke volume was increased in proportion to 173 ml. The large stroke volume, in turn, dictated a low pulse rate to match the frequency parameter Lf/U, where L is mitral ring diameter, f the frequency, and U is peak diastolic velocity. Since viscous effects are of secondary importance in mitral valve function, because viscous diffusion times are so much greater than the duration of diastole, no attempt was made to match the viscosity of blood or the Reynolds number Ud/v (where v is kinematic viscosity).

Evidence that vortices exist in the left ventricles of dogs and sheep has been presented by Taylor and Wade.[5] They used ciné-angiography and a radio-opaque dye in closed-chested animals, and endoscopic ciné-photography in open-chested animals; they observed stable vortices occupying the entire ventricle. They also noted that there was no evidence of flow reversal through the mitral valve at the time of valve closure, which implied that the mitral valve was closed, or nearly closed, by the end of diastole, in agreement with the experiments with the model mitral valve.

Movements of the anterior cusp of the mitral valve have been recorded by ultrasonic techniques in resting man by Pridie and Oakley.[1] Their measurements of anterior cusp position showed rapid opening, followed by movements towards closure, before partial reopening occurred at the onset of atrial systole. The cusps then returned towards the closed position by the end of diastole. These measurements, too, show close agreement with the results for the model mitral valve (Figs. 5 and 6). Since the cusps in the model valve were free to move in diastole, and followed so accurately the movements observed in man, the explanation that the cusps are tethered in diastole and moved by traction by the papillary muscles[2] is neither likely nor necessary.

CONCLUSION

The mechanism of the mitral valve has been analyzed with the use of a model left ventricle. The valve was seen to open wide early in diastole, then move steadily towards closure, and was almost closed at the end of diastole, whether atrial systole was present or absent. The effect of atrial systole was to cause partial reopening of the valve before resumption of closure. The anterior cusp tended to close before the posterior cusp unless the ventricle was dilated, in which case the cusps closed together.

The movements of the mitral valve cusps corresponded closely with ultrasonic measurements in man, and were shown to be due to:

1. a ventricular vortex concentrated in the outflow tract, tending to close the anterior cusp;

2. flow acceleration and deceleration through the mitral ring, deceleration helping to close both cusps; and

3. a Venturi effect which tried to keep the cusps parallel.

These three effects account for cusp movements when atrial systole is present or absent and whether the ventricle is normal or dilated.

REFERENCES

1. Pridie, R.B., Oakley, C.M. Mechanism of mitral regurgitation in hypertrophic obstructive cardiomyopathy. *British Heart Journal* 32:203, 1970.

2. Rushmer, R.F., Finlayson, B.L., Nash, A.A. Movements of the mitral valve. *Circulation Research* 4:337, 1956.

3. Bellhouse, B.J., Bellhouse, F.H. Thin film gauges for the measurement of velocity or skin friction in air, water or blood. *J. Scientific Instruments,* Series 2. 1:1211, 1968.

4. Bellhouse, B.J. Fluid mechanics of a model mitral valve and left ventricle. *Cardiovascular Research,* VI, No. 2. 199, 1972.

5. Taylor, D.E.M., Wade, J.D. The pattern of flow around the atrio-ventricular valves during diastolic ventricular filling. *Journal of Physiology* 207:71-72p, 1970.

10 Some Observations on the Motion of a Two-Dimensional Mitral Valve*

L. Talbot, Ph.D.
C. S. F. Lee, M. Sc.

As a part of an extensive model study on the fluid dynamics of the mitral valve now being carried out at the University of California, Berkeley, some tests have been conducted on a "two-dimensional" valve. The purpose of these tests was to study the valve closure process, particularly the role of flow deceleration, for the case of a very simple geometry, and hopefully to shed some light on the role of the chordae tendineae in the valve closure process.

The tests were conducted in a mitral valve rig very similar to that just described by Dr. Bellhouse. In the particular sequence of photographs reported here, the "cardiac output" was 1.25 l/min, with an end-diastolic volume of approximately 200 cc. The pulse rate was 20/min., with systole occupying 1.0 seconds or one-third of the period of a pulse, and diastole the remaining 2.0 seconds. The active period of diastole was 1.65 seconds. There was no atrial contraction, although the rig has provision for this additional feature. Water was used as the test fluid, and flow visualization was carried out by means

* This work was supported by the U.S. National Science Foundation.

111

112

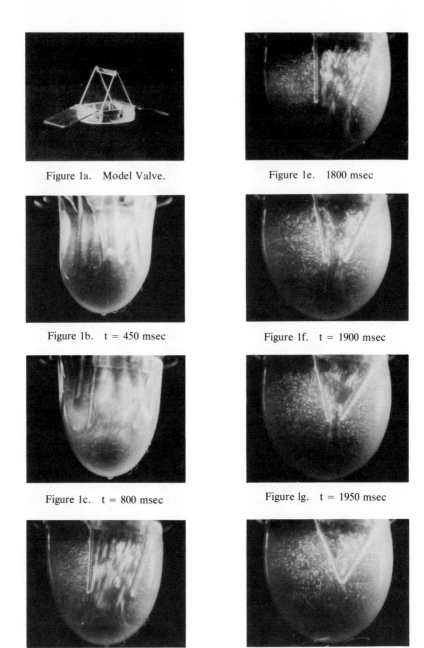

Figure 1a. Model Valve.

Figure 1e. 1800 msec

Figure 1b. t = 450 msec

Figure 1f. t = 1900 msec

Figure 1c. t = 800 msec

Figure lg. t = 1950 msec

Figure 1d. t = 1400 msec

Figure 1h. t = 2000 msec

Figure 1. Motion of a two-dimensional model mitral valve.

of the hydrogen bubble technique. Although the stroke volume chosen was rather small in comparison to the end-diastolic volume, this was done to facilitate observation of the valve motion and flow patterns in the early stages of diastole. Increasing the stroke volume (i.e., decreasing the end-systolic volume) produced increased wrinkling of the ventricular wall in early diastole, causing optical distortions which interfered with the viewing of its interior.

The "two-dimensional" valve used in the tests is shown in Fig. 1 a. It consisted of two rigid Plexiglas valve cusps, 2.5 cm long, which were mounted on a frame provided with parallel triangular side walls and containing an orifice 2.5 cm in diameter. In the closed position, the included angle between the cusps was 27°. The valve hinges were quite flexible, and permitted the cusps to open to well beyond an included angle of 180° (Fig. 1a). Apart from their hinges and the cross-support joining the vertices of the triangular side walls, the cusps were unconstrained.

Figs. 1b-1h show the sequence of events at successive instants of time after the onset of diastole, taken to be at t = 0. In Fig. 1b at t = 450 msec, the valve has partially opened. The fluid motion in the ventricle is predominately an outward displacement, due to motion of the valve cusps. In Fig. 1c, at t = 800 msec, one observes the formation of a vortex behind the aortic (anterior) cusp, which has opened fully, actually overshooting slightly its mid-diastolic position. The mural (posterior) cusp has also opened fully, but not as far as the aortic cusp. Fig. 1d shows the fully-developed diastolic flow pattern, at t = 1400 msec. The jet emerging from the valve is clearly evident, and the vortex motion behind the aortic cusp has become somewhat diffused. This pattern continues until the end of the period of active diastole, which occurred at t = 1650 msec. Figure 1e shows an early stage of valve closure, at t = 1800 msec. The mural cusp has undergone significant inward movement, while the aortic cusp has as yet been only slightly displaced. A strong jet through the valve is still evident. In Fig. 1f, at t = 1900 msec, one observes a later stage of the closure process. Both cusps have now moved close to apposition, with the mural cusp still leading the aortic cusp. The motion within the ventricle is generally inward, behind the cusps, although there is still a strong narrow jet issuing from the partially closed valve, and a vortical motion exists in the lower portion of the ventricle. The fluid contained within the upper portion of the valve has begun to move upward, and a stagnation point exists in the flow field within the valve. The closure is almost complete at t = 1950 msec (Fig. 1g). There is still a narrow jet issuing from the valve, and motion within the ventricle still displays a vortical character. There is a marked upward displacement of fluid within the valve itself. We see the valve completely closed, at t = 2000 msec, the moment of onset of ventricular systole (Fig. 1h).

Although the data displayed in these figures, as well as other measurements of pressure and velocity, are still under analysis, certain qualitative conclusions may be drawn from the results. First, it appears that the primary mechanism responsible for valve closure during diastole is the adverse pressure gradient associated with the deceleration of the fluid passing through the valve. This fluid deceleration is, of course, a result of the deceleration of the walls of the ventricle, which commences after the rate of expansion of the ventricle passes through its maximum value in the latter stage of diastole. In fact, although the details of the mitral valve geometry and flow field differ from those of the aortic valve, the mechanisms of flow-deceleration valve closure are essentially the same in the two cases.[1] The mechanism may be explained roughly as follows. The pressure field associated with the flow deceleration is such that the pressure in the jet, in the vicinity of the apex of the ventricle, exceeds that within the valve. Because the fluid motion in the ventricle, at least in the present case, is a low velocity flow as compared with the jet issuing from the valve, there is little pressure variation in this flow field. Consequently, the pressures behind the valve cusps are very nearly the same as that at the apex of the ventricle. Since this apex pressure exceeds the pressure within the valve when flow deceleration commences, so do the pressures behind the valve cusps, and the valve begins to close. The process may be modified somewhat in the case of substantially increased stroke volume, or decreased end-diastolic volume, with correspondingly higher velocities in the flow field in the ventricle and behind the valve cusps. In this event, some of the dynamic pressure associated with the motion may be recovered in the form of additional pressure increase behind the valve cusps, further contributing to the closure process. However, an order-of-magnitude analysis shows that the dynamic pressure recovery is generally small compared to peak deceleration pressure differences. It may be expected that this dynamic pressure contribution would therefore occur mainly in the early stage of valve closure, whereas the deceleration process is clearly the most important in the later stage of closure. We anticipate that further analysis of these data will enable us to provide more quantitative information in respect to these observations.

The second conclusion which can be drawn from these data is that the closure mechanism described operates efficiently without the need for forces applied to the free margins of the valve cusps, such as might be supplied by chordae tendineae. Nor do chordae tendineae appear necessary to prevent over-opening of the valve, since the valve cusps align themselves quite naturally with the boundaries of the essentially parallel jet issuing from the valve in mid-diastole. Indeed, the valve motion appears to reflect to a considerable extent the motion of the ventricular wall, so much so that it may in fact be possible to predict valve motion solely from knowledge of ventricular wall motion and vice versa. Of course, in the case of the physiological valve, the chordae tendineae are essential for the prevention of valve prolapse during ventricular systole, but we do not believe that they play an important role in diastole.

The rigid-cusped ''two-dimensional'' model valve whose motion we have described here can, at best, be considered as only a very crude approximation to the flexible and three-dimensional physiological valve, and the same is true with respect to comparison between the model and physiological ventricles. Despite this, we believe that the fluid-dynamical phenomena responsible for valve closure are qualitatively the same for both cases, although quantitative details of the pressure and velocity distributions may differ.

REFERENCE

1. Bellhouse, B.J., Talbot, L. The fluid mechanics of the aortic valve, *J. Fluid Mechanics*. Pt 4. 35:721-735, 1969.

11 The Use of Electromagnetic Flowprobes in the Mitral Valve Position—Principle, Advantages, and Limitations

Robert S. Reneman, M.D.

INTRODUCTION

Flowmeters based upon Faraday's law of electromagnetic induction have been developed independently by Kolin[14] and Wetterer.[30] Since the early sixties, these instruments have widely been used to measure blood flow through intact arteries and pressurized veins in animals (see, for example, references 12, 13, 17, 19, 20, 25) and in humans (e.g., 6, 10, 21, 26). More recently, electromagnetic flowmeters have been used to measure mitral valve flow in animal experiments (e.g., 8, 16, 18), and have even been used clinically in humans.[9]

It is generally accepted that the good results obtained with probes around arteries can be extrapolated to probes in the mitral annulus, but this is not necessarily the case. The aim of the present survey is to summarize the principle, advantages, and limitations of electromagnetic flowmeters and to show that some of the drawbacks of the method are more pronounced with probes in the mitral valve position.

PRINCIPLE

Electromagnetic flowmetry is based upon the principle that an electrical conductor moving in a direction perpendicular to a magnetic field induces a voltage proportional to the strength of the magnetic field and the velocity of the conductor. This voltage can be picked up with two electrodes.

Flowing blood is a moving conductor and will induce a voltage when a magnetic field is applied perpendicular to the direction of blood flow. Electromagnet, electrodes, and wires are built into a suitable material to form a probe which can easily be placed around a blood vessel. Special probes have been constructed for implantation in the left atrial side of the mitral annulus to measure mitral valve flow.[8]

Under ideal circumstances the induced voltage (E_f) equals:

$$E_f = B.D. \bar{v} \ 10^{-8}$$

in which B = the magnetic flux density (gauss)

D = the distance between the electrodes (cm)

$\bar{v}$ = the mean velocity over the cross-sectional area of the mitral ostium (cm/sec)

so that after calibration, volume flow of flow rate can be determined.

The first electromagnetic flowmeters made use of a constant magnetic field, generated by a permanent magnet or by energizing an electromagnet with a d-c current. In spite of the theoretical simplicity, this principle has been abandoned because the magnet and most of the non-polarizable electrodes are rather bulky. Close to the heart, it is difficult to eliminate the interference of the electrocardiogram with the flow signal.

Modern electromagnetic flowmeters are a-c flowmeters of the sine-wave[15,28] square-wave[7,11] or pulsed-field type.[5,29] In sine-wave flowmeters the magnet is energized by a sinusoidal alternating current, and in square-wave flowmeters by a rectangular alternating current. Pulsed-field flowmeters are characterized by rectangular magnetic fields of opposite polarity which are separated from each other by a brief period in which the magnetic fields equal zero. In these techniques the flow is sampled with a frequency (= carrier frequency) equal to that of the a-c current. The a-c methods deliver an amplitude-modulated signal and avoid the problem of polarization.

Moreover, unwanted signals, with a frequency significantly lower than the carrier frequency of the flowmeter, can largely be eliminated. A major disadvantage of the a-c method is the transformer effect, i.e., a voltage induced by the alternating magnetic field. This transformer voltage can be separated more easily from the flow-induced voltage in square-wave and in pulsed-field flowmeters than in flowmeters of the sine-wave type. Recently, however, the use of full wave demodulation and a stable phase adjustment seems to have improved the elimination of the transformer effect in sine-wave instruments.

Calibration of probes occurs by perfusing the probes at known-volume flows and correlating the flowmeter output in mv to the flow in ml/min. Since the calibration curves are linear, and the sensitivity remains equal when the polarity of the flow changes, only zero flow and one calibration point are required to determine the sensitivity of the probe. Calibration can be performed in vitro[4,31] or in vivo.[17,29]

Although the results obtained in in-vitro calibration are rather reproducible, the determined probe sensitivity usually differs from that assessed in vivo. The most common sources of differences between in-vitro and in-vivo calibrations are differences in conductivity of the perfusion fluid and the surrounding tissues and structures in both situations. In order to avoid the complicated procedure of in-vivo calibration, one normally makes use of in-vitro calibrated probes because most of the investigators are interested in relative changes in volume flow rather than in absolute volume flow values. If the latter information is required, in-situ calibration,[2,6,17,20] i.e., under the experimental circumstances, is necessary.

ADVANTAGES

The major advantages of electromagnetic flowmeters are:

1. The mechanical entity to be measured, i.e., blood flow, is directly transformed into an electrical signal.

2. Flow can be measured as an instantaneous function of time so that not only mean blood flow but also phasic blood flow, i.e., changes in blood flow during the cardiac cycle, can be recorded continuously.

3. The delay in the instrument is minimal and is mainly determined by the characteristics of the output filter.

For a 100 Hz filter with a roll-off of 6 db/octave, the delay is less than 1.6 msec. This minimal delay is especially important in phase-relation studies.

4. The calibration curves are linear.

LIMITATIONS

The proportionality of the induced voltage to the mean velocity over the cross-sectional area of the blood vessel or the mitral ostium, and, therefore, to volume flow, is based upon the assumption that the magnetic field is uniform and the velocity profile is axisymmetric, a situation which rarely exists under biological circumstances.

Nonuniformity of the field, especially its falling off upstream and downstream of the electrodes, causes the voltage-to-flow ratio to vary in response to variations in axisymmetric velocity profiles, i.e., deviations from the symmetry of the velocity profiles around the axis of the vessel or the mitral ostium.

In uniform magnetic fields, deviations from axisymmetric velocity profiles will also change the voltage-to-flow ratio, since the contribution of flow to the induced voltage varies over the cross-sectional area of the blood vessel or the mitral ostium. The ability of flow at each point of the cross section to contribute to the induced voltage is given by a weight function.[22,23] The form of the weight function depends on: (1) the geometry of the electrodes, (2) the conductivity of the vessel and the surrounding structures, and (3) the form of the magnetic field chosen.

In general the available probes for application in the mitral valve position have point electrodes in direct contact with the blood stream. In this situation the weight function is more unfavorable than with probes around blood vessels when the point electrodes are not in direct contact with the blood. In the latter situation the conducting vessel inside the probe gives less extreme weight function values, and therefore diminishes the variations in flowmeter sensitivity with changes from the axisymmetry of the velocity profile.[23] Figure 1 shows the weight function as determined in a model with nonconducting pipes, and the point electrodes in direct contact with the perfusion fluid. This type of weight function can give rise to large errors when the velocity profile is not axisymmetric. Concentration of flow near an electrode produces excessive voltages and misleading readings.

The weight function values presented in Figure 1 are obtained with transverse magnetic fields which are long in the flow direction, so that edge effects can be ignored.[24] In mitral valve probes, the transverse magnetic field is short in the flow direction, so that edge effects have to be taken into account. This will affect the weight function unfavorably. In addition, since the nonconducting pipes, proximal and distal to the electrodes, will influence the weight function values only insignificantly, the weight function given (Fig. 1) is not likely to be extreme for the situation with probes in the mitral valve position. Since model studies revealed that the anterior cusp of the mitral valve closes before the posterior cusp,[1] the velocity profile in the mitral ostium during the last part of diastole is not likely to be axisymmetric, which will result in inaccuracies in the determination of volume flow with electromagnetic flowmeters. Forward flow along the electrodes will give excessive volume flow readings, while in the case of a net forward flow across the mitral ostium, a simultaneously present

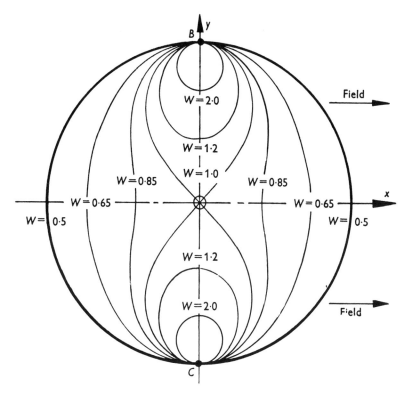

Figure 1. The ability of flow at various points of the cross-section to contribute to the induced voltage, when point electrodes are in direct contact with the perfusion fluid. After Shercliff (23).

eccentric back flow along the electrodes will disproportionally reduce the volume flow reading.

It is quite likely that the dependency of the flowmeter reading on the velocity profile can be diminished by using large electrodes and an elaborate magnetic field shape, which will decrease the variations in weight function over the cross-sectional area of the mitral opening.[3]

Additional inaccuracies in the determination of volume flow across the mitral valve result from differences between in-vitro and in-vivo calibration factors and the difficulty of obtaining a zero flow reference in vivo, especially in the presence of mitral valve regurgitation. Practically, in-situ calibration of probes in the mitral valve position can only be performed by comparing the flowmeter output with the cardiac output values as determined with dye, or thermodilution techniques, methods which are subject to errors themselves. For application in the mitral valve position, in-vitro calibration of the probes has to be performed with the electrodes in direct contact with the perfusion fluid, since the insertion of a vessel segment or synthetic tubing into the probe will influence the flowmeter sensitivity.[32] Because it is difficult to obtain a zero reference in vivo, one has to rely on the stability of the electronics. In spite of the excellent stability of modern electromagnetic flowmeters, some zero drift is still present, especially when changes at the surface of the electrodes, for instance due to clotting, occur.

Although both forward and back flow can be determined with electromagnetic flowmeters, these instruments only measure the net result of antegrade and retrograde flow; thus, these flow components cannot be recorded separately when present at the same time. The antegrade and retrograde components of flow can be measured separately with flowmeters based upon the Doppler principle.[27]

CONCLUSIONS

Electromagnetic flowmetry has proven to be an asset in studying phasic mitral valve flow. However, electromagnetic flow probes in the mitral valve position measure relative changes in volume flow rather than absolute volume flow values. This is mainly due to the unfavorable weight function and the nonaxisymmetric velocity profile across the mitral ostium, especially during the last part of diastole. Forward flow along the electrodes will give excessive volume flow readings, while in case of a net forward flow, a simultaneously present eccentric back flow along the electrodes will disproportionally reduce the volume flow reading. With large instead of point electrodes, and with an elaborate magnetic field shape, the dependency of the flowmeter reading on the velocity profile can probably be diminished.

REFERENCES

1. Bellhouse, B.J. Fluid mechanics of a model mitral valve and left ventricle. *Cardiovasc. Res.* 6:199, 1972.

2. Bergel, D., Makin, G. Experience with calibration procedures. In *New Findings in Blood Flowmetry*. Oslo: Universitetsforlaget, 1968.

3. Bevir, M.K. The theory of induced voltage electromagnetic flowmeters. *J. Fluid Mech.* 43:577, 1970.

4. Brunsting, J.R., Ten Hoor, F. Factors preventing accurate *in vitro* calibration of noncannulating electromagnetic flow transducers. In *New Findings in Blood Flowmetry*. Oslo: Universitetsforlaget, 1968.

5. Cannon, J.A. The design, characteristics, operation, and accuracy of pulsed field electromagnetic blood flowmeters. In *New Findings in Blood Flowmetry*. Oslo: Universitetsforlaget, 1968.

6. Cappelen, C., Hall, K.V. Electromagnetic blood flowmetry in clinical surgery. *Acta Chir. Scand. Suppl.* 368, 1967.

7. Denison, A.B., Spencer, M.P., Green, H.D. A square-wave electromagnetic flowmeter for application to intact blood vessels. *Circulat. Res.* 3:39, 1955.

8. Folts, J.D., Young, W.P., Rowe, G.G. Phasic flow through normal and prosthetic mitral valves in unanesthetized dogs. *J. Thorac. Cardiovasc. Surg.* 61:235, 1971.

9. Folts, J.D. Phasic transmitral blood flow in animals and man obtained without the use of cardiopulmonary bypass. This book, Chapter 14.

10. Greenfield, J.C., Rembert, J.C., Young, W.G., Newland Oldham, H., Alexander, J.A., Sabiston, D.C. Studies of blood flow in aorta-to-coronary venous bypass grafts in man. *J. Clin. Invest.* 51:2724, 1972.

11. Hognestad, H. Square-wave electromagnetic flowmeter with improved baseline stability. *Med. Res. Engn.* III. 28, 1966.

12. Joyce, E.E., Gregg, D.E. Coronary artery occlusion in the intact unanesthetized dog: intercoronary reflexes. *Amer. J. Physiol.* 213:64, 1967.

13. Khouri, E.M., Gregg, D.E. Miniature electromagnetic flowmeter applicable to coronary arteries. *J. Appl. Physiol.* 18:224, 1963.

14. Kolin, A. An electromagnetic flowmeter. Principles of the method and its application to blood flow measurements. *Proc. Soc. Exp. Biol.* 35:53, 1936.

15. Kolin, A. An a-c induction flowmeter for measurement of blood flow in intact blood vessels. *Proc. Soc. Exp. Biol.* 46:235, 1941.

16. Laniado, S., Yellin, E.L., Miller, H., Frater, R.W.M. Temporal relation of the first heart sound to closure of the mitral valve. *Circulation* 47:1006, 1973.

17. Noble, M.I.M., Gabe, I.T., Trenchard, D., Guz, A. Blood pressure and flow in the ascending aorta of conscious dogs. *Cardiovasc. Res.* 1:9, 1967.

18. Nolan, S.P., Dixon, S.H., Fisher, R.D., Morrow, A.G. The influence of atrial contraction and mitral valve mechanics on ventricular filling. A study of instantaneous mitral valve flow *in vivo. Amer. Heart. J.* 77:784, 1969.

19. Provan, J.L., Hammond, G.L., Austen, W.G. Flowmeter studies of internal mammary artery function after implantation into the left ventricular myocardium. *J. Thorac. Cardiovasc. Surg.* 52:820, 1967.

20. Reneman, R.S., Clarke, H.F., Simmons, N., Spencer, M.P. *In vivo* comparison of electromagnetic and Doppler flowmeters: with special attention to the processing of the analogue Doppler flow signal. *Cardiovasc. Res.* 7:557, 1973.

21. Reneman, R.S., Spencer, M.P. The use of diastolic reactive hyperemia to evaluate the coronary vascular system. *Ann. Thorac. Surg.* 13:477, 1972.

22. Shercliff, J.A. Relation between the velocity profile and the sensitivity of electromagnetic flowmeters. *J. Appl. Physiol.* 25:817, 1954.

23. Shercliff, J.A. *The Theory of Electromagnetic Flow-Measurement* London: Cambridge University Press, 1962.

24. Shercliff, J.A. The effects of nonuniform magnetic fields and variations of the velocity distribution in electromagnetic flowmeters. In *New Findings in Blood Flowmetry*. Oslo: Universitetsforlaget, 1968.

25. Spencer, M.P., Greis, F.C. Dynamics of ventricular ejection. *Circulat. Res.* 10:274, 1962.

26. Spencer, M.P., Denison, A.B. Pulsatile blood flow in the vascular system. In *Handbook of Physiology*. Section II. Circulation II. Washington, D.C.: American Physiological Society, 1963.

27. Strandness, D.E., Kennedy, J.W., Judge, T.P., McLeod, F.D. Transcutaneous directional flow detection: A preliminary report. *Amer. Heart J.* 78:65, 1969.

28. Westersten, A., Herrold, G., Assali, N.S. A gated sine wave blood flowmeter. *J. Appl. Physiol.* 15:533, 1960.

29. Westersten, A., Rice, E., Brinkman, C.R., Assali, N.S. A balanced field-type electromagnetic flowmeter. *J. Appl. Physiol.* 26:497, 1969.

30. Wetterer, E. Eine neue Methode zur Registrierung der Blutströmungsgeschwindigkeit am uneröffneten Gefäss. *Z. Biol.* 98:26, 1937.

31. Wolfson, S.K., Icöz, M.V., Surur, F., Pritchard, M. Semi-automatic calibration technique for electromagnetic flowmeter probes. *Med. Res. Engn.* IV. 37, 1968.

32. Wyatt, D.C. Dependence of electromagnetic flowmeter sensitivity upon encircled media. *Phys. Med. Biol.* 13:529, 1968.

12 Velocity Profile and Impedance of the Healthy Mitral Valve*

D.E.M. Taylor, F.R.C.S.
Joan S. Whamond

Investigations into the fluid dynamics of the mitral valve, normal, diseased and prosthetic, have necessitated the development of techniques for accurate, point-by-point estimation of pressure and flow within the heart. In addition, there is a need for methods of mapping the position and movements of the valve anulus and cusps during diastole for the normal valve, and of determining the position of occluders or leaflets in prosthetic valves. For the first of these we have developed a method which is equally applicable to experimental animals in the laboratory or to patients at the time of open cardiac surgery. The technique developed for the latter of intracardiac photography has only been applied in the acute experimental animal.

PRESSURE AND FLOW DETERMINATIONS

The flow patterns within the heart are complex in nature, particularly considering that we are never dealing with a uniform flow

* This work was carried out under grants from the Scottish Home and Health Department and the British Heart Foundation. The analog hybrid computer used was provided by the Wellcome Trust.

127

channel, either from one point in the flow path to another, or even from time to time during the cardiac cycle. The technique which we have developed, and which is now used routinely,[1] relies on a modification of the Pitot principle incorporated into an 18SWG needle with a depth indicator so that its positions within the heart at the time of measurement can be determined to a relative accuracy of 0.25 mm. The needle is double-barreled and has two eyes which face in opposite directions, so that in effect the pressure at a point is estimated along two vectors at 180° from one to the other; for obvious reasons of classical analogy the device has been named a Janus needle. If the needle is placed so that it lies directly in the line of flow, the eye facing the stream will act as an impact meter; it will convert the kinetic energy of flow into a static head of pressure, thus measuring the combined lateral pressure plus kinetic energy. The eye facing away from the flow will have a drag exerted on it by the flow away from the eye and, theoretically, this will also be equal to the kinetic energy; therefore, the downstream eye measures the lateral pressure minus the kinetic energy. By simple mathematics it is possible to derive from this the lateral and kinetic energy components and to work out the velocity of flow from the latter. If the direction of flow is not constant, then by the use of the needle in two positions at right angles to each other and by compounding a large number of consecutive cardiac cycles, it is possible to derive the flow with its vector at any time during the cardiac cycle. The calibration of these needles does not conform to the exact physical relationships expected from the Bernoulli equation, but each needle can be calibrated against known flows in vitro, and a characteristic curve can be produced which can be set for later computer processing of the records. The pressure tracings thus obtained with the Janus needle are recorded on F.M. analog tape. The transducers used each have simultaneously applied a zero and a full scale deflection, usually 200 mm Hg: no attempt is made to set the transducers relative to each other during the recording stage; this is carried out at the processing stage with computer assistance. Regardless of the number and types of needles being used for pressure and velocity, one transducer is always taken as the master and all other transducer outputs are adjusted relative to this by a null error method. Using the records obtained with the Janus needles and computer graphic techniques, it is possible to build up pictures of velocity profiles and of flow patterns within the heart. With the use of techniques requiring the Fourier transforms of pressure and flow, it is possible to determine whether the flow is basically stable or turbulent at any particular stage during the cardiac cycle; it is also possible to derive compound impedance and its resistive and reactive components.[2,3,4,5]

VALVE MOVEMENTS

The technique used for this relies on high speed ciné-photography using a cardiac endoscope which was developed for our use by Optec Limited.[6,7] The telescope system has a wide-angled lens, and the position of any point on a frame may be described as two angular coordinates, first, an angle of rotation round from the notch which is marked on the outer circumference frame, and second, an angle out from the center line. By taking photographs of the inside of the ventricle from two positions a known distance apart and again by overlaying 24 to 50 consecutive cardiac cycles and making measurements on these, it is possible by standard spherical geometry and computer graphic techniques to build up a three-dimensional picture of the valve and its movements, as well as the movements of the heart wall. The results to be described are a composite picture derived both from studies of patients at operation and from animal research over the past decade.

Normal Valve Movements

Before considering the flow profiles within the valve canal, we must first describe our interpretation of the dynamics of the valve cusps during diastole. The early pictures which we reported[6] have been confirmed by other workers.[8,9,10] These studies described the valve cusps as rapidly parting, with a partial approximation during mid-diastole after the rapid filling phase, followed by a widening again after atrial systole. The pictures of cusp movement which were produced differed markedly from what was seen with echocardiographic techniques, where there is extensive, rapid movement of the anterior cusp of the mitral valve, almost to the initial position after the rapid filling phase, rather than the lesser movement reported using either endoscopic or cineradiographic techniques.

However, it should be taken into account that in echocardiography the reference point used is the septal wall rather than the line between the two commissures which has been used as the reference point in endoscopic studies. As has been described by Tsakiris,[11] the mitral annulus moves during diastole, tilting posteriorly as filling progresses; therefore, we reprocessed our data using a reference point on the anteromedial ventricular wall and found that the extensive and rapid mid-diastolic movement of the anterior cusp observed on echocardiography was now seen. Measurements of the posterior cusp at this time showed that there was also some backward movement of the posterior cusp, which was confirmed on echocardiogram records where both anterior and posterior cusps of the mitral valve were recorded. Thus in mid-diastole, instead of the valves showing a marked approximation, there is only a partial approximation and the valves as a whole at their free margins both tend to move posteriorly. Studies in pure flow dynamics[12] show that when a jet is directed into a closed-ended cylinder, a condition analogous to flow through the mitral valve into the ventricle, a vortical system similar to that of the ventricle is produced; however, there is not one but two stagnation points, and the flow patterns oscillate between the two with a quite rapid movement from one to the other. During endoscopic studies, if one looks at the cusp movements in the heart and observes flow with small bubbles or with fine particles of calcium carbonate, it appears that a similar type of event is occurring in the normal mitral valve. During mid-diastole there is a switch of stagnation point within the ventricle from a position close to the apex near the septum to a more lateral and posterior position on the free wall of the ventricles.[13] The result of this is that during diastole the relative position or slope of the cusps to the valve ring changes and, indeed, the angle of the inlet of the mitral valve at the free cusp margin also changes. This has marked effects on the velocity profile, as will be demonstrated. The shape of the canal itself, as described by du Plessis and Marchand,[14] is an obliquely truncated conoid, but both the inlet at the valve ring and the outlet at the free cusp margin are ellipsoid, the eccentricity being less at the outlet of the mitral valve canal than at the inlet. Consequently, mean hydrolic depth is much less reduced as one proceeds through the mitral valve canal than would be anticipated from mere consideration of the relative areas at these two positions.[7]

VELOCITY PROFILES

At the inlet of the mitral valve, at the level of the annulus, the velocity profile is basically that of plug flow with both a flat profile throughout diastolic filling and a zone of high shear only near the margins of the valve (Figs. 1 and 2). In early diastole, during the rapid filling phase, the same type of flat velocity profile is also seen at the free cusp margin level. The stagnation point is near the apex, and there is the formation of the vortical system described previously.[9,10,15] As the flow begins to slow during mid-diastole and the posterior movement of the valve cusps occurs, the angle of the anterior cusp to the plane of the inlet becomes more acute, resulting in an acceleration in the velocity profile adjacent to the anterior cusp. Thus, rather than the flat profile of early diastole, as one goes through

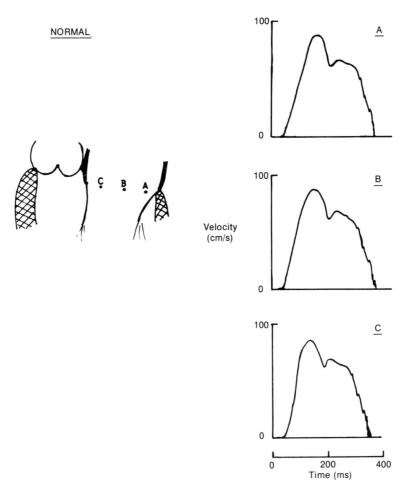

Figure 1. Velocity curves at three positions on an anteroposterior traverse at the level of the valve annulus. The curves are almost identical, indicating a flat velocity profile; they have little random fluctuation, indicating stable flow and show closure without regurgitation.

132

mid and late diastole, the profile becomes skewed with much more rapid velocities occurring anteriorly than are seen posteriorly (Fig. 3). This is reflected in different velocities, and therefore different energies, within the vortices, so that although the vortex behind the anterior cusp and going into the outflow region of the ventricle becomes more vigorous, the vortex associated with the posterior or mural cusp becomes smaller and less vigorous. The closure of the

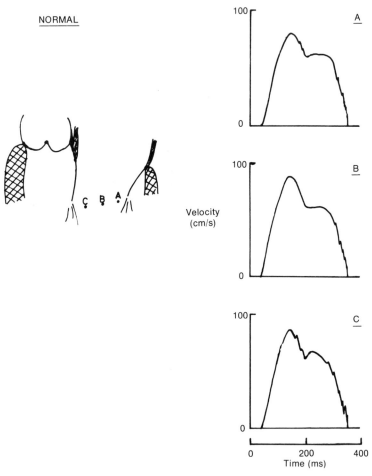

Figure 2. Velocity curves at three positions on an anteroposterior traverse across the left ventricle at a level just distal to the free cusp margins in the fully open position. The curves differ in shape in mid and late diastole because of the skewing of the velocity profile, but still show stable flow characteristics.

valve is rapid; it is associated with virtually no reflux and with only a minimal disturbance of flow pattern during this time.

TYPE OF FLOW OBSERVED

At all levels in the valve canal and also within the ventricle, there are only two transient periods of flow disturbance associated with diastolic filling. These take place during the deceleration phase when the switch in the stagnation point occurs and during terminal diastole around the the time of valve closure. Apart from this, flow patterns appear to be stable, but it is not possible to determine whether we are dealing with purely laminar flow or a mixed laminar/turbulent flow with stable patterns.

EFFECT OF HEART RATE

With an increase in heart rate, the major effect is that although the velocity during the rapid filling phase does not increase very much

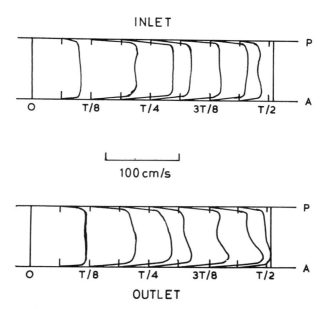

Figure 3. Velocity profiles at times in 1/16 (π/8 rad) of a cardiac cycle. Note the flat axiosymmetric profile at the level of the valve annulus, but the nonaxiosymmetric flow with acceleration of the laminae nearer to the anterior cusp in mid and late diastole at the level of the free cusp margins.

in proportion to the change in mean velocity across the valve, there is a very marked increase in flow consequent on atrial systole, with a flow velocity through the valve during atrial systole becoming almost as great as that during the early rapid filling phase, and with a consequent increase in the atrial supplementation.[2] The latter is not necessarily at variance with the results presented by other studies,[16,17] as our figures were obtained by extrapolating the filling curve and taking the area above it; if the method of dropping a vertical were adopted, we would also show a decrease in atrial contribution with increased heart rate. In terms of the velocity profile, the stagnation point switch still occurs, and the skewing of the velocity profile at the outlet of the mitral valve becomes much more accentuated. However, despite these changes, the occurrence of flow disturbance shows very little change, and a predominantly stable type of flow pattern remains. There were two reasons for this: first, the area at the cusp margins remained larger for most of diastolic filling, with less eccentricity;[13] and second, because of the changed pattern of filling, with the increase in the peak velocity of flow being less than the increase in mean flow, the increase in peak Reynold's number was approximately proportional to the change in Womersley's $\propto$. For the latter, taking the relationship proposed between the critical Re by Cotton,[18] the values we have observed for these variations in the normal heart would all have been below the critical Re for turbulence.

IMPEDANCE AND ENERGY LOSS

If the mitral valve is considered to be a simple orifice, using a DC analogue, the energy loss should be proportional to the square of the flow rate: this does not occur and the energy loss bears less than a square-law relationship to flow, although it is more than a linear relation.[2,3] If the pulsatile nature of the flow is also considered, a first approximation shows that the impedance change should depend both on the resistance, which will change in proportion to flow, and the reactance, which will change in proportion to heart rate.[5] Preliminary investigations indicate that neither of these predictions are correct for the normal mitral valve. The resistive behavior is less affected by flow than anticipated, possibly related to the changed geometry of the valve canal, and the reactance also shows less dependence on heart rate than predicted.[3] Therefore, the normal valve can adapt to changing cardiac output so as to optimize the increase in energy loss in a manner similar to that already reported for the aortic valve.[4]

SUMMARY

The flow through the normal mitral valve is predominantly stable at all heart rates. At the level of the valve ring, the velocity profile is flat and consistent with a plug flow such as one would anticipate at the inlet to a pipe system. At the free cusp margin, i.e., the valve outlet, although flow starts off with a flat velocity profile, following a movement of both cusps towards the posterior wall of the heart after the initial rapid filling phase, the velocity profile becomes skewed with more rapid flow adjacent to the anterior cusp. These changes in mid and late diastole are accentuated with increasing heart rate and are also associated with a marked increase in the peak velocity of flow during atrial systole. The stability of flow patterns and the changing valve geometry and filling pattern enable an increased cardiac output to be achieved without the square law increase in energy loss anticipated by flow across an orifice.

REFERENCES

1. Taylor, D.E.M., Whamond, J.S. Measurement of energy and flow distribution within heart chambers *in vivo*. Edited by D.J. Cockerell. In *Fluid Dynamic Measurement in the Industrial and Medical Environments*. Leicester: University Press, 1972.

2. Taylor, D.E.M., Whamond, J.S. The dynamics of left ventricular filling at high heart rates. *J. Physiol.* 225:40, 1972.

3. Taylor, D.E.M., Whamond, J.S., Tansley, J. Transvalvular impedance across normal, stenotic and prosthetic heart valves. In *Abstracts of 4th Conference on Recent Advances in Bioengineering*. University of Surrey, 1974.

4. Carnie, N., Mukhtar, A.I., Pollock, C.G., Taylor, D.E.M., Whamond, J.S. Impedance spectra change across the aortic valve at different heart rates in the sheep. *J. Physiol.* 238:48, 1973.

5. Eastell, R., Taylor, D.E.M., Whamond, J.S. Impedance change to differing heart rate and cardiac output across the acutely stenosed aortic valve. *J. Physiol.* 248:33, 1975.

6. Hider, C.F., Taylor, D.E.M., Wade, J.D. Action of the mitral and aortic valves *in vivo* studies by endoscopic cine photography. *Q. J. Exp. Physiol.* 51:372, 1966.

7. Taylor, D.E.M. Mitral valve geometry and flow dyanmics at varying heart rates in the dog. *J. Physiol.* 227:37, 1973.

8. Padula, R.T., Cowan, G.S.M., Jr., Camishion,

136

R.C. Photographic analysis of the active and passive components of cardiac valvular action. *J. Thor. Cardiovasc. Surg.* 56:790, 1968.

9. Bellhouse, B.J. Fluid mechanics of a model mitral valve. *J. Physiol.* 207:72, 1970.

10. Wieting, D.W., Hwang, N.H.C., Kennedy, J.H. Fluid dynamics of the human mitral valve. A.I.A.A. 9th Aerospace Sciences Meeting. New York, 1971, p. 25.

11. Tsakiris, A.G. Study of size and motion of the mitral annulus in normal and abnormal conditions. This book, p. 21

12. Malloy, N.A., Taylor, P.L. Oscillatory flow of a jet into blind cavity. *Nature* 224:1192, 1969.

13. Whamond, J.S., Taylor, D.E.M. The dynamic anatomy of the mitral valve. In *Abstracts of Euromech Colloquium on Cardiovascular and Respiratory Mechanics,* 1975.

14. Plessis, L.A. du, Marchand, P. The anatomy of the mitral valve and its associated structures. *Thorax* 19:221, 1964.

15. Taylor, D.E.M., Wade, J.D. The pattern of flow around the atrioventricular valves during diastolic ventricular filling. *J. Physiol.* 207:71, 1970.

16. Folts, J.D. Phasic transmitral blood flow in animals and man obtained without the use of cardiopulmonary bypass. This book, Chapter 14.

17. Nolan, P. Flow characteristics of mitral valvular prostehses: ball, disc and xenograft. This book, Chapter 25.

18. Cotton, K.L. The instantaneous measurement of blood flow and of vascular impedance. Ph.D. Thesis, University of London. Cited by D. McDonald. In *Blood Flow in Arteries*. London: Edward Arnold, 1960.

13 The Normal Mitral Valve: Patterns of Instantaneous Mitral Valve Flow and the Atrial Contribution to Ventricular Filling

Stanton P. Nolan, M.D.

Cardiac performance has been extensively characterized by studies of the hemodynamic events in the left ventricle. Less attention has been directed to the role of the left atrium, which serves both as an elastic reservoir and as an active booster pump, or to the function of the mitral valve, which controls the direction of, and impedance to, flow. These structures have an obvious and direct influence upon ventricular filling and ventricular performance.

METHODOLOGY

A method for measuring and recording the volume and pattern of instantaneous blood flow through the mitral valve was devised and utilized in the studies to be described. The experiments, carried out in normal calves, were designed to provide information concerning the atrial contribution to ventricular filling and the mechanical behavior of the mitral valve.

A specifically constructed electromagnetic flow transducer was used to measure mitral valve flow. A fabric fixation ring was applied to the transducer and this was sutured to the atrial wall above the mitral valve during cardiopulmonary bypass. The transducer has an inside diameter of 22 millimeters and an orifice area of 3.8 square centimeters. It was placed in such a way that it neither distorted nor obstructed blood flow. An extravascular flow transducer was placed on the ascending aorta and pressures were measured simultaneously in the left atrium, left ventricle, and aortic root. All data were recorded simultaneously on magnetic tape and later rerecorded photographically for analysis. Dynamic calibration of the pressure and flow measuring systems, from one to 25 cycles per second, demonstrated that the maximum and minimum differences in transit time between the two systems were 2.7 and 1.9 milliseconds, respectively. Calves were studied in the anesthetized, open-chest state. Continuous recordings were made during each experiment for periods varying from one to three hours, providing a total of 15 hours of recorded simultaneous pressure and flow. There were spontaneous variations in heart rate from 50 to 200 per minute; cardiac rhythm interpreted from the electrocardiogram ranged from normal sinus to low nodal rhythm. Premature ventricular contractions were produced by light mechanical stimulation of the heart, and cardiac output was varied by the slow infusion or withdrawal of blood from the femoral artery.

RESULTS

The normal pattern of instantaneous mitral valve blood flow was determined at heart rates of 70 to 100 per minute and with PR intervals between 0.12 and 0.18 seconds. Illustrated (Fig. 1) are simultaneous recordings of the electrocardiogram, the aortic blood flow, the mitral valve flow, and the aortic, left ventricular, and left atrial pressures. Under conditions of normal heart rate and PR interval, it was possible to define six separate phases of mitral valve flow and their relationships to the atrial and ventricular pressures. Phase I, as indicated in Figure 1, was a period of low rate and volume of flow that lasted 30 milliseconds during protodiastole. Phase II began with the onset of the positive atrioventricular pressure gradient and, during this period, flow accelerated rapidly and declined slowly. Phase III commenced with atrial contraction when flow again accelerated to a secondary peak. With reversal of the atrioventricular pressure gradient, although flow decelerated rapidly, forward flow persisted 15 milliseconds after reversal of the pressure gradient. Phase IV was the only period of reversed flow, and this occurred during isovolumetric ventricular contraction. Phase V varied in length from 15 to 40 milliseconds; it consisted of a small volume and low rate of flow that followed the atrial "c" wave. Finally, Phase VI extended throughout the remainder of systole, during which period there was no detectable mitral valve flow.

In all animals studied, Phases I, IV, V, and VI were consistent in amplitude and timing if the mitral valve was competent. Phase II and III, however, showed marked variations which were related to heart rate and the timing of atrial contraction.

Figure 2 illustrates the effect of heart rate on Phases II and III of mitral valve flow. Phase II, as stated before, represents the flow occurring passively during the initial part of diastole, while Phase III represents flow occurring during active atrial contraction. The effect of heart rate on flow during each of these phases is apparent. Each of

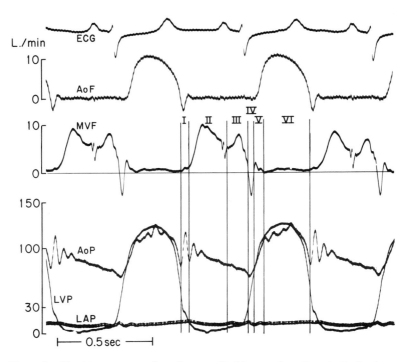

Figure 1. Simultaneous recordings from a calf with normal aortic and mitral valves. The electrocardiogram (ECG) shows normal sinus rhythm and a heart rate of 95. The P-R interval is 0.14 sec. The patterns of aortic (AoF) and mitral valve flow (MVF) are normal. The aortic (AoP), left ventricular (LVP), and left atrial pressures (LAP) are shown at the bottom. Vertical lines have been constructed to define the six phases of mitral valve flow, and each phase is labeled with a Roman numeral (see text).

140

the flows was recorded at comparable P-R intervals; however, the heart rate varied from 52 to 165 per minute. At the lower heart rates, there is very little blood flow during the latter part of Phase II, while at the higher heart rates there is a loss of the secondary acceleration of flow in Phase III.

Figure 3 demonstrates the effect of altering the P-R interval. These patterns of flow were recorded at heart rates of 92 to 95 per minute. The pattern at the top of the illustration occurred with a P-R interval of 0.14 seconds while the pattern shown at the bottom was recorded during nodal rhythm. It is apparent from the change in

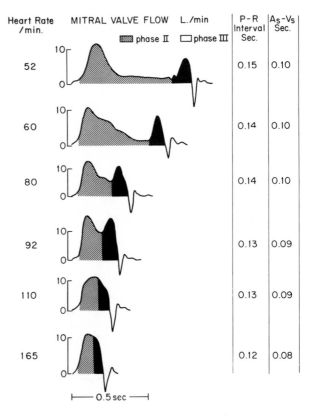

Figure 2. Effect of heart rate on mitral valve flow. Mitral valve flow recorded at six different heart rates from 52 to 165 beats per minute. The P-R and A_s-V_s intervals are normal for each heart rate. The area enclosed by Phase II flow is crosshatched, while the area under Phase III flow is solid. Above a heart rate of 92 beats per minute there is no secondary acceleration during Phase III.

pattern that the secondary acceleration in flow due to atrial contraction decreases with decreasing P-R interval, and that the volume of flow during atrial contraction likewise decreases.

A study of the variations in the Phase III flow with variations in heart rate or P-R interval suggests that atrial contraction makes a significant contribution to ventricular filling. However, from these patterns it is impossible to say what portion of the flow occurring during atrial systole was due to contraction, and what portion to the elastic qualities of the atrium.

More direct evidence of the effect of atrial contraction was obtained from several animals. Cardiac rhythm changed spontaneously from normal sinus to nodal rhythm without a change in heart

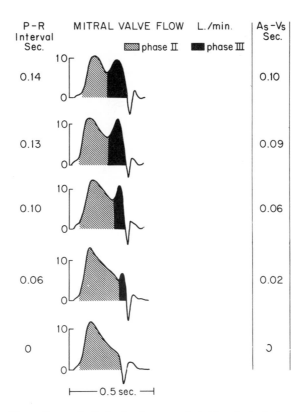

Figure 3. Five patterns of mitral valve flow recorded at heart rates between 90 and 95 beats per minute, but with progressive decrease in the P-R interval. The area enclosed by Phase II flow is crosshatched, and the area beneath Phase III flow is solid. As the P-R interval shortened, the amplitude and area enclosed by Phase III decreased.

rate. In nodal rhythm, Phase III flow disappeared and there was a 20% decrease in mitral and aortic stroke volume, and a 20% decrease in cardiac output. This would suggest that atrial contraction augments ventricular filling.

Premature ventricular contractions produced a barely detectable change in the Phase IV flow. Thus, with multiple observations, the increase in negative flow was only 0.2 ml. It is unlikely, therefore, that premature ventricular contractions are the cause of significant mitral regurgitation.

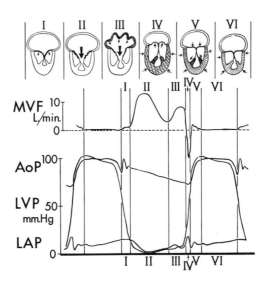

Figure 4. A graphic representation of the six phases of normal mitral valve flow (MVF) and their relationship to the aortic (AoP), left ventricular (LVP), and left atrial pressures (LAP). The behavior of the atrium, ventricle, papillary muscles, and mitral valve, which accounts for the changes in mitral valve flow, is shown at the top. Phase I: onset simultaneous with dicrotic notch of the aortic pressure pulse. Low rate and volume of flow lasting 30 to 40 msec. during protodiastole. As LVP falls, mitral leaflets descend toward the ventricle. Phase II: onset with positive LAP-LVP gradient. Flow accelerates rapidly, declines slowly. Passive filling of the ventricle determined by the volumes and elastic qualities of the atrium and ventricle. Phase III: onset with atrial contraction, rising to secondary peak, then decelerating rapidly. Forward flow persists 10 to 15 msec after reversal of the LAP-LVP gradient. This is the only period of active ventricular filling and varies with the timing and force of atrial contraction. Phase IV: the only period of reverse flow. This occurs during isovolumetric contraction, coinciding with the atrial c wave. It is caused by the closed mitral leaflets bulging into the atrium as LVP rises. Phase V: small volume and low rate of forward flow lasting 25 to 30 msec. This is caused by continued papillary muscle contraction which draws the mitral leaflets toward the ventricle. Phase VI: this period extends throughout the remainder of systole. There is no detectable flow until the onset of the succeeding Phase I.

COMMENTS

From our observations of mitral valve flow, we have developed a theory to explain the events that surround ventricular filling. A graphic summary of our theory is shown (Fig. 4). At the top of the illustration there is a schematic representation of the left side of the heart; in the middle is the mitral valve flow; and, at the bottom, the simultaneous pressures. Phase I is a period of low volume and rate of flow which occurs during protodiastole, when ventricular pressure falls and tension is released from the mitral leaflets. Phase II begins with the reversal of the mitral pressure gradient when the valve opens; this is a period of passive flow determined by the volumes and elastic qualities of the atrium and ventricle. In Phase III there is a secondary acceleration of flow with atrial contraction; however, due to the mass acceleration effects, forward flow persists for 15 milliseconds after reversal of the pressure gradient. Phase IV is a period of negative flow when the mitral valve bulges into the atrium. In Phase V the papillary muscles contract, increasing the tension on the leaflets and returning a small volume of blood to the ventricular side of the mitral flow probe. Careful measurement has shown that the sum of the volumes of flow during Phases I and V equals the negative volume in Phase IV. This is evidence that there is no net mitral regurgitation through the normal valve.

In summary, these studies indicate that: 1) with normal heart rates of 80 to 100 per minute, and with normal P-R intervals, six separate phases of mitral valve flow are apparent; 2) atrial contraction can augment ventricular filling by as much as 20%; 3) the mitral valve closes without regurgitation in sinus or nodal rhythm; 4) the regurgitation accompanying premature ventricular contractions is negligible; and 5) the major role of atrial contraction is the augmentation of ventricular filling—not the prevention of mitral regurgitation.

SELECTED READING

Nolan, S.P., Dixon, S.H. Jr., Fisher, D.H., Morrow, A.G. The influence of atrial contraction and mitral valve mechanics on ventricular filling—a study of instantaneous mitral valve flow in vivo. *Am. Heart J.* 77:784-791, 1969.

14 Phasic Transmitral Blood Flow in Animals and Man Obtained Without the Use of Cardiopulmonary Bypass

John D. Folts, Ph.D.

Phasic transmitral and tricuspid blood flow has been measured using circular electromagnetic flowmeter probes.[1-6] These are surgically placed in the atrium above the appropriate atrioventricular valve, utilizing cardiopulmonary bypass and hypothermia, and requiring a large atriotomy through which the flowprobe is sutured in place. With two exceptions[1,2] all hemodynamic measurements were made at the completion of the flowmeter implantation and shortly after the termination of the cardiopulmonary bypass. These were open-chest anesthetized animals which were recovering from the effects of cardiopulmonary bypass and a two to three hour surgical procedure.

A new flowprobe is described for obtaining transmitral volume flow which can be implanted without the use of cardiopulmonary bypass. It allows for acute placement of the probe in 10–15 minutes so that mitral flow studies can begin when the animal has received minimal anesthesia. In addition, this probe can be acutely placed in the atrium of man at the time of valvular surgery, prior to establishing cardiopulmonary bypass, for evaluating valve flow and any insufficiency that may be present. Finally this probe can also be chronically implanted in dogs in 20 minutes without significant damage to the atrium and without the use of cardiopulmonary bypass.

METHODS

Chronic flowprobe implantation

A C-shaped electromagnetic flow probe was constructed as previously described[7] and shown in Figure 1a. The probe has a layer of dacron cloth on the outer surface for placing sutures. This flowprobe is passed through a small hole cut in the tip of the atrial appendage, with bleeding controlled by a purse-string suture in the left atrial appendage. The entire probe is advanced into the left atrium, and the purse string is tightened around the flowprobe cable. The probe is then positioned in the left atrium over the plane of the mitral valve, and just above the atrioventricular ring by feeling through the atrial wall. It may then be sutured in place by passing 3-0 sutures through the left atrial wall, above the AV ring, and through the dacron sewing ring. Sutures are not placed in the area of the interatrial septum but may be placed three-fourths of the way around the left atrium. Sutures are sufficient to hold the probe in place chronically. The flowprobe cable is then brought out through the chest incision in a manner similar to placing any other flowmeter probe chronically. Five dogs were prepared with mitral flowprobes chronically implanted in this manner. Left atrial and left ventricular catheters for pressure measurement were also implanted as previously described.[8]

Acute experiments in dogs and man

The flowprobe (Fig. 1b) was designed in collaboration with Carolina Medical Electronics.* It has a special flexible handle which can be bent in any direction and will maintain that position until purposely bent to a new position. Probes are constructed in a range of sizes from 50–80 mm circumference to fit in the atria of dogs and man.

The probe is passed through the atrial appendage as previously

---

* Carolina Medical Electronics, Inc., P.O. Box 307, King, North Carolina 27021.

described, and positioned over the mitral valve. The flexible cable is then bent to an appropriate position to hold the flowprobe in place above the mitral ring. Left atrial and left ventricular pressure can be obtained with catheters passed through the atrial and ventricular walls and connected to equisensitive pressure gauges. Five open-chest anesthetized dogs were prepared, with the acute style flowprobe positioned above the mitral valve in an average of 18 minutes. The flowprobe could be left in place for up to three hours for continuous recordings of transmitral flow.

The larger human probe was used in a patient at the time of open heart surgery. The probe was positioned over the mitral valve before cardiopulmonary bypass was established, and again after the valve had been repaired and the cardiopulmonary bypass had been discontinued. Left atrial and left ventricular pressure was obtained with Angiocath catheters passed through the atrial and ventricular walls

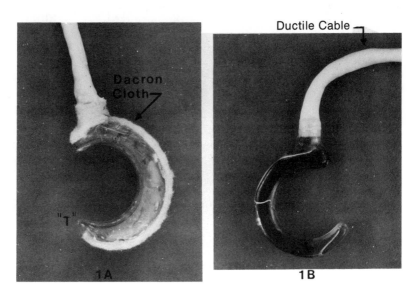

Figure 1a. On the left is the C-shaped electromagnetic flowmeter probe for chronic implantation. The tip "T" is passed through a hole cut in the atrial appendage and the probe advanced into the atrium. After positioning it over the mitral valve, the probe is sutured in place with 3-0 silk sutures passed through the atrial wall and into the dacron sewing ring.

Figure 1b. On the right is the flowprobe for acute implantation. The probe is advanced into the left atrium and positioned over the mitral valve by appropriate bending of the special ductile handle.

and attached to equisensitive pressure gauges. Flow and pressures were recorded on a direct writing recorder.*

RESULTS

A sample record obtained ten days postoperatively from one of the five dogs chronically instrumented is shown in Figure 2. The effect of atrial contraction on mitral inflow is marked AC. The left atrial and left ventricular pressure are obtained using indwelling catheters which have been previously described.[8]

---

* Hewlett Packard.

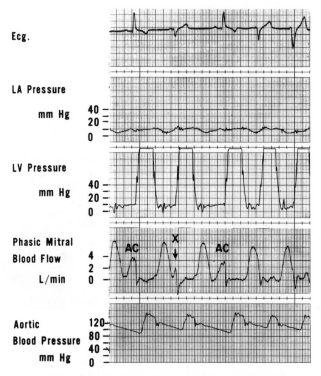

Figure 2. Phasic mitral blood flow in an unanesthetized dog. The atrial contribution to mitral inflow is shown at the point marked AC. In the second cardiac cycle a nodal beat occurs with shortening of the P-R interval, and the atrial component of mitral inflow is cut off at point X. There is flow below the zero flow line which indicates mitral regurgitation after point X. The last two cardiac cycles are produced by ventricular premature beats and there is no p wave, and no atrial contribution to mitral inflow.

The effect of nodal and ventricular arrhythmias on normal mitral inflow can be clearly seen in the electrocardiogram (Fig. 2). The first cardiac cycle is normal with normal sinus rhythm. The second beat is produced by nodal excitation, and the atrial contribution to mitral flow is cut off by the premature systole, at point x. Some systolic mitral regurgitation is noted. The third cycle is normal with a normal amount of mitral flow due to atrial contraction as indicated by AC. The fourth and fifth cardiac cycles are caused by ventricular premature beats as noted on the ECG. There is no p wave, and no atrial contraction to contribute to mitral inflow. The peak aortic blood pressure is decreased following the last two premature beats, presumably due to less ventricular filling.

The record obtained from another resting, chronically instrumented, unanesthetized dog is shown (Fig. 3), and the effect of increasing heart rate on mitral inflow due to atrial contraction is seen. Heart rate in the first panel is 95 beats/min and the atrial contribution to mitral inflow is 29%. In panel B, the dog has been aroused and heart

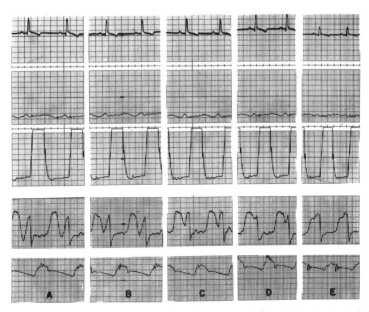

Figure 3. Phasic mitral flow at five different heart rates. In panel A the heart rate is 95 beats/min and the atrial contribution to total mitral inflow is 29% as measured by planimetry of 10 consecutive cardiac cycles. In panel C the heart rate has been increased to 114 beats/min and the atrial contribution to mitral inflow is 19% of total mitral flow. In panel E the heart rate has been increased to 134 beats/min and the atrial contribution to total mitral inflow is only 10%.

rate increased to 108 beats/min; the atrial contribution is reduced to 27% of total mitral inflow. In panels C and D, heart rate is increased to 114 and 125 beats/min respectively, with subsequent decreases in mitral flow due to atrial contraction. In panel E, the heart rate is 134 beats/min and the atrial contribution to mitral inflow is only 10%.

One can see (Fig. 4a) the mitral flow obtained in one of the open-chest anesthetized dogs with the flowprobe placed acutely in the left atrium. Left atrial and left ventricular pressure are recorded through indwelling catheters implanted as previously described.[8] Aortic pulse pressure was 135/105 mm Hg. This animal was given an acute, two-minute episode of aortic valvular insufficiency using a special catheter device designed to be passed down the carotid artery and into the left ventricle through the aortic valve.[9] Using this device, aortic insufficiency can be produced temporarily and then can be discontinued.

In Figure 4a the effects of 120 seconds of aortic insufficiency on phasic mitral flow may be seen. There are two places in the cardiac cycle where mitral regurgitation is produced. During diastole, at point

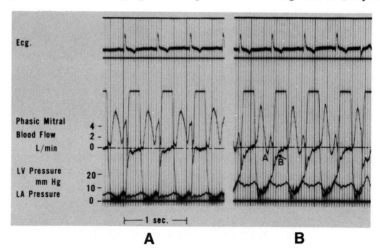

Figure 4a. Phasic mitral flow, left atrial and left ventricular pressure, and ECG recorded from an anesthetized open chest dog, using the acute style flowmeter probe. The left ventricular end diastolic pressure is 7 mm Hg and aortic pulse pressure (not shown) was 135/105 mm Hg.

Figure 4b. Hemodynamic changes which occur after 120 seconds of acute temporary aortic insufficiency. The phasic mitral flow is altered with two areas of mitral regurgitation produced at A and B by the induced aortic insufficiency. The left ventricular end diastolic pressure is elevated to 20 mm Hg and there is premature reversal of the atrial and ventricular pressures with subsequent regurgitant mitral flow. Aortic pressure is now 130/65 mm Hg.

A, reverse mitral flow is consistently noted. During systole, the shaded area marked B shows 38% of the total mitral flow regurgitating back into the left atrium. The left atrial and left ventricular end diastolic pressures are considerably elevated and the aortic pulse pressure is now 130/65 mm Hg. When the acute aortic insufficiency is discontinued, the heart recovers, LVEDP becomes normal again, and the mitral regurgitation disappears.

Patient Study

A 55 year old man was found to have severe mitral insufficiency at cardiac catheterization. Left ventricular angiography showed a thin, pliable, billowing mitral leaflet suggestive of ruptured chordae tendineae. The LVEDP was 24 mm Hg and the LA systolic pressure had a V wave with a peak pressure of 55 mm Hg.

At surgery, prior to establishing cardiopulmonary bypass, the mitral flow was measured using the C shaped flowprobe; LA and LV pressures were obtained with Angiocath catheters placed through the atrial and ventricular walls and connected to equisensitive pressure gauges. The mitral flow and pressures are shown (Fig. 5a). The flow below the zero flow line represents the mitral regurgitation and averaged 34% of the total mitral flow.

The large V wave may be seen in the LA pressure tracing, and this peak pressure averaged 50 mm Hg. The flow tracing on the left shows a forward flow above the zero line of 3.8 L/min with 34% of the left ventricular filling regurgitating back into the left atrium during systole. A high forward mitral flow would be anticipated in mitral insufficiency, which would be decreased when the mitral insufficiency is corrected. The valve was repaired by valvuloplasty and the insertion of a Carpentier ring. One hour after the bypass had been discontinued the record was obtained (Fig. 5b). There is no longer any mitral regurgitation and there is no longer any significant V systolic pressure wave in the LA pressure. The forward mitral flow is 2.5 L/min and there is no regurgitant fraction. This would indicate that the mitral insufficiency has been corrected.

DISCUSSION

The new flowprobe described in this paper avoids the need for cardiopulmonary bypass and the complications such as hypothermia, hypoperfusion, and hemolysis associated with its use.

In addition, chronically prepared animals can be prepared in less than an hour, rather than the two to three hours required when bypass is used. This increases the survival rate of the dogs prepared. The atrial contribution to mitral inflow increases significantly five to seven days after surgery when compared to that obtained at surgery. This is thought to be due to recovery of the atrial musculature from the effects of anesthesia and surgery. In addition, the new probe passed through the tip of the atrial appendage avoids an extensive atriotomy which must be surgically closed when mitral probes are placed in the usual fashion.

Human mitral and tricuspid flow can be evaluated at the time of surgery, before and after valvular repair. The flexible handle allows the surgeon to position the flowprobe over the mitral valve from any

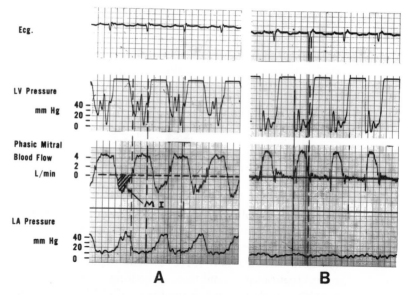

Figure 5. Phasic human mitral flow, measured at the time of surgery in a patient with severe mitral insufficiency is shown on the left (A). There is a large V wave in the systolic left atrial pressure which averaged a peak of 50 mm Hg. The area above the zero flow line represents total mitral forward stroke volume, and the area below the zero line represents the regurgitant fraction. After valvuloplasty and the insertion of a Carpentier ring, and one hour after the discontinuation of the cardiopulmonary bypass, the phasic mitral flow shown on the right (B) was obtained. There is no mitral regurgitation and the V wave has disappeared from the left atrial pressure. The forward mitral stroke-volume, as measured by the area above the zero flow line, has decreased and the total mitral flow is 2.3 L/min.

surgical approach. In some cases of aortic insufficiency, left ventricular angiography shows associated mitral insufficiency which is thought to be secondary to the aortic valve disease. In such a case, the mitral probe could be used to evaluate the mitral valve before and after aortic valve repair. Any residual mitral insufficiency remaining after aortic valve repair could be quantitated.

SUMMARY

A specially designed C-shaped electromagnetic flowmeter probe may be passed through the tip of the atrial appendage without the use of cardiopulmonary bypass. This allows for acute measurement of transmitral volume flow in animals and man at the time of surgery. These flowprobes can also be surgically implanted chronically in animals without the need for cardiopulmonary bypass. This simplifies the surgical procedure and increases postoperative survival, allowing for more investigators to study mitral blood flow in chronically instrumented animals.

Human valve flow may be evaluated at the time of surgery and the presence or absence of any mitral regurgitation readily detected.

REFERENCES

1. Folts, J.D., Young, W.P., Rowe, G.G. Phasic flow through normal and prosthetic mitral valves in unanesthetized dogs. *J. Thor. Cardiovasc. Surg.* 61:235, 1971.

2. Folts, J.D., Young, W.P., Ravnan, M.L., Rowe, G.G. Phasic tricuspid flow in chronic unanesthetized dogs. *J. Appl. Physiol.* 34:519, 1973.

3. Nolan, S.P., Dixon, S.H., Jr., Fisher, R.D., Morrow, A.G. The influence of atrial contraction and mitral valve mechanics on ventricular filling. *Am. Heart J.* 77:784, 1969.

4. Williams, B.T., Worman, R.K., Jacobs, R.R., Schenk, W.G. An *in vivo* study of blood flow patterns across the normal mitral valve. *J. Thor. Cardiovasc. Surg.* 59:824, 1970.

5. Yellin, E.L., Silverstein, M., Frater, R.W.M., Peskin, C. Pulsatile flow dynamics across the natural and prosthetic mitral valve. Proceedings 23rd ACEMB, p. 96, 1970.

6. Yellin, E.L., Laniado, S., Peskin, C.S., Frater, R.W.M. Atrioventricular pressure-flow dynamics and valve mo-

tion. Edited by A.S. Iberall and A.C. Guyton. In *Regulation and Control in Physiological Systems*. International Federation of Automatic Control, p. 311-314, 1973.

7. Folts, J.D. Electronic zero for chronic application of electromagnetic flowmeter probes. *J. Appl. Physiol.* 28:237, 1970.

8. Folts, J.D. Preparation of a chronic indwelling catheter using a commercially available infant feeding tube. *J. Appl. Physiol.* 30:417, 1971.

9. Folts, J.D., Rowe, G.G. Coronary and hemodynamic effects of temporary acute aortic insufficiency in intact anesthetized dogs. *Circ. Res.* 35:238, 1974.

15 Simultaneous Recording of Mitral Valve Echogram and Transmitral Flow*

Shlomo Laniado, M.D.
Edward L. Yellin, Ph.D.

INTRODUCTION

With the introduction of echographic techniques in clinical cardiology, the ultrasonic registration of mitral cusps' motion has led to a better understanding of the behavior of the normal and diseased valve.[1-5] The present study describes the dynamic relations between transmitral flow and valve echogram, with emphasis on the temporal relation between the events of flow, motion, and sound; correlation between quantitative changes in flow and the degree of cusp motion; and the role of the atrium in closure of the mitral valve.

* Supported by a grant from the Binational Science Foundation (BSF) Jerusalem. Investigation was done at the Cardiac Research Laboratory, Ichilov Hospital, Tel Aviv, Israel.

155

156

METHODS

Experiments were performed on open-chest dogs in which a squarewave electromagnetic flow cuff* was sutured in the left atrium above the mitral ring during open-heart surgery. Mitral valve echogram was obtained by placing 3.5 MHz 3 cm focused transducer† on the right or left ventricular surface, directing the beam to record the characteristic signals of the mitral echogram. Mitral flow and echogram were recorded simultaneously with the ECG; left ventricular, left atrial, and aortic pressures and phonocardiograms were recorded by techniques described previously.[6,7]

An original record demonstrating the relationship between mitral flow, cusp motion, and heart sounds is presented in Figure 1.

---

* Model 501 Carolina Medical Electronics.
† Series 100 Echocardiograph, Unirad Corporation.

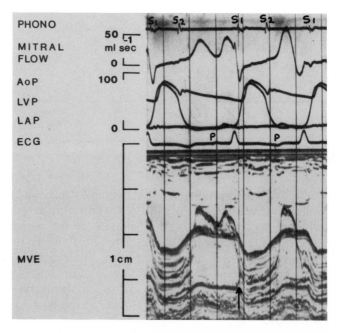

Figure 1. Original dog record taken at a paper speed of 75 mm/sec, demonstrating flow and cusp-motion relationship. The second beat is an atrial premature beat with a prolonged P-R interval. Arrow marks the time of valve closure. Time lines are 200 msec apart. AoP = Aortic Pressure. LVP = Left Ventricular Pressure. LAP = Left Atrial Pressure. MVE = Mitral Valve Echogram.

RESULTS

Motion Flow and Sound Correlation

Cessation of flow and closure of the mitral valve did not occur at the crossing point of left atrial and left ventricular pressures, but about 30 msec later, they coincided with the first major component of the first heart sound (Fig. 1). However, in the second beat (Fig. 1), which is an extra-systole with a prolonged P-R interval, and which was accompanied by a premature valve closure, S_1 did not come with the deceleration and cessation of flow, but at the time of the final closure and tension of the valve and its attachments, which followed ventricular contraction.

The Dynamic Relation of Cusp Motion to Mitral Flow

The experimental records demonstrate that there is a remarkable similarity in configuration between transmitral flow and the anterior cusp echogram (Figs. 1, 2, 3). However, while the opening movement of the anterior cusp started simultaneously with the onset of mitral flow, the cusp reached its full excursion of opening well before peak flow (with an average time interval of 0.044 sec), and immediately started its posterior diastolic movement (the E-F segment of the echogram), while flow was still accelerating. This time lag between the point of maximal valve opening and peak mitral flow was greater when peak flow was larger, or when it was delayed because the atrial augmentation coincided with the rapid filling phase (Fig. 1, second beat).

In contrast to opening, the closing movement of the cusp lagged behind the decelerating mitral flow. When flow reached zero, the cusp was still in midway position, reaching only 40–60% of its total posterior excursion. This phenomenon is even more obvious in the beats with prolonged P-R interval (Fig. 1), where at the time of zero flow the anterior cusp has reached only a third of its total backward excursion.

The Effects of Reduced Cardiac Output and Stroke Volume on the D-E Amplitude and on the E-F Speed of the Echogram

The maximal amplitude of opening of the anterior mitral cusp (the D-E amplitude) was not altered by a reduction of cardiac output and filling volume. A relatively small flow could achieve the same maximal amplitude of opening as large flow. This is shown in Figure 2, where due to atrial fibrillation and irregular rhythm, mitral flow varied significantly from beat to beat in amount and configuration, but the cusp still achieved the full opening excursion. However, reduced filling volume and cardiac output were found to be accompanied by decreased E-F slope. Eight dogs with an average cardiac output of 2.22 ± 0.06 l/min and filling volume of 24 ± 0.82 ml had E-F speed of 64 mm/sec. Nine dogs with an average cardiac output of 0.84 ± 0.04 l/min, and filling volume of 11.83 ± 1.0 ml had an E-F speed of 30 mm/sec.[7]

In animals with normal cardiac output, complete valve opening occurred with the amount of 17.6% of the total filling volume, and valve closure was achieved with relatively small amount of backflow—13.8% of total filling volume. In dogs with failing hearts and low output, the regurgitant flow at closure grew up to levels of 18–35% of the total filling volume.

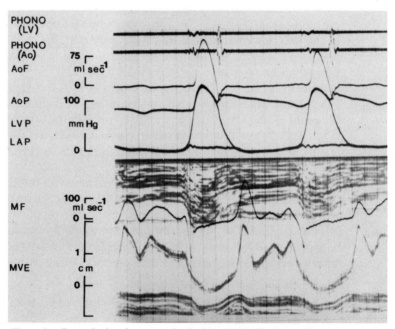

Figure 2. Record taken from an animal with atrial fibrillation and irregular ventricular rhythm. Note that despite the similarity between mitral flow and echo tracings, the anterior cusp has achieved a full amplitude of opening even in beats with a reduced filling wave. Time lines are 100 msec apart. (The ECG was omitted from this tracing for technical reasons.)

The Effects of Prolonged P-R Interval on the Mitral Flow and Echogram

With prolongation of the P-R interval, the atrial contraction coincided with the rapid filling wave and added to it. As a result of a transfer of a larger volume of blood from the left ventricle in a shorter time period, the atrioventricular pressure gradient reversed in mid-diastole. This started a rapid deceleration of mitral flow, followed by a premature apposition of the cusps. The final closure was completed with the onset of ventricular contraction and was always accompanied by larger regurgitant volume (Figs. 1, 3, 4).

The Effect of Atrial Fibrillation on Mitral Flow and the Echogram

In atrial fibrillation, and with long R-R interval, the A-V pressure gradient may repeatedly change its direction. This, in turn, may affect mitral flow which fluctuates, accelerates, or decelerates following

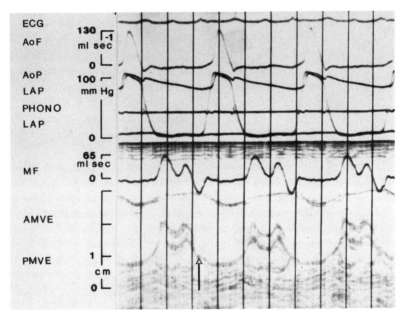

Figure 3. A record obtained in a dog with a P-R interval of more than 0.20 sec. In this dog a complete valve closure (arrow) was accomplished before the onset of ventricular contraction; however, this premature closure was accompanied by a considerable amount of regurgitant volume. AMVE = Anterior Mitral Valve Echogram. PMVE = Posterior Mitral Valve Echogram. Paper speed is 75 mm/sec. Time lines are 200 msec apart.

the oscilations in the pressure gradient. The anterior cusp may follow these fluctuations and demonstrate additional peaks of motion, occasionally resembling the A wave of the echogram (Fig. 2).

DISCUSSION AND CONCLUSIONS

The successful simultaneous recording of mitral flow, cusp motion, and heart sounds permitted us to examine the dynamic relations between all these variants under different conditions.

With the onset of a positive atrioventricular pressure gradient at the beginning of diastole, the mitral valve starts its opening simultaneously with the increase in flow across its ring. Complete valve opening always occurs before peak flow. The time from opening flow (corresponding to complete valve opening) to peak flow varies depending on the magnitude and configuration of the rapid filling wave, which in turn may be affected by the length of the P-R interval.

While valve opening can be associated with minor increases in flow, the closing motion of the cusp is delayed following the rapid deceleration of flow. The valve may stay open widely despite the fact that minimal or even zero flow has occurred. Closure of the mitral valve is not complete at the time of zero atrioventricular pressure gradient at the end of diastole, but only some time after the reversal of the pressure gradient, because of inertia of the blood flowing from the left atrium.[6] The first major component of the first sound was found to be related to the completion of the rapid process of closing and tensing of the valve and its attachments.

Our observations demonstrate that cusp motion grossly follows changes in flow; however, it cannot be considered a true reflection of those changes. Flow may vary over a large range and the cusps may still achieve the same maximal excursion. It is impractical, therefore, to quantify total mitral flow and cardiac output from the echographically derived valve-orifice area.[8]

In states of low cardiac output and decreased filling volume, there is a reduction in flow rate during the early filling phase, and a reduced flow deceleration. This is accompanied by a reduction of the E-F slope and may account for observations of a reduced E-F slope in patients who did not suffer from mitral stenosis but from other diseases, such as aortic stenosis, idiopathic hypertrophic subaortic stenosis, atrial myxoma, and mitral insufficiency, all characterized by reduced left ventricular compliance or low cardiac output.[3,5,9,10]

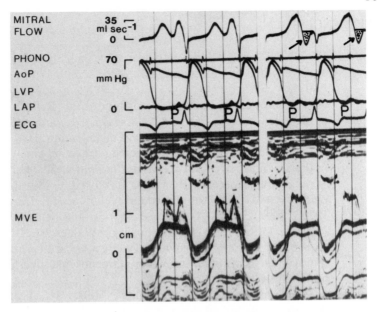

Figure 4. The panel at the left demonstrates flow-motion relationship with a normal P-R interval (0.12 sec). The panel at the right shows the effect of spontaneous prolongation of the P-R interval in the same animal (P-R interval of 0.20 sec), which was accompanied by a premature pressure-gradient reversal and partial valve closure, with an increased amount of regurgitant flow (arrows). Paper speed is 50 mm/sec. Time lines are 200 msec apart.

The optimal closure of the mitral valve—that is, with the least back flow—was found to occur in hearts which were in sinus rhythm and normal P-R interval. Under normal conditions and with the optimal interval between the atrial and ventricular systoles, mitral valve closure is brought about by the actions of flow deceleration, vortex formation, ring contraction, and shortening of the long axis of the ventricle. With prolonged P-R interval (Figs. 3 and 4), ventricular filling and atrial relaxation result in a reversed pressure gradient, not accompanied by axial shortening. This frequently leads to late diastolic regurgitation with incompetent valve closure. It has been suggested that the atrium helps in closure of the mitral valve by initiating the process of closure following atrial activity.[11] The present study indicates that a normal interval between atrial and ventricular activities is also important for adequate closure, by counteracting the effects of premature pressure gradient reversal, which is accompanied by an ill-timed incompetent closure.

REFERENCES

1. Edler, I. Atrioventricular valve mobility in the living human heart recorded by ultrasound. *Acta Med. Scand.* 170 (suppl. 370): 85, 1961.

2. Joyner, C.R., Reid, M.J., Bond, J.P. Reflected ultrasound in the assessment of mitral valve disease. *Circulation* 27:503, 1963.

3. Zaky, A., Nasser, W.K., Feigenbaum, H. Study of mitral valve action recorded by reflected ultrasound and its application in the diagnosis of mitral stenosis. *Circulation* 37:789, 1968.

4. Wharton, C.F.P., Lopez Bescos, L. Mitral valve movement: A study using an ultrasound technique. *Br. Heart J.* 32:344, 1970.

5. McLaurin, L.P., Gibson, T.C., Waider, W., Grossman, W., Craige, E. An appraisal of mitral valve echocardiograms mimicking mitral stenosis in conditions with right ventricular overload. *Circulation* 48:801, 1973.

6. Laniado, S., Yellin, E.L., Miller, H., Frater, R.W.M. Temporal relation of the first heart sound to closure of the mitral valve. *Circulation* 47:1006, 1973.

7. Laniado, S., Yellin, E.L., Kotler, M., Levy, L., Stadler, J., Terdiman, R. A study of the dynamic relations between the mitral valve echogram and phasic mitral flow. *Circulation* 51:104, 1975.

8. Fischer, J.C., Chang, S., Konecke, L.L., Feigenbaum, H. Echocardiographic determination of mitral valve flow. (Abstract). *Am. J. Cardiol.* 29:262, 1972.

9. Shah, P.M., Gramiak, R., Kramer, D.H., Yu, P.N. Determinants of atrial and ventricular gallop sounds in primary myocardial disease. *N. Eng. J. M.* 278:753, 1968.

10. Winters, W.L., Hafer, J., Soloff, L.A. Abnormal mitral valve motion as demonstrated by the ultrasound technique in apparent pure mitral insufficiency. *Am. Heart. J.* 77:196, 1969.

11. Zaky, A., Steinmetz, E., Feigenbaum, H. Role of atrium in closure of mitral valve in man. *Am. J. Physiol.* 217:1652, 1969.

16 Analysis and Interpretation of the Normal Mitral Valve Flow Curve*

Edward L. Yellin, Ph.D.
Shlomo Laniado, M.D.
Charles S. Peskin, Ph.D.
Robert W.M. Frater, M.D.

INTRODUCTION

Traditionally, left ventricular inflow has been calculated indirectly from measurements of volume derived from cardiometry, roentgenography, myocardial segment length, or internal dimension changes. Ventricular filling has also been inferred from hemodynamic parameters which reflect the state of ventricular function, e.g., cardiac output, left atrial pressure, and left ventricular diastolic pressure. Neither method is as precise as the direct measurement of phasic transmitral flow, which offers the possibility of more meaningful physiological studies in the experimental animal.

In this report we formulate a simple mathematical approach with which to analyze the pressure-flow relation in the chambers of the left

---

* Supported in part by the National Institutes of Health, Grant No. HL-16354 and the Cardiovascular Research Laboratory of the Department of Surgery, Albert Einstein College of Medicine.

163

heart and to present the results of such measurements. Our focus is analytical and our emphasis is conceptual rather than quantitative.

METHODS

Large mongrel dogs were anesthetized with pentobarbitol 30 mg/kg i.v. and placed on cardiopulmonary bypass. An intracardiac electromagnetic flow probe* was sutured to the mitral annulus in the supra-annular position and a cuff probe placed on the ascending aorta. Left ventricular, left atrial, and aortic pressures were measured with catheter-tip strain gauge transducers† and recorded along with the ECG, LV dp/dt, and intracardiac phono on an oscillographic recorder.‡

THEORY

Following the approach of Spencer and Greiss,[1] who studied aortic outflow, we describe the atrioventricular pressure difference in terms of resistance and inertance (Fig. 1, upper insert). That is, the total pressure difference is proportional to the sum of the rate of change of flow, and of the flow. In the lower insert, the differential equation is solved for the condition of no pressure difference, i.e., during diastasis, and it is seen that under these conditions flow decays exponentially toward zero. The properties of the first equation are well known and are shown schematically in the figure. The A-V gradient reversal and the start of inflow occur simultaneously; flow peaks after the pressure difference peaks and before it reaches zero; flow decelerates exponentially with equalization of pressure; and an atrial contraction imparts additional momentum to the fluid so that flow reaches zero after the A-V pressure crossover. Compliance is significant only during systole when energy is stored in the viscoelastic valvular appartus during closure and released during opening.

RESULTS

An oscilloagraphic record from a dog with moderate to rapid heart rates is shown (Fig. 2). At all three heart rates there is a rapid

---

* Carolina Medical Electronics.
† Millar.
‡ Electronics for Medicine.

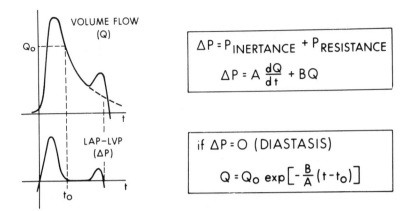

Figure 1. The equation of motion for the fluid as it crosses the mitral valve and its rationale in the upper right. The equation is solved for flow as a function of time during diastasis when the pressure difference is zero. The curves on the left are schematic depictions of a pressure-flow relationship which obeys the formulation of the equations.

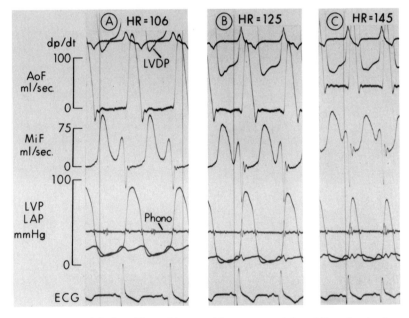

Figure 2. An original oscillographic record from a normal dog at three heart rates. AoF = Aortic Flow; MiF = Mitral Flow; HR = Heart Rate; LVP, LAP = Left Ventricular and Left Atrial Pressures; ECG = Electrocardiogram; Phono = Phonocardiogram; dp/dt = Derivative of LVP; LVDP = Left Ventricular Diastolic Pressure at high sensitivity (not used in this study).

rate of fall of ventricular pressure and a rapid early filling phase which peaks at the time the LVP reaches its nadir; the three mitral flow curves have a bicuspid wave-form with a clear atrial component; the diastolic filling period is greater than 50% of the total period; approximately 25% of the mitral inflow occurs by the time ventricular relaxation is completed; and the flow oscillation at valve closure coincides with the first heart sound and the atrial "C" wave.

In contrast with Figure 2 the hemodynamic data from another dog at equal or slower heart rates (Fig. 3) show a slowed rate of relaxation, particularly in the late isovolumic relaxation period; a depressed early filling phase; a LVDP which reaches its minimum as late as end diastole; a monocuspid mitral flow wave-form with an indistinguishable atrial component; and a shortened diastolic filling period (less than 30% of the total).

In Figure 4, the data illustrate the effect of a premature atrial contraction on an otherwise normal condition. The P wave in the ECG occurred before the completion of ventricular depolarization and the atrial contraction coincided with the early rapid filling so that

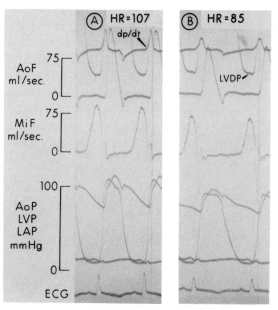

Figure 3. An oscillographic record at moderate and low heart rates from a dog with depressed contractility illustrating mitral wave-forms different from Figure 1. AoP = Aortic Pressure.

peak mitral flow increased. Because of the decreased filling period, however, the filling volume was reduced.

The atrial contribution to filling is analyzed (Fig. 5) in the record of a dog with a transient sequence of A-V dissociation, with regular sinus rhythm leading to some nodal and some ectopic ventricular contractions. The mitral inflow in beats 1 and 2 are similar in magnitude and duration, except that beat 2 has an atrial component and beat 1 does not. If the deceleration phase in beat 2 is extrapolated to follow the same shape as beat 1 (i.e., exponential), then the atrial contribution is the shaded area above the dashed curve. That area represents the difference in filling volume between the two beats and is clearly the area which would have existed if there were no atrial contraction in beat 2, and the filling period remained unchanged. Beats 6 and 7 also have an initially similar wave-form, except that in this case there is no atrial contraction in beat 7, and its diastolic period

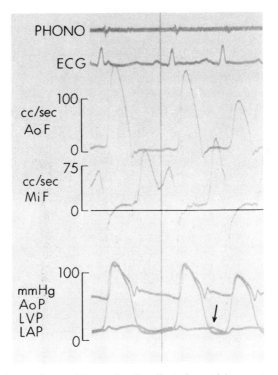

Figure 4. A normal record illustrating the effect of an atrial premature contraction.

is shortened. Thus, in contrast to 1 and 2, the difference in filling volume between beats 6 and 7 is the entire shaded area in beat 6, not just the area above the extrapolated curve.

Mid-diastolic reversal of the A-V pressure difference is illustrated in Figure 6. In Panel A, cinefluorograms of the delineated mitral

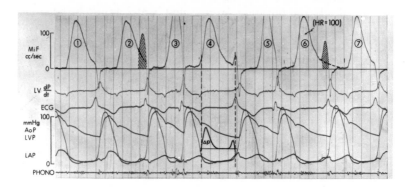

Figure 5. A record of a dog with A-V dissociation illustrating the differences between beats with and without an atrial contraction. The dashed curves are flow extrapolations based on the theory. They and the shaded areas are discussed in the text. In beat No. 4, the pressure difference has been superposed to illustrate the temporal relations between pressure difference and flow.

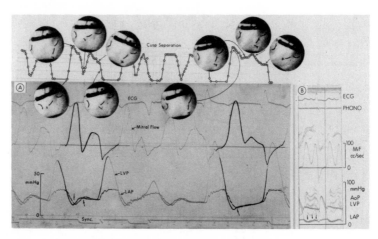

Figure 6. A record from a dog with a failing heart produced by volume overload (Panel A), illustrating the effect on mitral flow of reversal of the pressure gradient during diastole. Some of the traces have been darkened for illustrative purposes. The mitral cusps were delineated with radiopaque sutures. The effects of mid-diastolic gradient reversal under normal conditions are shown in Panel B. The arrows indicate the points of pressure cross-over.

cusps and a plot of cusp separation are superposed on the hemodynamic data. In the first beat the pressure difference becomes negative rather than zero during diastasis (between the two arrows) and flow decelerates rapidly, bringing the valve to closure. The gradient then becomes positive (second arrow) and forward flow resumes in the absence of an atrial contraction. The last beat in Panel A is similar to the first, except that the gradient does not oscillate during diastastis, there is no second wave of forward flow, and the valve remains widely open. In Panel B, we see another example of pressure oscillations where the second pressure cross-over coincides with an atrial contraction leading to an unusually large second peak. The long P-R interval in Panel B results in an atrial relaxation and pressure reversal (third arrow) before ventricular contraction, and a significant amount of backflow occurs during valve closure.

DISCUSSION

These results are consistent with those found in calves;[2] in the chronic unanesthetized dog;[3] in dogs and in humans with catheter tip probes in the mitral orifice;[4,5] and our previous work on dogs.[6,7] The data demonstrate clearly that the flow field has the resistive and inertial properties described in the equation (Fig. 1). The phasic pressure-flow characteristics at valve opening, valve closing, and during diastasis substantiate the fluid dynamic principles developed herein. Particularly impressive are those mid-diastolic events with exponential deceleration (Fig. 2, Panel A; Fig. 5, beats 1, 4, 6, 7), and with rapid deceleration due to an adverse gradient (Fig. 6, Panels A, B). Both are predicted by the theory. Particular emphasis should be placed on the finding (substantiated by theory) that mitral flow continues for approximately 25 msec after the A-V pressure crossover, so that the gradient reversal should not be used to infer cessation of flow and valve closure.

Figures 3-6 are not all "typical" results. Indeed, they have been selected as examples of pressure-flow relations which may not be normal or common, but which can be interpreted by a simple mathematical formulation. By presenting such diverse hemodynamic conditions, we have demonstrated that while the pressure-flow relations may change in pathology or unusual circumstances, the physical laws describing these events do not. Therein lies the power of analysis.

These results indicate that small pressure differences across the normal mitral valve (differences which might mistakenly be called artifacts) lead to large changes in the flow wave-form and valve motion. This suggests that mitral flow is a sensitive indicator of small variations in the left atrial or ventricular pressures, which, in turn, reflect the diastolic properties of the two cardiac chambers. Mitral flow measurements can thus be used to study ventricular properties.[8]

The finding that flow decays exponentially during diastasis (if $\Delta p = 0$) leads us to propose a new method for defining the atrial contribution to ventricular filling. In those beats where mitral flow has started to decelerate before atrial systole, an exponential extrapolation will divide the flow wave-form into a part which would have existed had the atrium not contracted, and a part due solely to atrial contraction (Fig. 5). This approach chooses each beat as its own control and assumes a constant filling period, but has the disadvantage of not considering the specific condition which led to the loss of the atrial contraction—for example, sinus vs. nodal rhythm.[2] With this approach, we calculate an average atrial contribution of approximately 10%. Choosing the entire area under the curve during atrial contraction (Fig. 5, shaded areas of beats 2 and 6) gives an average contribution of approximately 20%. The smaller figure leads us to speculate about reports concerning dramatic increases in cardiac output after the restoration of normal atrial rhythm. We suspect that it is not the atrial contribution which is important, but rather the elimination of asynchronous, ineffective ventricular ectopic contractions which lead to the improvement in cardiac output. More thought and work are certainly required here.

Other interesting questions which arise from the measurement of mitral flow include: the relation between ventricular relaxation rate and mitral flow rate; and the contractile properties of the left ventricle during isovolumic contraction, when, because of fluid inertia, a significant portion of the period is not actually isovolumic, and the ventricle is contracting against an increasing preload.

Finally, although the lumped parameter method cannot describe the distributed forces due to fluid motion, our results are consistent with those of others who have used different fluid dynamic approaches. The vortex system presented by Bellhouse,[9] and the stable flow patterns described by Taylor and Wade,[10] can exist only if the dissipative forces are viscous. Inertial losses are symptomatic of a highly disturbed or turbulent system. The exponential decay of flow during diastasis supports the finding of a stable vortex system. The breaking jet theory of Henderson and Johnson[11] is likewise consistent with our findings, because the closing volume tends to be minimized when the ventricle contracts while inflow is still occurring.

CONCLUSION

The successful measurement of phasic transmitral flow along with related hemodynamic parameters has revealed significant new insights into atrioventricular dynamics and has encouraged continued investigations in this area.

ADDENDUM

Inasmuch as good flowmeter frequency response is vital for the study of temporal relations and dynamic events, we include the following short addendum.

The damping characteristics of two Carolina Medical Electronics flowmeters are illustrated in the oscillographic record (Fig. 7). Records were taken during a steady state so that the stroke volume in each series was constant. "Time Constant" and "Hz Response" are terms used by the manufacturer to describe the damping characteristics; they are inversely proportional to each other. In the new flowmeter (Model 501), more high frequency components and noise were passed as the frequency response was increased, but the wave-forms were essentially unchanged in area and magnitude. In the older flowmeter (Model 322), on the other hand, there was unacceptable

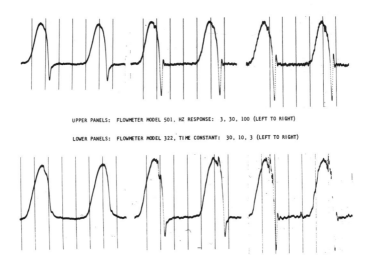

UPPER PANELS: FLOWMETER MODEL 501, HZ RESPONSE: 3, 30, 100 (LEFT TO RIGHT)

LOWER PANELS: FLOWMETER MODEL 322, TIME CONSTANT: 30, 10, 3 (LEFT TO RIGHT)

Figure 7. Oscillographic records illustrating the phasic flow patterns for different frequency-response characteristics of the flowmeter. Further discussion in the Addendum.

distortion at the highest time constant. These records also indicate that it is not always necessary to conduct elaborate frequency response tests. If, upon increasing the frequency response, the high frequency components appear in the trace, and there is no further change in shape of the wave-form, we can conclude that there is no distortion or frequency-dependent time delays in the flowmeter.

REFERENCES

1. Spencer, M.P., Greiss, F.C. Dynamics of ventricular ejection. *Circulation Research* 10:274, 1962.

2. Nolan, S.P., Dixon, D.H., Fisher, R.D. et al. The influence of atrial contraction and mitral valve mechanics on ventricular filling. A study of instantaneous mitral valve flow *in vivo*. *Amer. Heart J.* 77:784, 1969.

3. Folts, J.D., Young, W.P., Rowe, G.G. Phasic flow through normal and prosthetic mitral valves in unanesthetized dogs. *J. Thor. and Cardiov. Surg.* 61:235, 1971.

4. Kalmanson, D., Toutain, G., Novikoff, N., Derai, C. Retrograde catheterization of left heart cavities in dogs by means of an orientable direction Doppler catheter-tip flowmeter: A preliminary report. *Cardiovascular Research* 6:309, 1972.

5. Kalmanson, D., Bernier, A., Veyrat, C., Witchitz, S., Savier, C.H., Chiche, P. Normal pattern and physiological significance of mitral valve flow velocity recorded using transseptal directional Doppler ultrasound catheterization. *Br. Heart Journal* 37:249, 1975.

6. Laniado, S., Yellin, E.L., Miller, H., Frater, R.W.M. Temporal relation of the first heart sound to closure of the mitral valve. *Circulation* 47:1006, 1973.

7. Laniado, S., Yellin, E., Kotler, M., Levy, L., Stadler, J., Terdiman, R. A study of the dynamic relations between the mitral valve echogram and phasic mitral flow. *Circulation* 51:104, 1975.

8. Kennish, A., Yellin, E., Frater, R.W.M. Dynamic stiffness profiles in the left ventricle. *J. Appl. Physiol.* 39:665, 1975.

9. Bellhouse, B.J. Fluid mechanics of a model mitral valve and left ventricle. *Cardiovascular Research* 6:199, 1972.

10. Taylor, E.E.M., Wade, J.D. Pattern of blood flow within the heart: A stable system. *Cardiovascular Research* 7:14, 1973.

11. Henderson, Y., Johnson, F.E. Two modes of closure of the heart valves. *Heart* 4:68, 1912.

Dr. Wieting: There is only one question I would raise concerning Dr. Bellhouse's work: the rubber bag he showed us took on a more spherical configuration than I feel the natural ventricle has. Also, there is a small vortex which develops behind the posterior leaflet in all the studies I have done, both in a ventricular and in a cylindrical chamber.

Dr. Bellhouse: I don't think that small changes in the shape of the ventricle have much effect on the ventricular vortex. However, in one experiment, we shaped the ventricle so that there was a much bigger region behind the posterior cusp than behind the anterior cusp. In this case the main vortex strength lay behind the posterior cusp, with the result that the posterior cusp closed sooner than the anterior cusp.

Dr. Yacoub: I enjoyed Dr. Bellhouse's presentation. Can I ask him how he explains the fact that echocardiography shows simultaneous movement of the anterior and posterior cusps?

Dr. Bellhouse: The marked asymmetry of the vortex in my model of the left ventricle might be greater than in the physiological ventricle; this would tend to exaggerate differences in movements of the anterior and posterior cusps.

Dr. Gabe: Can I just ask Dr. Bellhouse what he feels is the influence the chordae have on the vortices? Do they reduce the energy of the vortices in any way?

Dr. Bellhouse: I think that any obstruction within the ventricle will reduce the strength of the vortex, but that the losses in vortex strength produced by the chordae tendineae and trabeculae carnae will be small.

Dr. Taylor: I think we can help resolve this apparent difference in the valve cusp movement observed by echocardiography, and those just demonstrated by Dr. Bellhouse in his model studies and older descriptions based on cineradiography. Unlike the models where a rubber 'ventricle' of uniform compliance is used, the left ventricle has a variable compliance, the septal region being stiffer than the free wall: this results in a rotation of the valve annulus relative to the anterior chest wall during diastolic filling. In our original measurements on cusp movement based on endoscopic cinephotographic records, we chose as our reference line the plane joining the commissures, and obtained pictures similar to those shown by Dr. Bellhouse. Because of the apparent inconsistency of these with echocardiographic data, we have recently remeasured our original endoscopic records using as a reference point the anteroseptal wall, which corresponds to the echo reference line: this had produced records similar to clinical echocardiograms. It is all a question of the reference plane from which measurements are made.

On the point raised by the previous speaker, using a side-viewing telescope with our endoscope, we have observed flow between the chordae feeding the vortex associated with the anterior cusp, and the chordae do not appear to have a major influence on disturbing flow patterns or in generating secondary vortex trains.

Dr. Wright: Dr. Bellhouse, if we consider the topography of the heart, the outside is smooth, the inside is covered with knobs and excrescences. Do you think these can act as dampers?

Dr. Bellhouse: Yes.

Dr. Yellin: I would like to offer the possibility of an alternate approach to the function of the chordae, the role of vortices, the movement of the cusps, and flow patterns. The following two slides are the results of studies done by Dr. Peskin of New York University. We see in Figure 1 a model of the left heart without an aortic valve, since we are looking only at events during diastole. The equation of motion for the fluid and the heart wall has been solved numerically with a digital computer. What you see is not a simulation but rather a mathematical solution which is presented in a simulated form.

With ventricular relaxation, a pressure difference is set up from the atrium to the ventricle and the valve cusps swing out widely towards the septum and posterior wall. Therefore, at the beginning of diastole, the fluid momentum is directed toward the walls of the ventricle rather than the apex. In the next frame the jet is forming, the valve is moving toward closure, and a vortex is forming at the tip of the valve before the fluid reaches the apex and sweeps up the walls. If this solution is accurate, then, the size of the ventricle will have little to do with early vortex formation. The vortex is due to friction at the cusp surface.

The existence of chordae which tend to restrain the cusp from swinging open too far will help the vortex pattern. In this solution you can see a slight indentation in the apex where unseen elastic chordae connect the valves to the ventricle. Later in time a very well developed vortex is seen and the valve moves toward closure. Flow measurements indicate that the time required for the fluid to reach the apex in the dog heart is long compared with echo observation of cusp motion, so that the valve moves toward closure in vivo before the large vortex forms.

There is a continuation of the flow patterns (Fig. 2). There is a long diastasis so that flow is dying down although a small vortex still exists. Now the atrial contraction accelerates flow again, strengthens the vortex, and brings the valve towards closure. Finally, with ventricular contraction, closure is completed. Note the stagnation point just above the cusp margins where the fluid on one side moves into the ventricle and on the other into the atrium so that there is no backflow. Fluid inertia is carrying it into the ventricle rather than allowing backflow in the atrium.

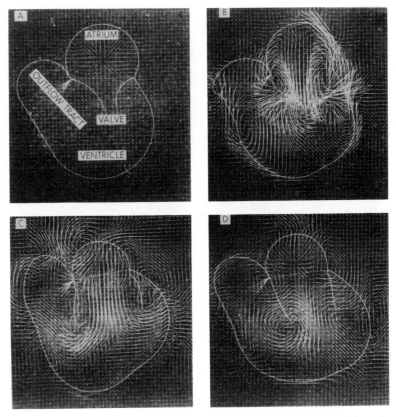

Figure 1. A mathematical solution to mitral flow dynamics and closure of the valve (see text).

Now this approach is admittedly speculative, but it is consistent with observations and should be given serious consideration. For example, the contraction of the jet as it goes through the valve indicates that the valve can move toward closure without in any way altering the movement of the main stream. This will not be seen in a model where the inlet is a straight tube such as Dr. Bellhouse has used, because there would not be any inward direction of the flow which has been directed by the tube toward the apex. This is one explanation for the vortices closing the valve in his model which may not be required in the natural valve.

Dr. Gabe: I wonder if I could ask Dr. Yellin a question about possible artifacts in this sort of flow measurement. It looks as if the flow through the mitral valve is going to be inertia-dominated. The

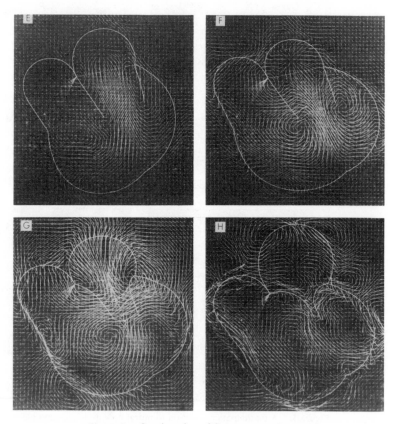

Figure 2. Continuation of flow patterns (see text).

method involves placing a rigid electromagnetic cuff above the valve which I suppose is about the length of the mitral valve. If the mitral valve inertance is roughly doubled in this kind of way, isn't it going to produce a significant artifact in the pressure gradient?

Dr. Yellin: I am not sure what you mean by inertance of the valve.

Dr. Gabe: In this context I mean the length of the valve multiplied by the density of the blood and divided by the cross-sectional area.

Dr. Yellin: It is a good question and the best answer I can give is that it is the inertia of the blood that dominates the system, not of the valve. In effect you are saying that we are creating a jet or tube of flow which is being accelerated and decelerated and, therefore, has inertia. You want to know whether a cuff probe would increase the size of the tube. The only way I can answer that is to say that we have done orifice flow studies and found that unless you get to a small diameter orifice (2,3,4 mm) the inertial term, except at opening and closing, is insignificant. We have also used electromagnetic probes at the mitral orifice as small as 12 mm diameter (i.e., much smaller than the annulus) and as large as 18.3 mm with the same initial pressure difference, so that we conclude that the probe does not increase the inertial term.

Dr. Rutishauser: Dr. Nolan, would you agree that the phases I, IV, and V may be due to the position of the probe above the valve and do not really mean that blood actually crosses from the left ventricle to the left atrium or vice versa?

Dr. Nolan: You have raised a point that disturbed us for several years. Phases I, IV, and V of mitral valve flow are always found with a normal mitral valve. These phases of flow correspond to fluctuations in the atrial and ventricular pressures. In addition, we discovered that certain pathological states, such as mitral regurgitation, could eliminate some of these phases. We concluded from these observations that these minor fluctuations in flow represent motion of the mitral leaflets when the valve is closed. Perhaps the problem is one of semantics. We do not believe that there is an actual flow of blood from ventricle to atrium during these phases but rather movement of the leaflets which in the closed position serve to partition the two chambers.

Dr. Yacoub: I have a question for Dr. Nolan. In phase III, forward flow is ascribed to atrial contraction, and this interpretation has been commonly used by all speakers. Yet, Dr. Yellin has shown that this forward flow wave or hump can occur in the absence of atrial contraction. In one of Dr. Laniado's slides where the dog had atrial fibrillation, there was still a late hump simulating phase III or atrial contribution. One of our patients in London who was in atrial fibrillation had a definite phase III. Are we right in ascribing this forward flow during end diastole to atrial contribution?

Dr. Nolan: Several of the other participants may also wish to answer your question. I did not refer to phase III as the atrial contribution to mitral valve flow, but I did state that phase III flow occurs during atrial contraction. Our experiments did not allow us to determine the percentage of ventricular filling which can be attributed to atrial contraction. However, we were able to demonstrate one situation in which atrial contraction augmented ventricular filling by 20%.

While I have the floor, I would like to ask Dr. Yellin a question. In the last slide that you showed, you interpreted the secondary accelleration of mitral flow as having occurred in the absence of atrial contraction. However, I had thought that the electrocardiogram demonstrated an early nodal rhythm, in which case the secondary accelleration may have been due to an abbreviated atrial contraction.

Dr. Yellin: In the last slide there is nothing on the electrocardiogram to indicate any electrical activity of the ventricle. We often see it in failure states of our dogs when we overload them with volume in order to maintain cardiac output. We also see it in late states of massive mitral regurgitation, and I think this is one of the areas that has good clinical application. I think it is worth further discussion.

Dr. Laniado: Dr. Yacoub's observation that some patients who are in atrial fibrillation demonstrate in the echocardiogram an "A" wave (resembling an atrial contribution to mitral flow) is true. We have often seen, in dogs with atrial fibrillation, that during long diastole the pressure gradient across the mitral valve may reverse following a rapid transfer of blood from the left atrium into the left ventricle during the early filling phase. The reversal of the pressure gradient rapidly decelerates mitral flow and in some cases may even induce reversal of flow through the open mitral valve. This in turn will induce a second pressure-gradient reversal now in favor of the atrium, coming at the end of diastole and simulating atrial contraction in its effect on flow and cusp motion.

Dr. Yellin: Let me add just one thing to that. Just because the mitral valve was open, and the atrium and the ventricle are one chamber, does not mean that there cannot be pressure oscillations between the two of them, and that these pressure oscillations will not produce flow. In fact what sometimes happens is that the ventricle can be a resonating system of very low frequency and the gradients can reverse and can cause flow to go back and forth. We occasionally see flow reversal as regurgitation during these conditions because these are acutely dilated ventricles and the valve is held open during the time the gradient reverses; therefore, you can get regurgitation. If the ventricle is not distended, the valve will close during that period of time and you won't get regurgitation.

Dr. Kalmanson: I'd like to answer Dr. Yacoub's question. We have carried out a series of recordings of mitral valve flow velocity in patients in sinus rhythm and in patients with atrial fibrillation. In patients in sinus rhythm, we consistently found a temporal relationship between the end diastolic forward flow wave and the P wave of the ECG. This holds true also for patients with a long P-R interval. On the other hand, in patients with atrial fibrillation, during diastoles of short length, there is no spur of end-diastolic forward flow waves. These only occur during long diastoles. Furthermore, contrary to what happens in patients with sinus rhythm, the shape or pattern as well as the duration of these waves varies from one diastole to the other. It is, therefore, logical to discriminate between regular and stereotyped end-diastolic forward-flow waves of patients in sinus rhythm, which can reasonably be ascribed to atrial contraction, and anarchical and intermittent humps that occur during long diastoles of atrial fibrillation. These may well be due to pure oscillations caused by pressure-gradient reversal as Dr. Yellin just suggested. Evidence which supports this hypothesis is given by the frequent occurrence of flow reversal between the two successive diastolic forward flow waves and even after the end-diastolic A wave in case of prolonged P-R interval.

Now, I would like to put a question to Dr. Folts. First Dr. Folts is to be warmly congratulated for having shown his recording of mitral flow volume in patients, obtained preoperatively, since it is the very first time that such data have been determined in man. I was a little disconcerted, however, when I saw the postoperative recording in your patient with mitral regurgitation. Indeed, as expected, the systolic-regurgitation flow wave disappeared after operation, but the diastolic-filling flow wave failed to decrease, as it is known to do after surgical cure. Do you think there might be some artifact due to your technique?

Dr. Folts: If so, I don't know where it would be, since the same probe was used before and after, and put in the same position. The only alteration has been the repair of a portion of the torn commissure and the insertion of a mitral ring. So, if it is an artifact, I don't know where it would come from.

Dr. Reneman: I should like to ask Dr. Folts two questions. First of all do you have any idea about the uniformity of the magnetic field in this C-shaped probe you showed us? We have noticed that the magnetic field is usually not uniform in C-shaped probes, so that they are more sensitive to changes from axisymmetric velocity profiles than can be expected from the weight function alone. Therefore, differences in the velocity profile before and after surgery can easily lead to unexpected volume flow readings after the operation. Secondly, can you give us some information about the sensitivity of your probe and the amperage with which you are feeding it? I expect the sensitivity to be low because of the large air gap.

Dr. Folts: I don't know exactly what the amperage is. Carolina Medical Electronics flowmeters have a constant current source for probes of that size that is the same for aortic probes and this mitral probe. It is calibrated by using dialysis tubing. Another way is to make a clay mold around it as some people have done for calibration purposes. The iron filing field distribution seems pretty uniform and is very comparable to a flowprobe constructed for a cuff around an aorta or some other large bore vessel.

Dr. Angell: I wonder whether the formation of vortices discussed in the earlier papers has any influence on the occurrence of that forward flow phase or whether it has anything to do with ventricle compliance.

Dr. Yellin: I am not sure I understand how the compliance question relates to the vortices. I know nothing about vortices in the intact heart; we just haven't measured them. Dr. Taylor has and he sees a stable pattern as he described. I'll make one comment on compliance, since you raised the question. In the studies we have done in the dog, roughly 25% of the ventricular inflow occurs while the ventricle is still relaxing, i.e., down to what the cardiologist calls the 0 point, 25% of the volume has already entered the ventricle and, therefore, I caution you against using the stroke-volume as determined from cardiac output to measure compliance. That is number one. Number two—the ventricle is a visco-elastic chamber and more force is required for rapid distension, so slow filling or filling in mitral stenosis which is uniform will give you a different calculation for volume compliance than rapid filling. There are several other problems which we really can't go into at the moment.

SUMMARY: PART III

Edward L. Yellin, Ph.D.

Cardiologists, engineers, physicists, physiologists, and surgeons employing a variety of technical and analytical skills have reported on both in-vivo and ex-vivo investigations of pressure flow relations and motion of the normal mitral valve. Using two different models, Dr. Bellhouse and Dr. Talbot separately demonstrated the relationship between mitral valve movements and the fluid mechanic effects of vortex formation and of the acceleration and deceleration of flow. Whereas Dr. Bellhouse, and later in the session Dr. Taylor (using ciné-endoscopy) both described a large vortex which forms by virtue of fluid sweeping up the ventricular walls after striking the apex, Dr. Yellin, during the discussion, offered an alternative approach which describes a vortex forming due to shear forces at the valve surface and is thus independent of ventricular size or geometry.

Dr. Taylor then described stable flow patterns and velocity profiles in vivo such that the energy losses were proportional to less than the square of the flow. Particularly important is his observation that the velocity profile at the mitral annulus is blunt, thereby allowing the investigator to convert velocity to flow (see Kalmanson, chapter 20); and his observation of skewness in the profile at the valve tips. As Dr. Reneman pointed out in the next presentation, the users of cuff type electromagnetic flow probes must be alert to the fact that nonaxisymmetric flow may give distorted volume flow measurements. This very important point cannot be overemphasized and should be implemented by investigations devoted to quantifying the effects of flow asymmetries on electromagnetic flow measurements.

In presenting his pioneering work on the measurement of mitral flow in calves, Dr. Nolan described the six phases of mitral flow, discussed the atrial contribution to filling, showed that because of fluid momentum, flow ceased after the A-V pressure cross-over, and indicated that there was only an insignificant amount of regurgitation following a VPC. These results were substantiated by Dr. Folts, who studied the pressure-flow relations in the chronic unanesthetized dog—a major achievement. Another first by Dr. Folts was his description of a method of introducing the mitral flow probe without cardiopulmonary bypass and a presentation of pre- and post-operative records from a patient with mitral regurgitation.

Dr. Laniado then presented his records of simultaneous measurement of mitral flow and mitral valve echogram, concluding that the valve opening was not correlated with flow, the E-F slope was proportional to cardiac output, mid-diastolic reversal of flow and cusp movement could occur with prolonged P-R interval, and significantly, the anterior mitral cusp starts its closing movement while flow is still accelerating. These data suggest that flow deceleration may not be required for the onset of cusp movement toward closure. If this is so, an early vortex formation may initiate inward movement and/or the chordae tendineae may be under tension at the maximum cusp opening and thus exert an inward force. Clearly, the role of the chordae deserves investigation.

And finally, Dr. Yellin's in vivo results substantiate the findings of the others. He analyzed the normal phasic flow dynamics in terms of resistance, inertance, and compliance, and formulated a simple mathematical approach with some predictive value. He defined the atrial contribution to filling differently than did Dr. Nolan, and thereby raised the question of arriving at an appropriate definition in the face of the complexities of different arrhythmias.

The quantity and quality of the data presented at this session clearly demonstrated the viability and the physiological value of measuring mitral blood flow. While there was general agreement and uniformity among the raw data, there was not always agreement on its interpretation. The session was exciting because the data were new; it was an order of magnitude more exciting because in opening up this new approach towards studying atrioventricular dynamics, it also inevitably generated controversy, and this is the stuff of which progress is made.

PART FOUR

FLOW DYNAMICS IN DISEASED VALVES

17 Fluid Dynamics of the Diseased Mitral Valve*

Joan S. Whamond
D.E.M. Taylor, F.R.C.S.

Investigations into the fluid dynamics of the stenotic mitral valve have been carried out on patients with either pure stenosis or stenosis with incompetence, who were undergoing surgery for valvulotomy.[1] This was described earlier (Chapter 12). In an operating theater, studies of this nature present difficulties with regard to sterility of equipment and the speed with which records have to be taken so as not to interfere with surgical procedures and put the patient at unnecessary risk. Because of this, all calibration of transducers, particularly balancing one against the other, and the conversion of pressure differences into velocity, were carried out retrospectively from analog magnetic tape records using hybrid computer methods.

The results on patients indicated that the stenotic valve showed marked differences in flow patterns and pressure/flow relationships from the normal: the indications were that these differences were similar to those already reported between the normal and stenotic

* Supported by grants from the Scottish Home and Health Department and the British Heart Foundation.

aortic valve.[2,3] It was not feasible for this to be fully established in patients; therefore, an animal preparation was developed to permit much more detailed fluid dynamic studies, with a range of different heart rates and cardiac output on an individual valve. The animal used was the sheep, and variable and controllable mitral stenosis was produced.

The animal experiments were carried out on anesthetized sheep. After a left thoracotomy, the mitral stenosis was produced by inserting a finger into the left auricle and inverting it to identify the level of the valve ring. Mattress sutures with Teflon washers were passed through the myocardium, at the commissures of the valve from the posterior to the anterior cusp, and held by snares. Care, however, had to be taken so that the coronary vessels would not be included in the sutures. The snares could then be drawn up, which allowed varying degrees of stenosis to be produced without making the valve significantly incompetent. It was found that two or three sutures produced the degree of stenosis required: usually a reduction of 75-85% in the valve area. A greater degree of acute stenosis tended to cause pulmonary edema and right heart failure.

The animal was allowed to rest for 30 minutes after the stenosis was produced, and between each set of recordings. Heart rate and cardiac output were varied by means of isoprenaline, administered by a slow infusion pump into a catheter passed down the external jugular vein, with the end sited in the pulmonary artery. The recordings were carried out in the same manner as in the patients. However, in addition, stroke volume was measured by an electromagnetic flowmeter cuff placed around the ascending aorta, and it was possible for more than one Janus needle to be used simultaneously. Phonocardiograms taken after the production of the stenosis showed the typical mid-diastolic murmur seen in patients.

The combined results of the patient studies and the animal experiments have enabled a picture to be developed which shows velocity profile and distribution across the valve and in the left ventricle, as well as the associated energy loss. We have begun to divide the latter into the resistive and reactive components of impedance. As there exists no standard method for dealing with this in a valved system, these results can be regarded as no more than tentative.

VELOCITY PROFILE AND FLOW PATTERNS

Velocity profile at the stenotic valve (Fig. 1), although basically flat with a zone of high shear adjacent to the wall as in the normal valve, showed a very irregular front, indicative of established turbulence. Dependent on the degree of stenosis, the peak velocity was in excess of 200 cm/sec, but peak volume flow was less than that seen in the normal valve (Fig. 2). The shear gradient adjacent to the wall was much greater than in the normal, depending on the degree of stenosis. The rate of change of shear at the onset of diastolic filling was also much higher than that seen in the normal valve, the latter being associated with a decreased rate of acceleration in volume flow as compared to the normal (Fig. 3). The high velocity stream passing through the stenosed valve acted as a jet in the left ventricle, its point of impact on the ventricular wall depending on the anatomical nature of the stenosis. Apart from the jetstream, there was no constant flow pattern within the ventricle; established turbulence rather than stable flow pattern occurred for most of diastolic filling.

The filling patterns observed were much flatter; the maximum rate of flow was still in early diastole. We have not observed the maximum rate of flow in late diastole as described by Kalmanson[4] in

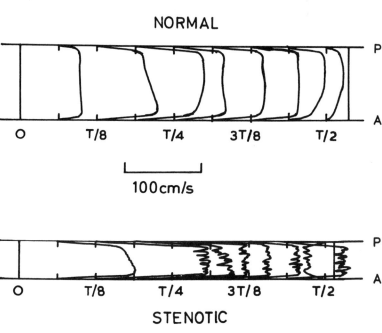

Figure 1. Flow profile at the level of the annulus in a normal and a stenotic mitral valve. Note the higher velocities occurring in the stenotic valve and the associated irregularity due to turbulence. The shorter relative duration of diastolic flow in the stenotic valve can be seen, and also the period of reversed flow preceding valve closure. In these examples, neither of the flow profiles are axiosymmetric: nonaxiosymmetry is common in diseased valves, but rare in the normal valve at the level of the annulus.

severe mitral stenosis, but in neither patients nor sheep have we yet studied the severity of stenosis reported.

A difference observed between patients and experimental animals is the extent of atrial supplementation. In patients in sinus rhythm, atrial supplementation can be significant, accounting for 30% or more of stroke volume, but this appears to be quite variable and dependent on the degree of atrial hypertrophy. In contrast to this, in all animals, atrial supplementation was small, usually less than 10% of stroke volume, and the pressure-drop record did not show a marked second pressure-drop peak during atrial systole as was observed in the normal (Fig. 3).

Visual observation of the atrium in the acute animal preparation showed that when the valve area was reduced by 75%, the atrium distended, with only a poor mechanical action. It is probable, therefore, that the animal preparation does not give an entirely accurate reproduction of the pressure and flow during atrial systole which occurs in human mitral stenosis where the lesion is slowly progressive and accompanied by atrial hypertrophy.

Because of the reduced mean hydraulic depth of a stenotic as compared to a normal valve, the peak Reynolds number was only

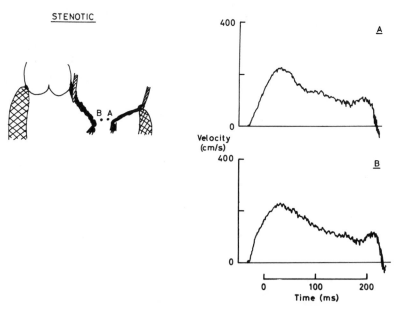

Figure 2. Velocity tracings at two points across a stenotic mitral valve. The initial acceleration is slower than that of the normal valve, and flow is turbulent except for a short period after flow starts. Despite the high velocities, peak flow is less than that seen in the normal. In this patient, atrial supplementation was only small.

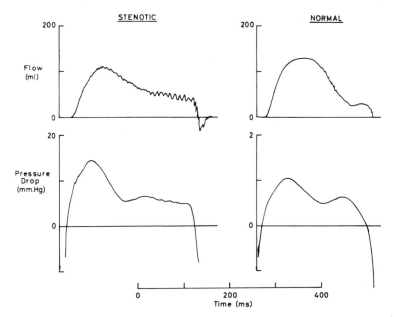

Figure 3. Flow and pressure difference across a normal and experimentally stenotic valve. Note the much flatter flow curve with stenosis, and the short period of reversed flow. Note, also, the minimum atrial contribution to flow, and loss of the atrial systolic peak in the pressure drop in the experimental stenosis.

slightly increased, in the range of 4,500 to 7,000 as compared to the normal range of 4,000 to 6,000.[5] There was a marked increase, however, in the mean Reynolds number owing to the changed pattern of filling from 1,500 to 2,500 in the normal valve to 3,000 to 4,000 in the stenotic.

PRESSURE/FLOW RELATIONSHIP

In the stenosed valve energy loss $\left\{ \dfrac{\int P + Q.dt}{\int dt} \right\}$ showed an approximately square law relationship to cardiac output, unlike the normal valve, where some adaptation to varying rate and flow occurred. The duration of diastolic filling as a proportion of the total cardiac cycle length was decreased in the stenotic as compared to the normal. For example, at a pulse rate of 70 to 90/min, where flow from atrium to ventricle took place for an average of 53% of the cardiac cycle in patients with a normal valve, this was reduced to 42% of the cycle in patients with moderately severe mitral stenosis. This appeared to be due to an increasing stiffness in the valve, with the time becoming longer from the point where the pressure in the atrium exceeded that in the ventricle, to the point at which flow commenced. The increase in opening pressure of a stenosed as compared to a normal valve was proportionately greater than the increase in either peak or mean pressure drop across the valve.

Valve closure was also affected. All stenotic valves showed some degree of incompetence, closure occurring in response to reversed flow. Valves which were not clinically incompetent, nevertheless, showed regurgitant fraction of 3 to 10% (Fig. 3).

As would be expected from the behavior of energy loss, impedance showed a dependence on cardiac output, and also on heart rate: this would suggest that both resistive and reactive components were involved. The relationship of resistive and reactive components of impedance to flow and heart rate was similar to that which would be anticipated from a simple orifice model, and thus resembles the behavior of the stenotic valve.[3] The impedance spectrum showed a much greater contribution by the higher order harmonics than did that of the normal valve, and, unlike the normal, no impedance matching was apparent with changing heart rate.[6,7]

SUMMARY

The stenotic mitral valve shows marked differences in behavior to that of the normal valve.

(a) Associated flow patterns are turbulent; they are consequent on high rates of shear and high mean Reynolds numbers.

(b) The filling profile occupies a shorter proportion of the cycle; it has a lower peak flow rate and initial acceleration, and it is much more evenly distributed over the filling period.

(c) The valve is slow to open with a high opening pressure, and closure follows reversed flow with a degree of valve incompetence.

(d) The pressure difference/flow relationships show a dependence on cardiac output and heart rate similar to that which would be predicted by a rigid orifice analogue.

REFERENCES

1. Taylor, D.E.M., Whamond, J.S.   Measurement of energy and flow distribution within heart chambers *in vivo*. Proceedings of

the DISA Conference. Edited by D.J. Cockerell. In *Fluid Dynamic Measurement in the Industrial and Medical Environments*. Leicester: Leicester University Press, 1972.

2. Carnie, N., Mukhtar, A.I., Pollock, C.G., Taylor, D.E.M., Whamond, J.S. Impedance spectra change across the aortic valve at different heart rates in the sheep. *J. Physiol.* 238:48, 1973.

3. Eastell, R., Taylor, D.E.M., Whamond, J.S. Impedance change to differing heart rate and cardiac output across the acutely stenosed aortic valve. *J. Physiol.* 248:33, 1975.

4. Kalmanson, D., Veyrat, C., Bernier, A., Witchitz, S. Mitral valve flow velocity tracings in patients with mitral valve diseases. Transseptal Doppler catheterization. This book, Chapter 20.

5. Taylor, D.E.M., Whamond, J.S. The dynamics of left ventricular filling at high heart rates. *J. Physiol.* 225:40, 1972.

6. Tansley, G., Taylor, D.E.M., Whamond, J.S. Energy loss, flow rate and impedance spectra across normal and diseased heart valves at varying heart rate. In *Abstracts of Euromech Colloquium on Cardiovascular and Respiratory Mechanics*. No. 32. Imperial College, London, 1973.

7. Taylor, D.E.M., Whamond, J.S., Tansley, J. Transvalvular impedance across normal, stenotic and prosthetic heart valves. In *Abstracts of 4th Conference on Recent Advances in Bio-engineering*. University of Surrey, 1974.

18 Flow Studies of Experimental Mitral Stenosis and Regurgitation*

Edward L. Yellin, Ph.D.
Shlomo Laniado, M.D.
Charles S. Peskin, Ph.D.
Robert W.M. Frater, M.D.

INTRODUCTION

Our understanding of the hemodynamics of valvular pathologies has been hampered by an inability to measure phasic transmitral flow directly. With the development of this technique, new possibilities for the growth of our physiological understanding have opened up.

In this presentation we follow the same general approach as in our previous discussion of the normal mitral valve. Our goal is to elucidate dynamic relations by providing a simple but useful mathematical formulation with which to analyze and quantify mitral stenosis, and by providing a conceptual approach to regurgitant dynamics.

* Supported in part by the National Institutes of Health, Grant No. HL-16354, and the Cardiovascular Research Laboratory of the Department of Surgery, Albert Einstein College of Medicine.

196

METHODS

Mitral Stenosis

Placement of the transducers is as described previously in Chapter 16, except that prior to the insertion of the flow probe, the commissural margins of the mitral cusps were sutured together to create a fixed, pliable, and competent mitral stenosis. The diameter of the stenotic orifice was measured at surgery and again at autopsy. The accuracy of the LA-LV pressure difference was checked at intervals during the experiment by matching the catheter-tip records with records from the same chambers using Statham gages. When possible, a complementary method was used: Vagal stimulation or cardiac arrest brought both pressures to a common value.

Mitral Regurgitation

Graded degrees of reversible acute mitral regurgitation were created either by inserting a plastic basket catheter into the mitral orifice, or by applying tension to a length of string which restricted the motion of the posterior cusp.

The determination of zero flow may be difficult since the heart,

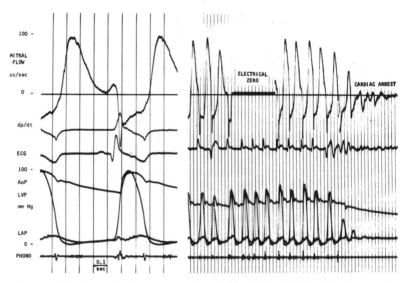

Figure 1. The determination of zero flow during mitral regurgitation. Left panel: exponential decay of flow toward zero during diastasis. Right panel: zero flow at cardiac arrest.

unlike an artery, cannot be occluded to give "mechanical" zero. With a competent mitral valve, the flow baseline can be determined with reasonable accuracy during systole when mitral flow is indeed zero. If there is regurgitation, however, one can slow the heart or create transient periods of prolonged diastasis and observe the exponential decay of the flow toward zero (Fig. 1, left panel); or a true baseline can be obtained by arresting the heart (Fig. 1, right panel).

THEORY

Mitral Stenosis

Because the high velocity jet issuing from the mitral orifice is pulsatile and is dissipated in the left ventricle via turbulent mechanisms, the equation of motion consists of an accelerative term and a term proportional to the square of the flow. Figure 2 presents this formulation and schematically depicts the anatomy of mitral stenosis. The mean of this equation when taken between the two points of zero flow eliminates the accelerative component and leaves the pressure-flow relation as shown in Figure 2. The rationale for this approach can be found in Yellin and Peskin,[1] where we prove that

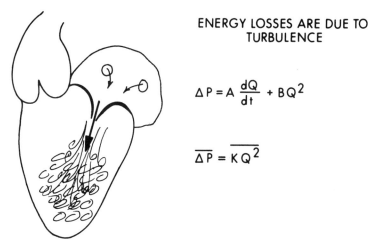

MITRAL STENOSIS

ENERGY LOSSES ARE DUE TO
TURBULENCE

$$\Delta P = A \frac{dQ}{dt} + BQ^2$$

$$\overline{\Delta P} = \overline{KQ^2}$$

Figure 2. Schematic of the anatomy of mitral stenosis and the equation (upper right) which describes the pressure-flow relation in this geometry. The time averaged equation is in the lower right.

except for some insignificant theoretical errors, it is the equivalent of the Gorlin equation:[2]

$$A_o = \overline{Q}/(0.7 \times 44.5 \sqrt{\Delta p}).$$

Mitral Regurgitation

We have not been successful in deriving a quantitative treatment of the regurgitant path, probably because the orifice changes its size too much during systole. We will, however, analyze mitral regurgitation in a *qualitative* manner, employing the principles developed for the normal and stenotic valves.

RESULTS

Mitral Stenosis

Figure 3 is an oscillographic record from a dog whose stenotic mitral orifice measured 0.8 cm². In contrast to the normal valve, the flow tends to remain constant throughout diastole, so that only at onset and at cessation of flow will any significant force be required to accelerate and decelerate the blood. As a consequence, resistance dominates the pressure-flow relations across the stenotic valve, and flow at any time other than onset and cessation is determined primarily by the pressure gradient at that time. Thus, peak flow occurs early in diastole, regardless of the rate of ventricular relaxation. Augmentation of flow by an atrial contraction is small, approximately 5% (shaded area, Fig. 3, beat 2). Were the diastolic period to be shortened by a premature contraction occurring just prior to what would have been the atrial contraction, then flow would be decreased by approximately 30% (Fig. 3, beat 3). Diastolic periods were chosen for analysis from stable beats at various heart rates, from premature contractions, and from post-extrasystolic periods. Using the Gorlin approach,[2] the calculated orifice area was remarkably close (Avg. 5%) to the measured area.

Mitral Regurgitation

Figure 4 is an oscillographic record which has been chosen because it dramatically illustrates the salient features of regurgitant dynamics under conditions of moderate incompetence. The results are presented in the lower portion of Figure 4 as the change in ratio of regurgitant to stroke volume (RV/SV). (Note that in this paper, stroke volume refers only to the forward volume flow.) In Panels A and B, beats numbered 1 are the last of a series of controls; beats numbered 2 are ventricular premature contractions (VPC); and beats numbered 3 are post-extrasystolic contractions (PESC). In Panel A, the VPC fails to open the aortic valve; it is followed by a prolonged diastolic period; there is a decreased aortic end diastolic pressure leading to an early opening of the valve; and the PESC is potentiated, leading to an increase in LVP, stroke volume, and dp/dt. In Panel B, the VPC occurs later so that the aortic valve opens, but stroke volume and dp/dt are reduced. The PESC (beat No. 3) is only slightly potentiated and the aortic end diastolic pressure only slightly reduced.

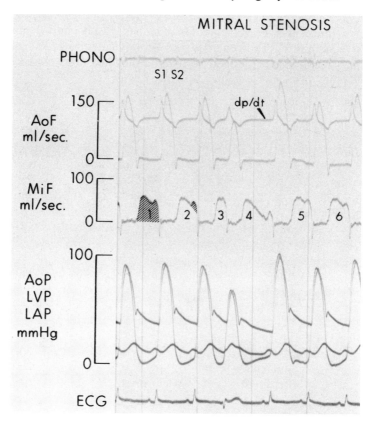

Figure 3. An oscillographic record from a dog with mitral stenosis created by suturing the commissural margins together during cardiopulmonary bypass. Phono = Intracardiac Phonocardiogram; AoF = Aortic Flow; MiF = Mitral Flow; AoP, LVP, LAP = Aortic, Left Ventricular, and Left Atrial Pressures; ECG = Electrocardiogram; dp/dt = Derivative of LVP. Time lines at one/sec.

Under these conditions, in both panels of Figure 4 the absolute value of the regurgitant volume and the RV/SV ratio both increase during the VPC. In Panel B, the regurgitation during the PESC remains the same as normal, but since there is a small potentiated increase in stroke volume, there is an insignificant decrease in the relative regurgitation.

DISCUSSION

Mitral Stenosis

The dynamic pressure-flow relations in mitral stenosis are characterized by the equation of motion in Figure 2. Most important, the time-averaged equation, which is closely equivalent to the Gorlin equation, has been shown to be applicable to mitral stenosis under conditions of induced arrhythmias and heart rate changes, i.e., under

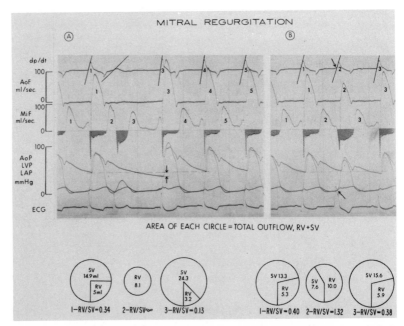

Figure 4. An oscillographic record from a dog with mitral regurgitation (shaded). In the upper trace the slope of dp/dt is emphasized with the solid line. Vertical broken lines indicate the amount of regurgitation occurring between mitral valve closure and aortic valve opening. Note that most of it is due to a closing volume artifact. Horizontal broken lines emphasize aortic end diastolic pressure differences. In Panel B, the arrows point to a period of slow ventricular contraction, resulting in a large regurgitant volume. The lower part of the figure illustrates the changes in the ratio of regurgitant to stroke volume. Time lines at one/sec.

various flow conditions. A reasonably good approximation to the orifice area can be calculated, and it is clear that the average pressure difference required to fill the ventricle is proportional to the square of the flow. Our work, therefore, supports the clinical application of the Gorlin equation as an adequate first approximation to the orifice area.

Mitral Regurgitation

The incompetent mitral valve presents an interesting study in dynamics because during ventricular contraction two paths are available for flow. Each path has its own impedance and each is under the action of a different driving force. Our data, of which Figure 4 is representative, are consistent with the work of others (Wiggers and Feil,[3] Rodbard and Williams,[4] Braunwald et al.,[5] Ross et al.[6]), but the following interpretation is not always in agreement with theirs. While these results are not comprehensive (not all conditions of acute and chronic regurgitation have been studied) and should be considered speculative, they present for the first time an experimental model which is truly in vivo and preserves the system characteristics completely. There are no analogs, external shunts, or internal paths that change the intrinsic properties of the system.

The conclusions presented below are based on the analysis of records with the heart in normal sinus rhythm; with peripheral resistance modified by vasoactive drugs; and with ventricular function modified by inotropic agents and volume loading. Particularly interesting is the analysis of extrasystolic and post-extrasystolic beats (Fig. 4).

Following ventricular contraction and reversal of the A-V gradient, mitral inflow is decelerated, and in normal sinus rhythm the mitral valve closes approximately 10 msec before the aortic valve opens. During this short time, flow is accelerated along the regurgitant path. When the aortic valve opens, there is an additional path for flow. The distribution of the filling volume along these two paths then becomes a function of the relative driving forces and impedances.

The two impedances are apparently highly dependent on frequency, so that flow can cross the aortic valve and enter the systemic circulation more readily than it can cross the incompetent mitral valve. Thus, the aortic end diastolic pressure influences the flow distribution in two ways: via the time to valve opening, and via the compliance characteristics of the aortic "windkessel." The value of the former is clear: forward flow will begin sooner. Regarding the latter, at low pressures the aortic compliance increases and hence the impedance decreases. More important, however, the initial rate of rise of left ventricular pressure (that is, its contractility and synchrony of contraction), will determine the distribution of flow between the forward and regurgitant paths, because the impedance of the compliance path decreases with increasing frequency.

The regurgitant orifice, on the other hand, in addition to resistive properties, also has inertial characteristics which lead to an increase in impedance with increasing frequency. Because inertance is dominant at acceleration, the regurgitant path during isovolumic contraction has its largest impedance. Hence regurgitation is less than expected at that time (note the vertical broken lines in Fig. 4).

The data and analysis suggest that in mitral regurgitation the regurgitant fraction can be decreased and the forward fraction increased by the use of peripheral vasodilators in conjunction with positive inotropic agents and anti-arrhythmic therapy. This conclusion is based on hemodynamic considerations; its clinical applicability is, of course, subject to other medical considerations.

INTRA-AORTIC BALLOON PUMPING FOR MITRAL REGURGITATION

The results presented above and the favorable clinical experience of Gold et al.,[7] have led us to undertake a study of the dynamics

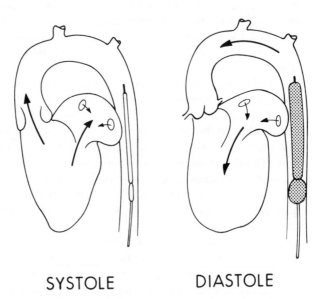

SYSTOLE   DIASTOLE

Figure 5. Schematic of the deflation and inflation of an intra-aortic balloon during systole and diastole.

of IABP in dogs with mitral incompetence. Our rationale was that this procedure would serve a two-fold purpose. 1) During systole, deflation of the balloon (Fig. 5) would lower aortic pressure, thereby increasing its compliance and lowering the impedance to outflow; a well-timed deflation would also decrease the time to aortic valve opening. The decreased afterload might also result in a reduced LVP

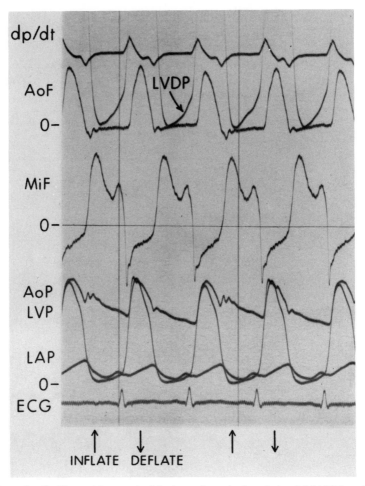

Figure 6. Oscillographic record of the hemodynamic data during 1:2 IABP in a dog with mitral regurgitation. Note that diastolic pressure augmentation during inflation is quite small, but the increase in negative aortic flow indicates an increase in coronary perfusion. There is an 11% increase in stroke volume during balloon deflation. Time lines at one/sec.

204

and thus a reduced driving pressure for regurgitation. Balloon deflation should, therefore, decrease RV/SV ratio. 2) During diastole, inflation of the balloon (Fig. 5) would increase the aortic diastolic pressure and augment coronary flow. Myocardial performance should improve, LVdp/dt should increase, and by the reasoning discussed previously, systemic flow would also increase.

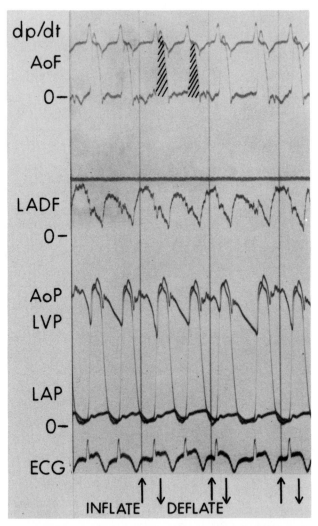

Figure 7. As in Figure 6, but the mitral flow is replaced by the Left Anterior Descending Coronary Artery flow (LADF). Pumping in the 1:2 mode illustrates the clear augmentation of coronary flow and improvement of stroke volume (shaded areas). Time lines at one/sec.

Some preliminary results are shown in Figures 6 and 7. In order to elucidate the dynamics of IABP on a beat-to-beat basis, the pump was operated in the 1:2 mode, so that the transient dynamic effects were observed before they became masked by reflex control mechanisms. In Figure 6, balloon deflation increased stroke-volume by 11%; regurgitant volume did not change, so that the RV/SV ratio decreased by 10%. This increase in stroke volume with IABP is normal, but unless there is a decrease in LVP, the regurgitant volume does not change. The effects of IABP on coronary flow are shown in Figure 7. The augmentation of coronary flow is clearly seen during balloon inflation and the increase in stroke volume is evident during deflation.

These data substantiate the physical analysis of the dynamics during mitral regurgitation, and they therefore indicate the desirability of further investigation. It must be pointed out, however, that these studies in dynamics are by no means definitive, because in both acute and chronic mitral regurgitation other physiological factors must be taken into consideration.

CONCLUSION

The methodology presented here is admittedly highly invasive and traumatic. Nevertheless it has enabled us to elucidate atrioventricular dynamics in a way not possible by less invasive means. We are now able to interpret the results of cardiac catheterization and noninvasive clinical methods more meaningfully.

REFERENCES

1. Yellin, E.L., Peskin, C.S.   Large amplitude pulsatile water flow across an orifice. *J. of Dynamic Systems, Measurement and Control.* Trans. ASME, Series G. 97:92-95, 1975.

2. Gorlin, R., Gorlin, S.G.   Hydraulic formula for calculation of the area of the stenotic mitral valve, other cardiac valves, and central circulatory shunts. I. *Am. Heart J.* 41:1-29, 1951.

3. Wiggers, C.J., Feil, H.   The cardio-dynamics of mitral insufficiency. *Am. Heart J.* 9:149-183, 1921-1922.

4. Rodbard, S., Williams, F.   The dynamics of mitral insufficiency. *Am. Heart J.* 48:521-539, 1954.

5. Braunwald, E., Welch, G.H., Sarnoff, S.J.   Hemodynamic effects of quantitatively varied experimental mitral regurgitation. *Circulation Research* 5:539-545, 1957.

6. Ross, J., Jr., Cooper, T., Lombardo, C.R. Hemodynamic observations in experimental mitral regurgitation. *Surgery* 47:795-803, 1960.

7. Gold, H.K., Leinbach, R.C., Sanders, C.A., Buckley, M.J., Mundth, E.D., Austen, W.G. Intra-aortic balloon pumping for ventricular septal defect or mitral regurgitation complicating acute myocardial infarction. *Circulation* 47:1191-1196, 1973.

19 Flow Dynamics in Mitral Regurgitation

Stanton P. Nolan, M.D.
Luis M. Botero, M.D.
Robert Rawitscher, M.D.

Clinically, the hemodynamic assessment of mitral regurgitation has been limited by the lack of a method for the measurement of instantaneous blood flow across the mitral valve. Our studies have been carried out in the experimental laboratory and have been limited to two areas: 1) the measurement of flow dynamics in acute mitral regurgitation, and 2) the study of diastolic mitral regurgitation occurring with aortic valvular regurgitation.

Calves were prepared with electromagnetic flow transducers in a manner similar to that used in studies of the normal mitral valve. Instantaneous ventricular volume was determined by integrating the differential flow—the mitral flow minus the aortic flow—and extrapolating this measurement to absolute volume by gauging the left ventricular compliance at the end of the experiment. Acute mitral regurgitation was produced by the serial division of chordae tendineae in order to produce approximately 40% mitral regurgitation. Aortic regurgitation was produced by rupture of a single aortic cusp.

Figure 1 is a recording from a calf with approximately 40% mitral regurgitation. The simultaneous aortic flow and the left ventricular

207

volume are also shown. The pattern of mitral valve flow in mitral regurgitation demonstrates a diastolic pattern quite similar to the normal flow. In each cardiac cycle, mitral regurgitation begins at the point where the negative Phase IV flow would have been expected in the normal valve. The regurgitation persists throughout systole and finally ends with the onset of the positive atrioventricular pressure gradient. It should also be noted that the rate of regurgitant flow decreases slowly throughout systole. Multiple recordings similar to this were made from 10 calves with 40% acute mitral regurgitation.

In these experiments, the heart rate and aortic pressure were

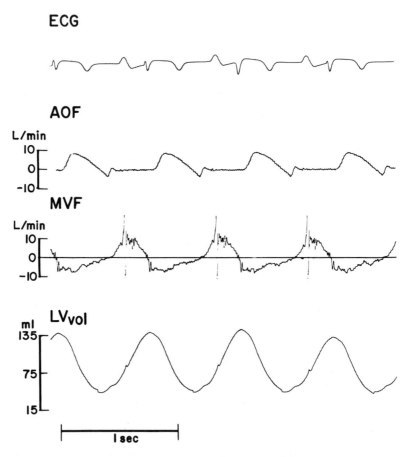

Figure 1. Simultaneous recordings from a calf with acute mitral regurgitation. The electrocardiogram (ECG) demonstrates a heart rate of 76 per minute. Ascending aortic blood flow (AoF); mitral valve blood flow (MVF) with 40% regurgitation; and left ventricular volume (LVvol) indicating a 70% ejected fraction.

	CONTROL	MITRAL REGURGITATION	P
LAP mean mmHg	10.3 ± 1.3	14.0 ± 1.3	0.1
LAP systolic mmHg	10.6 ± 2.0	15.5 ± 1.5	0.05
LVEDP mmHg	8.7 ± 1.2	9.5 ± 0.9	0.6
LVSW forward GM-M	36.0 ± 6.0	29.0 ± 3.0	0.2
LVSW regurgitant GM-M	----	2.9 ± 0.5	---
LVSW total GM-M	36.0 ± 6.0	32.0 ± 3.0	0.4

Figure 2. Values based on observations from seven calves with acute mitral regurgitation. LAP = left atrial pressure; LVEDP = left ventricular end-diastolic pressure; LVSW = left ventricular stroke work; GM-M = gram-meters.

maintained within a narrow range before and after the production of mitral regurgitation. The total blood volume showed no change. However, there was a marked decrease in the cardiac output and the aortic ejection time, as well as a slight lengthening in the mitral valve forward flow time. The aortic stroke volume decreased while the mitral valve forward stroke volume increased. There was no significant change in the left atrial pressure and only a slight rise in the left atrial sytolic pressure (Fig. 2). The left ventricular end-diastolic pressure was unaltered, and the left ventricular stroke work remained the same despite mitral regurgitation.

From the measurement of left ventricular volume, significant alterations were noted. As seen in Figure 3, left ventricular end-

	CONTROL	MITRAL REGURGITATION	P
Aortic SV ml.	55 ± 6	39 ± 3	< 0.01
Mitral SV ml.	55 ± 6	70 ± 4	< 0.05
% Mitral Regurg.	0	41 ± 4	----
LVED Vol. ml.	89 ± 5	87 ± 5	0.8
LVES Vol. ml.	34 ± 4	16 ± 2	< 0.001
Ejected Fraction %	60 ± 4	80 ± 2	< 0.001

Figure 3. Values based on observations from seven calves with acute mitral regurgitation. SV = stroke volume; LVED Vol = left ventricular end-diastolic volume; LVES Vol = left ventricular end-systolic volume.

210

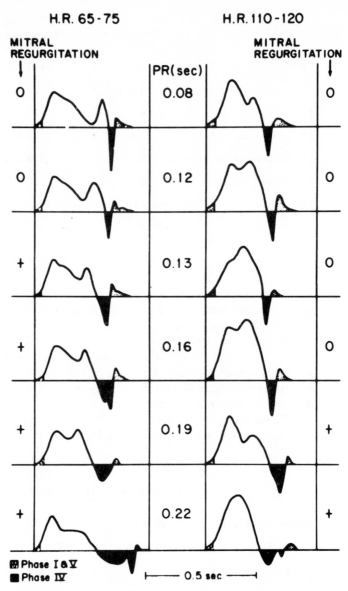

H.R. 65-75

H.R. 110-120

MITRAL
REGURGITATION

MITRAL
REGURGITATION

PR(sec)

0		0.08		0
0		0.12		0
+		0.13		0
+		0.16		0
+		0.19		+
+		0.22		+

⊞ Phase I & Ⅴ
■ Phase Ⅳ

⊢———— 0.5 sec ————⊣

Figure 4. Representative patterns of mitral valve flow in the presence of aortic regurgitation with P-R intervals from 0.08 to 0.22 seconds. At heart rates of 65 to 75 per minute (left), mitral regurgitation was present when the P-R interval was greater than 0.12 seconds. At heart rates of 110 to 120 per minute (right), mitral regurgitation occurred when the P-R interval was greater than 0.18 seconds.

diastolic volume was unaltered; however, left ventricular end-systolic volume was decreased. When the ejected fraction was calculated on the basis of the comparison of the end-systolic and end-diastolic volumes, it was found that 40% acute mitral regurgitation produced a 35% increase in the ejected fraction.

From these studies it appears that the immediate compensation for acute mitral regurgitation is achieved by a marked reduction in the left ventricular end-systolic volume. This reduction in end-systolic volume was so extreme in these experiments, i.e., an average end-systolic volume of 16 ml, that it must be assumed that any further compensation would require an increase in the end-diastolic volume.

The diastolic mitral regurgitation accompanying aortic regurgitation was studied in another series of experiments (Fig. 4). In the presence of aortic regurgitation, it was found that: 1) with heart rates of 110 to 120 per minute and P-R intervals greater than 0.18 seconds, there was a reversal of the diastolic pressure gradient across the mitral valve; 2) with diastolic reversal of the atrioventricular pressure gradient, diastolic mitral regurgitation occurred; 3) the occurrence of mitral regurgitation was independent of left ventricular end-diastolic pressure and the volume of the regurgitant flow ranged from 5 to 19% of the forward mitral valve flow; and, 4) due to aortic regurgitation the reversed diastolic mitral flow did not decrease ventricular volume.

The volume of diastolic mitral regurgitation that occurs with aortic regurgitation, and through an anatomically normal mitral valve, is small and apparently causes no alteration in ventricular volume. Care must be exercised, however, in the interpretation of left ventricular cineangiocardiograms in patients with aortic regurgitation, since diastolic mitral regurgitation might be mistaken for evidence of organic mitral valve disease.

SELECTED READING

Nolan, S.P., Fisher, R.D., Dixon, S.H., Jr., Williams, W.H., Morrow, A.G. Alterations in left atrial transport and mitral valve blood flow resulting from aortic regurgitation. *American Heart Journal* 79:668-675, 1970.

20 Mitral Flow Velocity Tracings in Patients with Mitral Valve Disease

Diagnostic use of the transseptal Doppler catheterization

D. Kalmanson M.D.
Colette Veyrat, M.D.
A. Bernier, M.D.
S. Witchitz, M.D.

INTRODUCTION

None of the techniques presently used in clinical cardiology provides information on the instantaneous flow across the mitral valve. Yet the paramount importance of the knowledge of instantaneous flow velocity profile and flow pattern for our understanding of the physiology and pathophysiology of the mitral valve has been clearly stressed by previous authors of this book (Bellhouse, Taylor, Talbot, Nolan, Yellin, Laniado). Unfortunately, the pressure gradient technique and the electromagnetic blood flow measurements remain merely experimental, except for the procedure proposed by Folts, which can be peroperatively applied to patients, but not during a routine cardiac catheterization.

The recent advent of intracardiac flow velocity measurements using the directional Doppler ultrasonic velocimeter catheter-tip[1]* provides a unique possibility of gathering flow velocity information at the site of the mitral valve. Such a technique was previously used at

---

* Sonicaid Ltd, Bognor Regis, Sussex, England.

the site of the tricuspid valve; it offered a valuable approach to the study of tricuspid flow physiology and to assessing tricuspid valve disease.[2]

Technique

We have been using the directional Doppler velocimeter Sonicaid 180, the performance and use of which have been published elsewhere.[3] The Doppler probe consists of one single piezoelectric crystal, acting successively as emitter and receiver, operating at 8.4 MHz. The size of the catheter is 7 French. According to the Doppler principle, the frequency shift between the ultrasound emitted to, and scattered back from, the red blood cells is directly proportional to the velocity of these red cells, which can be considered in first approximation as representing the blood flow velocity fairly well. An acrylic lens is placed at the end of the transducer and focuses the beam approximately 5 mm ahead of the tip. Experimental calibration of the velocimeter has demonstrated a satisfactory linearity up to velocities of 1.20 m/sec. The probe is directional, i.e., it can distinguish forward from backward flow. Time constant of the device has been shown to range between 10 to 15 msec.

In order to facilitate the intracardiac use of the catheter, the transducer has been mounted on a catheter-controller,* which enables the tip to be bent in any given direction. This allows a precise positioning of the tip parallel to flow, a prerequisite to obtain correct Doppler intracardiac records.

Method

The procedure was always carried out during a conventional transseptal catheterization, during which the precise site of the mitral annulus was localized using a pull-back maneuver from the left ventricle to the left atrium. (Fig. 1). After the pressure catheter had been withdrawn, the sheath leading through the interatrial septum into the left atrium being left in situ, the previously sterilized Doppler catheter was inserted into the proximal orifice of the sheath and pushed forward into the left atrium. The tip was then localized under fluoroscopy at the site of the mitral annulus, and its direction aligned with that of transmitral flow, using the loud speaker giving a sound translation of the Doppler shift, according to a previously described technique.[2]

---

* Meditech Inc., Watertown, Mass.

Recordings were made in the center of the mitral ring, and at the anterolateral, and whenever possible, at the posteromedial commissure. The curves were recorded during quiet respiration in unanesthetized patients on a 4-channel or 7-channel Mingograf recorder. ECG lead II and frequency-selecting phonocardiogram were simultaneously inscribed on the chart. The chart speed was 25 or 50 mm/sec. Distance between two successive spikes of the upper row equals one second.

Subjects

Two groups of patients were studied: 1) a control group of 10 patients in whom an organic lesion of the mitral valve was ruled out by the pressure catheterization, together with other conventional investigations. The detailed findings and diagnosis of these patients have been described elsewhere;[4] and 2) A group of 33 patients with mitral valve disease, including 15 patients with pure stenosis, 8 with pure regurgitation, and 10 with associated stenosis and regurgitation. In all

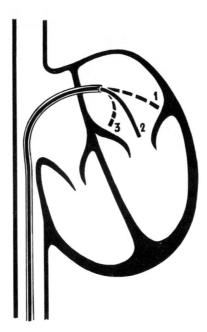

Figure 1. Velocimetric exploration of mitral blood flow. The Doppler catheter is pushed forward into the sheath leading to the left atrium, and its tip is localized under fluoroscopic control at various points of the mitral ring. Main points of interest are the anterolateral commissure (1), the center (2), and the posteromedial commissure (3).

patients both atrial and ventricular pressures were recorded simultaneously, allowing the determination of the LA-LV pressure gradient. Cardiac output and mitral regurgitation were measured by the indocyanine green dilution technique using the Waters apparatus.* Mitral valve area was calculated according to the Gorlin formula. The patients were classified according to the severity of their lesion on a four grade scale (0:no lesion, 1:mild, 2:moderate, 3:severe). This classification was based on the clinical picture and time course, as well as on the hemodynamic data which have been published elsewhere.[5] In particular, for mitral stenosis, the mitral valve area was greater than 1.5 cm² for grade I, ranged between 1.5 and 1.00 cm² for grade 2, and was less than 1.00 cm² for grade 3. For mitral regurgitation, the assessment of severity was based on the clinical presentation, as well as the pressure, dye dilution, and angiocardiographic data; for both lesions, assessment of severity was based on the surgical findings, when appropriate.

Results

It is worth mentioning that no complication was encountered, apart from transient atrial or ventricular arrhythmias. In three patients not included in this study, the procedure failed, and in two others it had to be stopped due to an increasingly severe bradycardia, which was considered an absolute indication to withdraw the catheter.

All recorded curves represent the flow velocity, calibrated in cm/sec, of blood flowing through the mitral valve. By convention, positive velocities correspond to blood flowing from the left atrium into the left ventricle, and negative velocities correspond either to blood flowing from the ventricle into the atrium or to a simple upward displacement of blood remaining in the atrium, right above the mitral leaflets.

NORMAL PATTERN AND PHYSIOLOGICAL SIGNIFICANCE OF MITRAL VALVE FLOW VELOCITY

The curve (Figs. 2 and 3) starts with a brief, precipitous, negative deflection of large amplitude, labelled *ic*, lining up with the first vibrations of the first heart sound. It is simultaneous with the isometric contraction period, and can be ascribed to the sudden backflow wave originated by the bulging of the dome-like closed mitral floor

---

* Waters, Rochester, Minnesota

known to occur during this short period. Whether this deflection reflects actual backflow from the ventricle into the atrium, or simply the upward displacement of the mitral floor, is subject to controversy. It lasts from 0.05 to 0.08 sec, and its magnitude is partly dependent on the distance of the catheter-tip from both the surface of the leaflets and the ridge of the annulus. In some patients this deflection could not be recorded.

Thereafter, the curve rapidly rises and rejoins the zero line, keeping close to it until the end of systole, where it often shows a small angulation synchronous with the second aortic sound. Then the curve presents a brief and small segment—positive, diaphasic, or negative (B-MO in Fig. 3), which corresponds to the isometric relaxation period of the left ventricle. At the MO point, the tracing suddenly rises and describes two successive positive, triangular, diastolic waves: the first labelled D, or initial filling flow velocity wave, followed by an end-diastolic wave, labelled A, larger or smaller than the D wave depending on the heart rate. The peak of the D wave occurs from 0.13 to 0.20 sec after the aortic second sound, whereas the A wave reaches its peak from 0.16 to 0.20 after the onset of the electrical P wave. For a given patient, there is a constant time relationship between the onset of the ECG P wave and the flow velocity A wave.

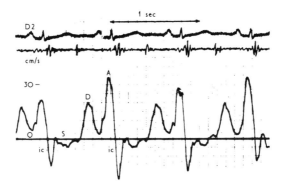

Figure 2. Normal flow velocity trace of the mitral valve. The curve is calibrated in cm/s. Velocities above the zero line refer to flow passing from the left atrium into the left ventricle; those below the zero line refer to flow directed from the left ventricle toward the left atrium. The curve starts with a brief percipitous negative deflection (ic) lining up with the first heart sound. During the remainder of systole, the S segment runs along the zero line (no flow). Note a minute notch lining up with the second heart sound. Then the curve crosses the baseline (opening of the mitral valve), and shows an initial positive, triangular, and almost symmetrical D wave. This is followed by an end-diastolic, larger, A wave, of shorter duration, whose timing bears a constant relation to the P wave of the electrocardiogram.

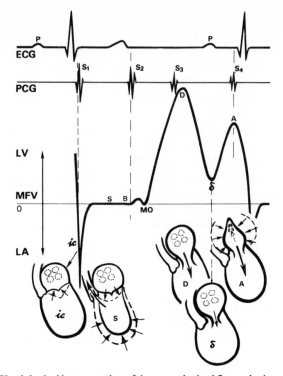

Figure 3. Physiological interpretation of the normal mitral flow velocity pattern of the mitral valve. The initial negative deflection (ic) is caused by the bulging of the mitral valve into the left atrium during isometric contraction, provoked by the contraction of the papillary muscles and completing the apposition of the leaflets. The S segment along the zero line indicates the absence of flow through the closed mitral floor. The small segment B-MO extending from the notch, synchronous with the second heart sound, to the onset of the D wave delimits the isovolumic relaxation period. The D wave represents the initial diastolic filling of the left ventricle, and the A wave, the end-diastolic filling caused by atrial contraction.

This A wave may therefore be logically ascribed to the atrial contraction. It is worth mentioning that we rarely found a so-called "diastasis" wave between the D and A waves, which in all our records joined together at a precise and single point labelled δ, which usually, but not always, is above or at the level of the zero line. In case of prolonged P-R interval, the descending limb of the A wave overrides the zero line before the occurrence of the first heart sound.

Discussion

The physical and physiological interpretation of intracardiac flow velocity recording raises many difficult problems. Some of them, such as those involving the displacement of the catheter-tip by blood flow or cardiac structures, the recording of echoes from valves or from wall, and the production of flow disturbances by the presence of a catheter, have been discussed at length elsewhere.[3] Such problems may limit the method, but by and large they do not really affect its practical validity. On the other hand, the representativity of the intracardiac flow velocity tracings and their relationship to mitral flow volume curve deserve to be discussed.

The physiological significance of the curve is closely dependent on the velocity profile and on the instantaneous size of the mitral annulus. 1) From their experimental pressure-gradient measurements across the mitral valve, Taylor and co-workers[6,7] demonstrated that the velocity profile across the valve region was flat, except for a zone of high shear very close to the valve surface. Therefore, a punctual measurement of the velocity at one point of the ring, as can be determined by the Doppler technique, may be considered as representative of the velocity profile of the ring. 2) Furthermore, our curves of mitral flow velocity are strikingly similar to those of mitral flow volume showed by Nolan[8] and Yellin[9] in the preceeding chapters. Such a similarity can be more precisely specified in the light of the studies of Tsakiris and colleagues.[10,11,12] These authors showed that there was a continuous increase in mitral ring area from the onset of the isovolumetric relaxation period until mid-diastole, so that the area is maximum before the atrial contraction (Fig. 4). Thereafter, the shrinkage of the mitral annulus is initiated to a great extent by the

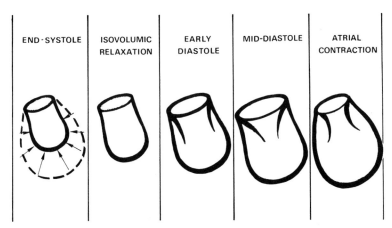

| END-SYSTOLE | ISOVOLUMIC RELAXATION | EARLY DIASTOLE | MID-DIASTOLE | ATRIAL CONTRACTION |

Figure 4. Variations in size of the mitral valve annulus during the cardiac cycle (after Tsakiris). There is a progressive increase in mitral ring area during isovolumetric relaxation, and above all during early and mid-diastole. Before the atrial contraction, the area is maximum. The shrinkage of the mitral annulus is, to a large extent, initiated by atrial contraction, and completed by ventricular systole. The total decrease in the area in dogs was found to range from 20 to 34% of the mid-diastolic maximum value. (Tsakiris).

atrial contraction and completed by ventricular systole. From their figures it can be deduced that flow velocity and flow rate do not vary linearly but that for a given mitral ring area, blood flow rate from blood flow velocity would be underestimated by a factor less than 34% during the initial filling phase of diastole, and overestimated by a factor less than 22% during the atrial contraction period. In spite of these nonlinearities, and taking into account the striking similarity of velocity and flow rate curves, the flatness of the velocity profile across the mitral ring, and the direction and the limited rate of change in size of the mitral annulus, it can be assumed that the flow velocity traces recorded by the Doppler technique provide valuable information on the timing and general pattern of mitral valve blood flow; they are therefore endowed with great clinical significance. In particular, they offer a valid reference system for the study by means of a pattern-recognition method of pathological tracings.

PATTERNS OF MITRAL FLOW VELOCITY IN PATIENTS WITH MITRAL VALVE DISEASE

Pure Mitral Stenosis

In all our 15 cases, the initial filling D wave showed characteristic anomalies (Figs. 5 and 6). These anomalies consisted of indentations, more or less large and irregular, giving a saw-tooth appearance to its ascending limb, its peak, and even the descending limb depending on the severity of the stenosis. As a whole, the earlier their onset and the greater their amplitude, the more severe the stenosis. The slope of the ascending limb and the timing of the peak were normal or almost normal in mild stenosis. In severe stenosis, this slope was decreased, the peak delayed, and the summit more or less decreased and flattened. All these anomalies were more pronounced near the commissural areas than near the center of the mitral annulus, where the velocities tended to be higher, the ascending limb steeper, and the onset of indentations delayed. In all cases the systolic S wave was found to be normal.[5]

Pure Mitral Regurgitation

In all our patients, a negative systolic S wave (Figs. 7 and 8) was found either at all sites of recording or only at one particular point. The deeper the systolic wave, the more severe was the mitral regurgitation.

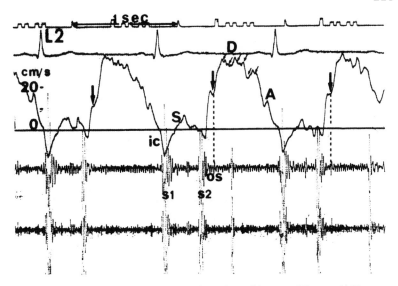

Figure 5. Mitral valve flow velocity trace in patient with pure mild stenosis. From top to bottom; electrocardiogram lead II, flow velocity trace, and phonocardiogram. The systolic velocity component is normal: negative deflection (ic) during isometric contraction, S segment along the zero line. The diastolic filling wave D rises abruptly but is interrupted by a small conspicuous notch (arrow) synchronous with the opening snap (os), then continues to rise with a steep slope up to the peak. Small indentations occur, giving the peak an appearance of an irregular and slightly descending plateau. The indentations proceed on the descending limb of the D wave. Heart rate is low, 54/min, and the A wave is small (calculated mitral area: 1.9 cm²).

Associated Mitral Stenosis and Regurgitation

In all 10 cases (Fig. 9) the tracings showed the association of a more or less deep, negative systolic S wave with somewhat pronounced, early indentations on the ascending limb of the diastolic D wave. The deeper the S wave, the more severe the regurgitation; the earlier the diastolic indentations and the more decreased the slope of the ascending limb of the D wave, the more severe the stenosis. An interesting and important finding is the fact that the velocity pattern may not be the same at different points of recording, as is the case shown in Figure 9. At the anteromedial commissure, the pattern is that of a rather severe stenosis, whereas at the center, it is that of a mild one. This indicates that the velocity profile across the mitral ring, for the most part, is not likely to be flat. Such variation of the recorded pattern from one point of the mitral annulus to the other stresses the sensitivity of the method but also necessitates a careful investigation of the ring before assessing the diagnosis and respective severity of the lesions.

222

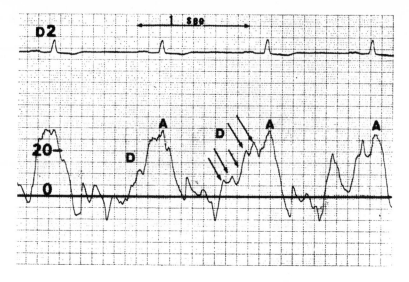

Figure 6. Mitral valve flow velocity trace in a patient with a pure, severe mitral stenosis (recording at the anterolateral commissure). The D wave is replaced by a very irregular ascending curve, with a gradual slope; the A wave is of higher amplitude than the D wave (calculated mitral area: 1 cm²).

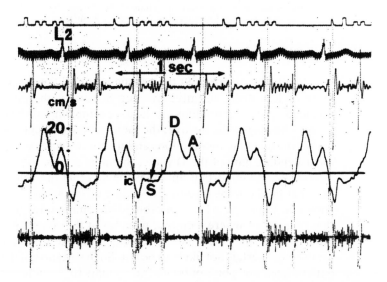

Figure 7. Flow velocity trace in a patient with a pure, mild mitral regurgitation. After the initial negative deflection (ic), the S segment of the curve rises again, without, however, reaching the zero line, and consistently remains slightly below that line throughout systole. The diastolic A and D waves remain normal.

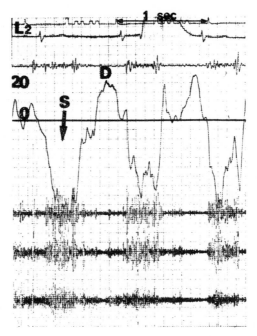

Figure 8. Flow velocity trace in a patient with pure, severe mitral regurgitation. The S wave is replaced by a very deep negative wave throughout systole (volume of regurgitation: 50% of cardiac output).

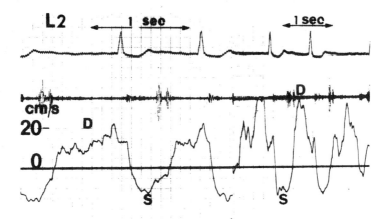

Figure 9. Flow velocity trace in a patient with severe stenosis and moderate regurgitation in atrial fibrillation. Left: at the commissural areas. Right: at the center of the mitral annulus. In both tracings, the S wave is negative throughout systole and of moderate depth. The D wave is cut off near the commissures; it is of much higher amplitude at the center of the annulus, and shows much less pronounced indentations (calculated mitral area: 1 cm²: volume of regurgitation: 10% of cardiac output).

Comments

The transseptal Doppler catheterization is the first of all clinical methods presently used in cardiology to provide unique information about the essential phenomenon, i.e., the beat-to-beat instantaneous transmitral flow disturbances. Our finding that, in all cases, characteristic anomalies of the tracings were noted, namely, anomalies of the S wave for regurgitation, anomalies of the D wave for stenosis, and both types of anomalies for associated stenosis and regurgitation, indicates that this method is a reliable one for assessing the diagnosis of mitral valve disease. Furthermore, in some patients whose pressure data or dye dilution did not confirm a mitral regurgitation which was clinically most probable, a small negative S wave was found; this suggests that the Doppler method might be more sensitive to small lesions than the classical methods of pressure measurements or dye dilution. In addition, there was a constant correlation between the intensity of the anomalies and the severity of the lesions as evaluated by the conventional techniques. In other words, the Doppler method can also be used to assess the severity of mitral valve disease, particularly in cases of associated lesions.

Interpretation of the Curves

Mitral Stenosis   It is most likely that the characteristic indentations of the ascending limb of the D wave are provoked by the turbulence generated by the impedance to transmitral blood flow, a consequence of the stenosis. They start with and sometimes after the opening snap, and are synchronous with the vibrations of the diastolic rumble of the phonocardiogram. This interpretation is consistent with Taylor's[13] finding of a very irregular front of the velocity profile. However, there is a discrepancy between some of our results and Taylor's findings.

First, the peak velocities were decreased in our tracings, a quite unexpected result since they may logically be assumed to be notably increased. This result might be explained by the loss of linearity of the Doppler technique for turbulent flow, which has been demonstrated to occur by Tunstall-Pedoe,[14] and also in some cases, by the severely decreased cardiac output. On the other hand, in patients with sinus rhythm, we usually noted a large A wave. This increased amplitude of the A wave is likely to be due to the fact that an amount of blood larger than normal remains in the atrium after the initial filling period of the ventricle; hence, the more severe the stenosis, the larger the remaining blood, and the higher the flow velocity of atrial evacuation toward the ventricle.

Mitral Regurgitation It results from the directionality of the Doppler probe that the systolic negative S wave provides a direct record of the regurgitant flow. By and large, the deeper and broader the negativity, the more severe the regurgitation. In other words, the Doppler technique offers a reliable method for assessing the diagnosis of mitral incompetence and also for evaluating its severity. Some reservation, however, is necessary in cases where regurgitation may be limited to a narrow jet, such as those associated with papillary muscle dysfunction or abnormal chordae tendineae. In these cases, as well as those of mild regurgitation, the diagnosis and assessment of severity can only be made after careful exploration of the mitral ring with the Doppler probe. On the other hand, the method may be very sensitive to small, isolated leaks of blood through the valve that otherwise cannot be detected by the conventional investigative procedures.

An unexpected finding is most certainly that of normal or even decreased diastolic velocities in patients with severe regurgitation, in whom they can be predicted to be increased. This discrepancy is likely to be due to the fact that the direction of the catheter-tip (and therefore of the ultrasonic beam) is not parallel to that of transmitral blood flow, a condition which induces a loss of linearity. Technical improvement of the technique appears to be desirable before quantitative measurements can be considered in such cases.

Associated Mitral Stenosis and Regurgitation In most cases, the characteristic anomalies for each lesion, according to its severity, show up on the same record: typical indentations for the stenosis and a negative systolic wave for the regurgitation. However, this may not always be the case; therefore, before assessing the diagnosis and the respective severity of each type of lesion, it is essential to explore carefully the mitral ring (center and commissural areas), since one type of anomaly may be conspicuous or even present only at one particular site of recording.

Limitations of the Method

With present catheters, Doppler catheterization is not always possible. In some patients in sinus rhythm who have hyperkinetic hearts, achieving a satisfactory immobilization of the catheter-tip may be very difficult and time-consuming, if not impossible. Insufficient exploration of the mitral ring may cause a lesion to be overlooked. It may be hoped that future improvements of the present catheters will reduce these shortcomings.

Regarding the loss of linearity of the probe for highly turbulent flow, as is the case in mitral stenosis, it should be stressed that the diagnostic value of the Doppler catheterization is not the least affected, since it is based on a pattern recognition method, rather than on the quantitative accuracy of the velocity measurements.

Conclusion

Despite some shortcomings and limitations, the transseptal Doppler catheterization of the mitral valve provides a reliable method for establishing the diagnosis and evaluating the severity of mitral valve disease. Moreover, it offers a wealth of information and knowledge regarding instantaneous transmitral blood flow, and this appears to be essential for a better understanding of mitral valve pathophysiology.

REFERENCES

1. Kalmanson, D., Toutain, G., Novikoff, N., Derai, C., Chiche, P., Cabrol, C. Le cathétérisme vélocimétrique du coeur et des gros vaisseaux par sonde ultrasonique directionnelle à effet Doppler. Rapport préliminaire. *Annales de Médecine Interne* 120:685, 1969.

2. Kalmanson, D., Derai, C., Novikoff, N. Le flux tricuspidien étudié chez l'animal et chez l'homme par cathétérisme vélocimétrique directionnel. Aspect normal, variations physiologiques et applications diagnostiques. *Archives des Maladies du Coeur et des Vaisseaux* 64:854, 1971.

3. Kalmanson, D., Toutain, G., Novikoff, N., Derai, C. Retrograde catheterization of left heart cavities in dogs by means of an orientable directional Doppler catheter-tip flowmeter: a preliminary report. *Cardiovascular Research* 6:309, 1972.

4. Kalmanson, D., Bernier, A., Veyrat, C., Witchitz, S., Savier, C.H., Chiche, P. Normal pattern and physiological significance of mitral valve flow velocity recorded using transseptal directional Doppler ultrasound catheterization. *British Heart Journal* 37:249-256, 1975.

5. Kalmanson, D., Veyrat, C., Bernier, A., Savier, C.H., Chiche, P., Witchitz, S. Diagnosis and evaluation of mitral valve

disease using transseptal Doppler ultrasound catheterization. *British Heart Journal* 37:257-271, 1975.

6. Taylor, D.E.M., Wade, J.D. Flow through the mitral valve during diastolic filling of the left ventricle. *Journal of Physiology* 200:73P, 1969.

7. Taylor, D.E.M., Whamond, J. Velocity profiles and impedance of the healthy mitral valve. This book, Chapter 12.

8. Nolan, S.P. The normal mitral valve: patterns of instantaneous mitral valve flow and the atrial contribution to ventricular filling. This book, Chapter 13.

9. Yellin, E.L., Laniado, S., Peskin, C., Frater, R. Analysis and interpretation of the normal mitral valve flow curve. This book, Chapter 16.

10. Tsakiris, A.G., Von Bernuth, G., Rastelli, G.G., Bourgeois, M.J., Titus, J.L., Wood, E.H. Size and motion of the mitral valve annulus in anesthetized intact dogs. *Journal of Applied Physiology* 30:611, 1971.

11. Tsakiris, A.G. The physiology of the mitral valve annulus. This book, Chapter 3.

12. Tsakiris, A.G., Gordon, D.A., Mathieu, Y., Lipton, I. Time-motion of both mitral leaflets early in diastole. This book, Chapter 4.

13. Whamond, J., Taylor, D.E.M. Fluid dynamics of the diseased mitral valve. This book, Chapter 17.

14. Tunstall-Pedoe, D.S. Diagnosis of aortic incompetence using directional Doppler blood velocity measurements—problems of quantitation. Edited by D.J. Cockrell. In *Fluid Dynamic Measurements in the Industrial and Medical Environments*. Leicester: Leicester University Press, 1972.

DISCUSSION: PART IV

Dr. Gabe: Mr. Taylor, I can't help being rather skeptical about the impedance results which you showed concerning the normal mitral valve, in which the moduli decreased inertially. One would expect the moduli to rise with frequency. Also, in the mitral stenotic valve one has a very nonlinear element, for its resistance is going to be something like a square law and the idea of impedance, then, is under great difficulty. I would like to know how you measured the impedance and what you think about this.

Mr. Taylor: The impedance spectra were obtained in the usual manner by dividing the Fourier moduli of pressure by the equivalent flow modules and the division into resistive and reactive components by the standard Fourier transform technique: in addition, we have looked at the shape and harmonic components of the curve of P/Q. We have been very surprised by our results so far, but as I stressed in our chapter, these results are only preliminary and we would by no means as yet regard them proven. Our intention in presenting this work at an early stage was to arouse interest, rather than to establish dogma. In both the normal and the stenotic valve, we are dealing with nonlinear systems and as yet nobody has produced a satisfactory mathematical analogue or a method of analysis of such a system which does not have theoretical limitations.

Dr. Gabe: I see. Did you actually take the whole flow and the whole pressure difference over the total heart cycle?

Mr. Taylor: We have carried out the analysis two ways, both by considering only the period of flow, as have several other groups, and also by considering the whole cardiac cycle, but regarding the period when the valve is closed as one of no information, rather than of zero flow.

Dr. Gabe: I am not too sure that's valid, is it?

Mr. Taylor: Neither are we, but this is the best our applied mathematics has been able to produce and implement. We are dealing with a type of fluid dynamics for which there is not, at present, a recognized standard method of analysis, and until the mathematicians and applied dynamicists produce standard techniques, we can only be guided by them in their own theoretical research.

Dr. Braimbridge: As I am a surgeon, I have a practical question. We have the Gorlin formula calculated for every case of mitral

stenosis on which we operate. We find that the stenosis is overestimated in the milder cases, and what I would like to ask is: Does the
shape of the mitral valve orifice affect the calculations? We see three
types of orifice—a circle, an oval, and a slit—and the surgeon's estimate of the stenosis does not agree with the physiologist's estimate. Is
it a shape phenomenon?

Dr. Yellin: First, in moderate stenosis, I suspect that the measured pressure gradient is subject to some error and thus gives you an
error in the calculated area. Fortunately, I guess, it does not matter
too much in moderate stenosis. Second, I cannot answer the question
as it relates to the in vivo situation, but I have studied orifice flow on
the bench with different shapes—elliptical, circular—and in fact at
one point I made six small holes, the total cross-sectional area being
equal to the original circle in the one orifice. I found that the pressure
difference was the same in all of those situations, so that it is my
opinion that the shape of the orifice or even the amount of calcification
will not influence the calculated area.

Dr. Fawzy: Dr. Kalmanson, in the flow profile curve, the up-
stroke of the curve occurred prior to the opening snap. I understand
that the opening snap is due to the opening of the mitral valve as
shown by simultaneous phonocardiogram and mitral echogram (ultra
sound) in mitral stenosis and mitral valve prosthesis. How do you
explain this phenomenon?

Dr. Kalmanson: The opening snap doesn't coincide with the
onset of the opening of the valve, but occurs afterward. In a series of
15 patients with mitral valve disease, we determined the true onset of
the opening of the valve as the time of the onset of the ascending limb
of the initial filling flow velocity wave, corrected for the transmission
delay. The opening snap determined on the simultaneously recorded
surface phonocardiogram consistently occurred well after this onset.
It was almost synchronous with a small notch appearing on the flow
velocity trace. This notch indicates a brief, transient deceleration of
flow, and its occurrence supports the hypothesis that the opening
snap is due to the sudden halting of the leaflets by fibrous, shrunken
chordae tendineae. Thus the opening snap does not indicate the true
onset of mitral valve opening but the point of maximum overture of
the valve leaflets, restrained by the chordae.

Dr. Folts: I would like to first compliment Dr. Kalmanson on the
excellent quality of his mitral velocity tracing with regard to the one
patient with severe mitral insufficiency. If we were to take your
tracing and superimpose it on my tracing (see Chapter 14), they would

be almost identical, so if there is artifact, it occurred in two different patients with two different techniques. They are almost exactly the same. Finally, have you had any occasion to recatheterize any of these patients after surgery and after correction of the valvular defect?

Dr. Kalmanson: For reasons you will easily understand, we did not dare carry out recatheterization after surgery. However, to pick up your objection, I don't think that two faulty results obtained by two separate teams are valid, just because they are consistent with one another. It is a well established fact that the ventricular filling is consistently increased in patients with mitral regurgitation, and the fact that this increase cannot be recorded by two different techniques just doesn't prove it doesn't exist. On the contrary, in my opinion, it is most likely that both techniques are tainted with artifacts. Additional evidence is the fact that in patients with tricuspid regurgitation, in whom it is far easier to position correctly the Doppler flow probe, we consistently found a largely increased filling velocity wave during diastole.

Dr. Tunstall-Pedoe: I'd like to congratulate Dr. Kalmanson on this very exciting use of the Doppler technique, but I think that he would agree that there are one or two cautions that I perhaps might amplify from my use of the technique, particularly for high velocity turbulent flow. The linearity of the technique that he demonstrated on calibration up to 120 cm/sec does not apply necessarily in high velocity turbulent flow, and I suspect from the actual calibrations that he had on his curves that, in some instances at least, he underestimated the true velocity. If you calculate the valve area present in mitral stenosis, the velocities that he demonstrated would be inconsistent with a reasonable cardiac output. I wonder if he would like to make any comments on this.

Dr. Kalmanson: This is indeed a very pertinent objection. There is no doubt that we do underestimate the true velocity in highly turbulent flow such as that occurring in mitral stenosis. However, since the diagnostic method we showed is primarily based on pattern recognition, in other words is qualitative rather than quantitative, this loss of linearity doesn't interfere with the practical value of the Doppler technique, as far as diagnosis is concerned.

Dr. Barlow: As I see it, the negative deflection which Dr. Kalmanson marks *ic* and which takes place during the isovolumetric phase of ventricular systole, must coincide with the *c* wave of the left atrial pressure. The peak of the *c* wave, in turn, coincides with the major left-sided component of the first sound. Could I ask you whether there is any correlation between the size of that negative deflection and the mobility of the leaflets in mitral valve disease? In other words, the negative deflection should be greater when the leaflets are mobile than when they are rigid or calcified.

Dr. Kalmanson: I think your presumption is most likely to be very true. However, we did not study this point, and I would like to add that it might not be an easy task, since the magnitude of the deflection is partly dependent on the position of the catheter tip with respect to the leaflets.

Dr. Reneman: I should like to come back to Dr. Folts' remark that he feels rather comfortable when similar curves are obtained with different techniques. He is perfectly right as far as qualitative measurements are concerned, but I want to stress that we are after objective information, i.e., quantitative information regarding the amount of regurgitation or the degree of stenosis. The point is that both electromagnetic and Doppler flowmeters are subject to inaccuracies of some magnitude, so that quantitative information is difficult to obtain.

Dr. Folts: I have been using electromagnetic flowmeters now for about 12 years and am quite familiar with the difficulties and inaccuracies encountered with the device. I did not say there was no error in that technique, only that I was encouraged by the fact that two separate techniques showed similar results.

Dr. Reneman: I have a question for Dr. Yellin. Don't you think the determination of the degree of stenosis depends on the localization of the stenosis? The velocity profile, after all, will be different, and, therefore, so will your flowmeter reading, when the stenosis is around the electrode or in the center of the ostium.

Dr. Yellin: Since the flow probe was far away from the orifice, there was no question about whether or not flow was axisymmetric. We are dealing with the dissipation of a turbulent jet, and if the kinetic energy which is to be dissipated is equal from one jet to the next, the shape of the orifice does not matter. To get back to my original answer to Mr. Braimbridge, we cannot evaluate, in the Gorlin equation, the rate of opening and closing of the valve during the time the orifice area changes. So essentially, we are calculating an effective area and not a true area; therefore, there is bound to be an error which we cannot estimate.

Dr. Reneman: Dr. Yellin, I do not have any objection to your determinations in vitro, but I was referring to the in vivo situation.

Dr. Mendel: I'd like to ask Dr. Yellin to expand on his conceptive dp/dt and impedance changes.

Dr. Yellin: The initial rate of rise of left ventricular pressure is determined by the intrinsic properties of the ventricle and not by impedance. Now, when I say that the impedance is frequency-dependent I am referring to the frequency which is seen by the flow paths when the aortic valve and the regurgitant orifice open, and that is the early rate of change of pressure, not the maximum. One of the problems, especially in depressed contractility and in arrhythmias, is that the early rate of rise is very slow. During the period when the ventricle sees the atrium rather than the aorta, if the compliance of the aorta results in a higher impedance because the rate of rise is slow, then the distribution will preferentially go to the atrium. However, I am not a physician and do not want to prescribe drugs, but I would like you to think about giving inotropic agents in addition to those for vasodilating, so that you can improve the initial contractility of the ventricle. This allows it to eject more into the aorta than into the atrium, because if you have a rapid rise of pressure, the aorta has a reduced impedance and will accept flow more rapidly.

Dr. Kalmanson: I've a question for Dr. Yellin. I was surprised by your finding that reducing the aortic pressure by means of a pump increases mitral regurgitation. Such results are in contradiction with well proven clinical facts. Could you please comment on this?

Dr. Yellin: I agree that reducing the aortic pressure improves the stroke volume and, therefore, when you measure cardiac output clinically you find it increases. But unless your measurements were also able to quantify regurgitation, I do not see how you can say that regurgitation goes down. You can only say that cardiac output goes up.

Dr. Kalmanson: You don't quite satisfactorily answer my question. What I meant was that when you ask patients with mitral regurgitation to inhale amyl nitrate—which is known to substantially decrease their aortic pressure—the mitral systolic murmur consistently and often considerably decreases. Although I admit that such a finding is qualitative rather than accurately quantitative, it does prove that the mitral regurgitation also decreases. In other words, a reduction in aortic pressure does induce a decrease in mitral regurgitation.

Dr. Yellin: I cannot answer all the points definitively, but I can say you are probably correct. If you have reduced both the end diastolic aortic pressure and the left ventricular systolic pressure, then you have created a situation where regurgitation will decrease because the driving pressure from the ventricle has decreased so the murmur would go down somewhat. But let us all think some more about it, because the murmur also is not only related to the amount of flow, but to the velocity. Dr. Laniado, who has done some work in this area, would like to comment.

Dr. Laniado: I just want to add that in the record of the dog which was presented today, the balloon augmentation to diastolic aortic pressure was not very impressive. This can explain why, in some animals, the reduction in mitral regurgitation was only moderate. We have noticed better results in patients. This may be a consequence of bigger effect on aortic pressure, as well as improvement of the total function of the left ventricle, following the increase in coronary flow.

SUMMARY: PART IV

D.E.M. Taylor, F.R.C.S.

This session has been of great interest in that discussion of flow dynamics across diseased mitral valves has been possible in great detail. We have heard three methods for velocity and flow measurement, all of which have produced reliable results, and the authors are to be congratulated on their expertise in instrumentation and on their discussion of a difficult subject.

Despite the dissimilarity of the three techniques—electromagnetic, ultrasonic, and differential pressure—the results have been remarkably similar. The characteristic of turbulent flow patterns with diseased valves, rather than the stable patterns of flow seen in the normal valve, has been firmly established together with its implications on the pressure-drop/flow relationship across the valve.

Despite the agreement between the various authors on the flow dynamics during the early diastolic phase, there are disagreements as to what occurs consequently on atrial systole. The results obtained by Dr. Kalmanson and his colleagues, with a large atrial supplement, are fascinating when compared to the results of the Charlottesville and the Edinburgh studies. It will be of great interest to see whether further research will show this difference to be due to the tightness of the stenosis, as the Paris team has obtained records from far more severe mitral stenosis than the others. On the other hand, the other two groups of workers have been studying a more acute experimental stenosis which does not have sufficient time for atrial hypertrophy to occur in these patients, atrial volume may be an additional factor. There is great scope for further study of atrial supplementation in the diseased heart, and this may prove to be as varied and important a phenomenon as it has been in the healthy heart.

Another important point in the discussion was the usefulness of the various valve-area formulas, particularly the most commonly used formula of Gorlin and Gorlin. Cardiologists and cardiac surgeons have known for years that these formulas are most accurate as predictors in tight stenosis, which is easily diagnosed clinically, but are of far more limited value as predictors in cases where clinical doubt exists already. The discussions have done nothing to modify this opinion. It may well be, as has been suggested, that valve shape is a factor, for the formulas assume a circular orifice, but in addition, the results presented have shown a gradation of types of flow and of time distribution of flow. We are not yet able to explain these factors fully.

234

Flow across a constriction is a well known problem to engineers and applied mathematicians. The shape of the orifice and the slope into and out of the constriction are important factors in pressure-drop/flow relationships in these simple analogues. We have not yet seriously studied the diseased mitral valve in such a rigorous way. Unfortunately, as with so many biomedical problems, we do not have a simple system: it is complicated by being valved or semivalved and by opening into a closed visco-elastic chamber. Here is a fertile ground for the pure researcher to pursue further studies on the diseased mitral valve. For this session, although providing many answers, has posed even more questions about fluid dynamics.

The clinician may not be familiar with the mathematics involved, but much can be learned from these studies. The reports have given a clear insight into both the disability of transfer of blood from atrium to ventricle in mitral valve disease, and of the mechanisms by which the body attempts to compensate. We should all view our patients' atria with much greater respect.

To appreciate fully the significance of these chapters and discussion, we will need to wait until we have heard about the dynamics of prosthetic valves, for I suspect from the abstracts and the work of my own group that the prosthetic valves in current clinical use are far closer in their dynamics to the stenotic and diseased valve than to the normal valve which they attempt to emulate.

PART FIVE

FLOW
DYNAMICS
IN
ARTIFICIAL
VALVES

21 Flow Dynamics across the Björk-Shiley Tilting Disc Valve in the Mitral Position

Viking Olov Björk, M.D.
Axel Henze, M.D.

INTRODUCTION

There are two types of artificial heart valves available for mitral valve replacement, namely the high-profile caged ball valves and the low-profile disc valves. The low-profile disc valves are preferred in the mitral position, since they do not protrude into the left ventricular cavity as the caged ball valves may. This protrusion may cause arrhythmia due to interference with the ventricular septum and obstruction of the left ventricular outflow tract.

There are two types of prosthetic closing mechanisms, the overlapping and the nonoverlapping (Fig. 1). An overlapping occluder hits the valve seat on closure at every heart beat, as in the Starr-Edwards ball valve or in the Lillehei-Kaster pivoting disc valve. The nonoverlapping occluder fits within the valve ring but does not hit the seat on closure, as in the Smeloff-Cutter ball valve or in the Björk-Shiley tilting disc valve.

There are two types of prosthetic occluders. The central occluder obstructs the central forward flow, as in different types of ball valves or in the Kay-Shiley disc valve. The tilting or pivoting disc occluder permits a central forward flow, as in the Björk-Shiley or Lillehei-Kaster disc valves.

The Björk-Shiley tilting disc valve for mitral valve replacement combines: 1) a low profile, 2) a nonoverlapping closing mechanism, and 3) a tilting disc occluder, permitting a central forward flow (Fig. 2).

RESISTANCE TO BLOOD FLOW

The gradient across the Björk-Shiley prosthesis was studied by heart catheterization in 50 patients within one year of mitral valve replacement. Recordings were made at rest and during exercise; the transprosthetic mean diastolic pressure difference, which was obtained by planimetration, was related to the transprosthetic mitral valve flow or cardiac output.

The best results were obtained if the mitral valve disc, which opens to 60°, was oriented with its bigger portion against the diaphragmal surface of the left ventricular cavity. With this orientation, the mean diastolic pressure difference was in average 4.7 mm Hg at

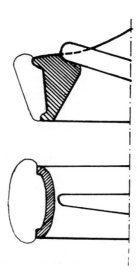

Figure 1. Overlapping closing mechanism (top). The occluder hits the valve seat at every heart beat. Nonoverlapping closing mechanism (bottom). The occluder fits within the valve ring and does not hit the seat on closure.

rest and 8.4 mm Hg during exercise, at a highest mitral valve flow of 450 ml/sec or cardiac output of 12 liters/min for the valve sizes 27, 29, and 31 mm tissue diameter (Böök[1]).

The orientation of the prosthesis mentioned above has long been routine at our clinic. This orientation can be obtained even after completed mitral valve replacement, as the prosthetic valve can be rotated within its sewing ring, but only by using the valve holder. Precautions should be taken against rotation by clamps or other surgical instruments which may injure the valve struts and disc, and cause malfunction of the prosthetic valve.

REGURGITATION

A prosthetic valve with a nonoverlapping closing mechanism is slightly regurgitant after valve closure, as some blood escapes between the occluder and the valve ring. The magnitude of this regurgitation is determined by the geometry of the circular slit between the occluder and the valve ring, and by the driving pressure. For example, the mean systolic pressure difference between the left ventricle and left atrium acts as the driving pressure upon the closed prosthetic valve in the mitral position (Fig. 3).

There is at present no method available for evaluating this regurgitation in patients. Recent experimental studies have, however,

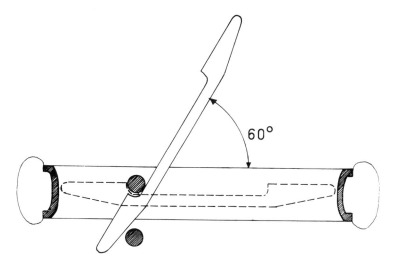

Figure 2. Cross-section of a Björk-Shiley tilting disc valve. Note low-profile with the nonoverlapping disc on closure. The disc tilts open 60° and permits a central forward flow.

shown that the regurgitation through the nonoverlapping closing mechanism of the Björk-Shiley prosthesis is slight and of little hemodynamic significance. The apparatus employed for this evalua-tion is briefly described in the following paragraphs.

The closed valve prosthesis formed the base of a column of test fluid of variable height, which represented the driving pressure (ΔP_s, mm Hg). The tube and reservoir were rigid. Pressure was measured directly above the valve level, and regurgitation ($\dot{V}_R$, ml/sec) was calculated by means of a graded cylinder and a stopwatch (Fig. 4). A biological situation was simulated by using human whole blood as test fluid. (Water has a much lower viscosity than blood, and therefore increases regurgitation.) The driving pressure (ΔP_S, mm Hg) and regurgitation ($\dot{V}_R$, ml/sec) formed a linear plot for valve sizes 25, 27, 29, and 31 mm diameter; the linear regressions are shown in Figure 5.

The in vivo driving pressure, i.e., the mean systolic pressure

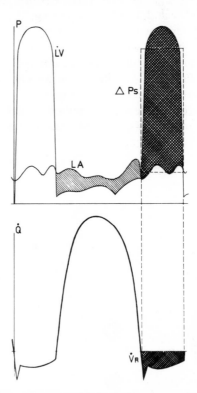

Figure 3. Diagram showing simultaneous recordings of pressures (P) in the left ventricle (LV) and left atrium (LA) and the flow across the Björk-Shiley prosthesis in the mitral position ($\dot{Q}$). The driving pressure (ΔP_s) or mean systolic pressure difference between LV-LA generates regurgitation after valve closure ($\dot{V}_R$).

difference between the left ventricle and left atrium, was obtained from our postoperative catheterization data at rest and during exercise.[2] Thereafter, the in vivo regurgitation was derived from the regressions in Figure 5 and related to the postoperative forward stroke volume, heart rate, and duration of systole from the catheterization data.

In summary, the in vivo regurgitation was low but proportional to the valve size, and in no case did it exceed 5% of the forward stroke volume at rest and during exercise.

HEMOLYSIS

The nonoverlapping closing mechanism was evaluated with respect to red blood cell destruction by means of a recently constructed test chamber.[3] This apparatus permitted a normal valve function in a minimal volume of human whole blood exposed mainly to the

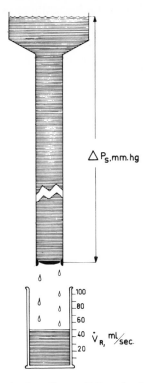

Figure 4. Experimental evaluation of regurgitation. A column of test fluid of variable height (ΔP_s) generates regurgitation through the closed valve prosthesis ($\dot{V}_R$).

244

occluder movements. Nonoverlapping occluders were found to cause much less red cell destruction than overlapping occluders. Converted to in vivo conditions, the red cell production rate of the bone marrow must increase by 10% in order to compensate for the red cell destruction caused by the nonoverlapping closing mechanism of the Björk-Shiley prosthesis. The corresponding value was 22% for the overlapping mechanism of the Lillehei-Kaster valve.[3] These results were confirmed by comparison of the nonoverlapping Smeloff-Cutter and overlapping Starr-Edwards ball valves.[4] The low rate of red cell destruction calculated for the Björk-Shiley prosthesis is in accordance with our clinical findings. Hemolysis was mild and without clinical significance.

HEMODYNAMIC IMPROVEMENT

The central hemodynamics before and after mitral valve replacement with the Björk-Shiley prosthesis were evaluated at rest and during exercise by cardiac catheterization in 50 patients.[1]

The stroke volume was low in relation to sex, age, and body size

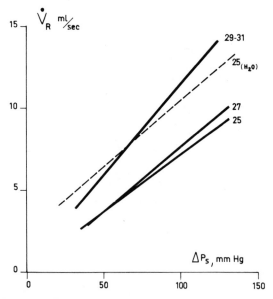

Figure 5. Relationship between driving pressure (ΔP_s, mm Hg) and regurgitation after valve closure ($\dot{V}_R$, ml/sec). Thick lines = linear regressions obtained on evaluation with human whole blood for valve sizes 25, 27, 29 and 31 mm tissue diameter of the Björk-Shiley prosthesis. The regression obtained on evaluation with water of the 25 mm valve is indicated by the broken line.

before operation, and amounted to 48.6 ± SD11.6 ml at rest and 46.5 ± SD11.4 ml during exercise. Following mitral valve replacement, the stroke volume remained basically unchanged at rest (53.4 ± SD15.1 ml) but increased significantly to 71.5 ± SD23.6 ml during exercise, an increase of 54% of the preoperative value. This improvement in the stroke volume during exercise was accompanied by a significant decrease in arteriovenous oxygen difference, indicating a less hypokinetic or more normokinetic central circulation after surgery.

The left atrium was decompressed by the mitral valve replacement, as indicated by a significant reduction in the left atrial mean pressures at rest (22.6 ± SD4.8 − 16.9 ± SD8.9) and during exercise (35.2 ± SD8.9 − 25.8 ± SD9.4). In addition, the pulmonary hypertension was normalized or at least reduced at rest and during exercise. The end-diastolic pressures of the right and left ventricles were slightly elevated and were not significantly changed by the operation.

CONCLUSION

The Björk-Shiley tilting disc valve combines a low profile, a non-overlapping closing mechanism, and a tilting disc permitting a central forward flow. Its resistance to blood flow is low. Its regurgitation is negligible and it causes a low degree of hemolysis. It has proven its efficiency in unloading the left atrium and pulmonary circulation at rest and during exercise in mitral valvular disease. The Björk-Shiley prosthesis is therefore considered to be a suitable substitute for the diseased mitral valve.

REFERENCES

1. Böök, K. Mitral valve replacement with the Björk-Shiley tilting disc valve. A clinical and haemodynamic study in patients with isolated mitral valve lesions. *Scand. J. Thor. Cardiovasc. Surg.* Suppl. 12, 1974.

2. Björk, V.O., Böök, K., Holmgren, A. Significance of position and opening angle of the Björk-Shiley tilting disc valve in mitral surgery. *Scand. J. Thor. Cardiovasc. Surg.* 7:187, 1973.

3. Henze, A., Fortune, R.L. Regurgitation and haemolysis in artificial heart valves. An experimental study of overlapping and non-overlapping closing mechanisms and of paraprosthetic leakage. *Scand. J. Thor. Cardiovasc. Surg.* 8:167, 1974.

4. Fortune, R.L., Henze, A. Haemolysis in ball valves with overlapping and non-overlapping closing mechanisms. An experimental study. *Scand. J. Thor. Cardiovasc. Surg.* 9:1, 1975.

22 Fluid Mechanic Performance of Five Prosthetic Mitral Valves

B.J. Bellhouse, M.A., D.Phil.
F.H. Bellhouse

INTRODUCTION

The natural mitral valve cannot easily be copied when designing a prosthetic valve, partly because of the limited fatigue life of existing blood-compatible, flexible materials, but also because of the structure of the valve. Precise positioning and tensioning of chordae tendineae would present considerable surgical and engineering problems. Thus prosthetic mitral valves differ greatly from the natural valve, varying widely in choice of materials and design.

The purpose of this chapter is to report studies of five prosthetic mitral valves tested in the model left ventricle used previously for studies of models of the natural mitral valve.[1,2] Two centrally occlusive valves (Starr-Edwards and Beall), one hinged disc (Björk-Shiley), one stented heterograft (Hancock), and a prototype three-cusp valve with sinuses (Oxford) were evaluated (Fig. 1). We examined valve competence and pressure drop across the valve when

248

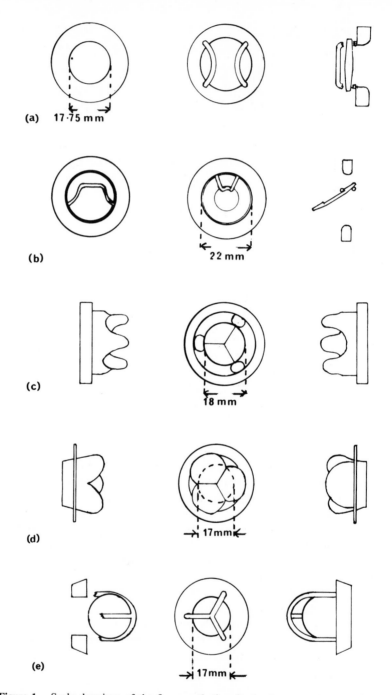

Figure 1. Scale drawings of the five prosthetic mitral valves tested. (a) Beall (b) Björk-Shiley (c) Hancock (d) Oxford (e) Starr-Edwards.

it was open as a function of cardiac output; we also observed flow patterns within the model left ventricle.

METHODS

Valve competence was measured in a rig in which the valve was subjected to a constant pressure on the ventricular side (produced by a static column of water) and exposed to the atmosphere on the atrial side. The valve sewing rings were impregnated with silicone rubber to eliminate leakage at the rings, and the leak rates through the valves were measured, using a graduated cylinder and stopwatch, for pressure differences across the valves ranging from 44.8 to 179.3 mm Hg.

The model left ventricle (Fig. 2) consisted of a rigid base (A) containing an aortic valve (B) and the mitral valve (C) under test. The moving part of the ventricle (D) was a transparent rubber diaphragm. The ventricle was placed in a rigid water-filled Perspex box, which was connected to a piston pump. When water was pumped into the box the ventricle contracted; when water was pumped out of the box the ventricle filled. The ventricle discharged through a 19 mm bore pipe (E) to a constant-head tank (1.58 m above the base of the ventricle), which overflowed to a second constant-head tank (0.95 m above the base of the ventricle) and was connected to the left ventricle by a pipe (F), of bore 25.4 mm. Provision was made for viewing the mitral valve from its atrial aspect, down the pipe (F), and for viewing the ventricular aspect of the valve through the transparent rubber ventricle and the walls of the Perspex tank surrounding the ventricle.

Pump output was measured by intercepting the flow between the two constant-head tanks, and collecting the discharge over a given time. Pump frequency was recorded with a stopwatch. Pump output Q is plotted against pump frequency (Fig. 3). Instantaneous velocity just upstream of the mitral valve was measured with a heated thin-film gauge,[3] and pressure difference across the valve was measured with a Kistler quartz-crystal differential pressure gauge. The two signals were stored on an oscilloscope screen, and were recorded photographically. End-systolic volume of the ventricle was 109 ml, and the valves were tested at four different flow rates: 2.6, 5.1, 8.2, and 12.4 l/min.

RESULTS

Static leak rate

The leak rate (ml/min) through the five mitral valves is plotted against pressure difference (mm Hg) across the valves (Fig. 4). The same results are shown in Table 1. The Oxford valve was the most competent (23 ml/min maximum leak rate) and the Björk-Shiley valve was the least competent (720 ml/min maximum leak rate). There was little to choose between the Starr-Edwards and Beall valves in this test; both these valves had roughly half the degree of incompetence of the Björk-Shiley valve. The Hancock valve produced results about four times as good as the Björk-Shiley valve. The leak rate through the Oxford valve varied little with pressure difference, and was only 3% of the Björk-Shiley valve leak rate when the maximum pressure difference was applied.

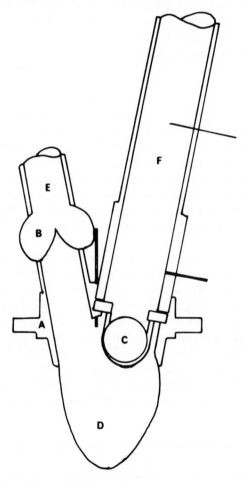

Figure 2. Drawing of the model left ventricle, showing the rigid base of the ventricle (A), the aortic valve (B), a mitral valve under test (C), and the rubber diaphragm (D) forming the moving part of the ventricle. The aorta is marked (E), and the inlet pipe to the mitral valve is marked (F).

The very high leak rates at physiological pressure differences (120 mm Hg) for the three mechanical valves imply that potentially-traumatic shear rates occur in the high-velocity flow between the valve seat and the occluder. It was not possible to measure these velocities directly, but they were obtained indirectly using standard hydraulic formulas.

The discharge Q through an orifice is related to the pressure difference across the orifice, Δh, by the formula[4]

$$Q = C_D A \sqrt{2g\Delta h} \qquad (1)$$

where A is the orifice area, g the acceleration due to gravity, and C_D the discharge coefficient, which is assumed to be constant and equal to 0.6. The broken curves in Figure 4 are derived from equation (1) for the Björk-Shiley, Beall, and Starr-Edwards valves. The experimental results for the two cusp-type valves do not conform to the parabolic shape predicted by equation (1), probably because the much smaller

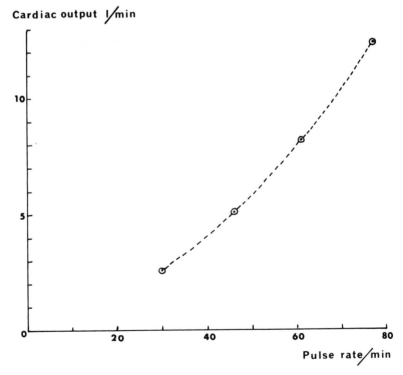

Figure 3. Cardiac output (1/min) plotted against pulse rate (min⁻¹) for the model left ventricle.

252

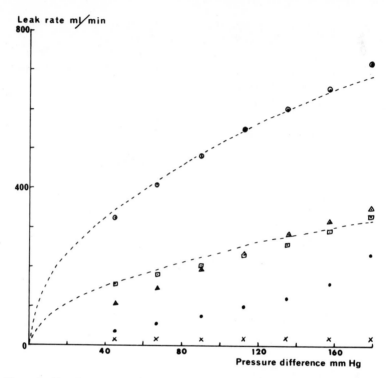

Figure 4. Results of static leak-rate test of the mitral valves. The leak rate (ml/min) for each valve is plotted against the pressure difference across the valve (mm Hg). The parabolas are drawn to fit the results obtained with the three rigid prosthetic valves (□ Beall, ⊙ Björk-Shiley, and △ Starr-Edwards). The leaflet valves have smaller leak rates, and the results do not fit parabolic curves (· Hancock, × Oxford).

Table 1.

Leak rate through the mitral valves when ventricular pressure is constant.

Constant ventricular pressure (mmHg)	Leak rate (ml/min)				
	Beall	Björk-Shiley	Hancock	Oxford	Starr-Edwards
179.3	330	720	182	23	355
156.9	290	655	156	22	320
134.5	260	610	122	21	285
112.1	230	550	100	20	228
89.6	204	485	76	18	188
67.2	182	410	57	18	147
44.8	156	325	37	18	107

leak rate between the flexible cusps of these valves does not produce high-energy jets through sharp-edged gaps; equation (1) is based on this assumption.

The area of the leakage orifice, A, for the Björk-Shiley valve is calculated from formula (1) to be 2.8 mm². The orifice is an annular gap between the disc and the inner diameter of the sewing ring, of perimeter 69 mm. Thus the gap width, w, is 0.04 mm, a little larger than the figure obtained by direct measurement.

The corresponding leakage orifice, A, for the Starr-Edwards and Beall valves is found to be of area 1.3 mm², which corresponds to annular rings of width w = 0.023 mm and w = 0.024 mm respectively.

Dividing the leakage flow rate, Q, by the leakage-orifice area, A, gives the jet velocity $\bar{u}$ at the orifice. The shear rate at the edge of the orifice can be estimated from equation (2) which was derived for flow in a long narrow channel.[4] For short, narrow channels, boundary layers on the walls will be thinner and shear rates higher than for long channels. Equation (2) will therefore underestimate shear rate.

$$\text{Shear rate at orifice edge} = \frac{6\bar{u}}{w} \qquad (2)$$

However, even these shear rates in the Björk-Shiley, Beall, and Starr-Edwards valves, at ventricular pressure of 120 mm Hg, are all in excess of 5×10^5 s^{-1}, and are therefore well within the range where mechanical lysis of red blood cells is predicted by Blackshear.[5]

Dynamic testing of the mitral valves

The considerable variation in competence of the mitral valves observed in the static leak tests did not have a big effect on the pumping efficiency of the model left ventricle. Even the substantial leak rate of the Björk-Shiley valve, corresponding to 285 ml/min in pulsatile flow, if systole and diastole are of equal duration, is only 5.7% of a cardiac output of 5 l/min.

Measurements of velocity just upstream of the mitral annulus (Fig. 2) showed that all the mitral valves closed with very little reversed flow. This was confirmed by observation of particles suspended in the water. The three rigid valves closed with considerable impact, which was easily audible, while the two leaflet valves closed silently.

Measurements of pressure drop across the mitral valves in diastole at pulse rates of 30, 46, 61 and 77/min showed pressure differences increasing with velocity squared through the mitral valve. The peak values occurred at mid-diastole, since the velocity-time curve

254

was sinusoidal. The greatest pressure differences occurred, of course, when the pump output was at its greatest value.

The results are shown in Table 2 and Figure 5.

Table 2

Measurements of peak pressure difference across the mitral valves (Δp) for four pulsatile flow-rates.

Pulse Rate /min	Flow Rate 1/min	Measured Peak Δp (mm Hg)				
		Beall	*Björk-Shiley*	*Hancock*	*Oxford*	*Starr-Edwards*
77	12.4	52.5	12.0	27.0	16.5	21.0
61	8.2	31.5	7.5	15.0	11.1	10.5
46	5.1	9.0	4.8	12.0	8.4	10.5
30	2.6	4.5	2.4	5.4	2.4	4.8

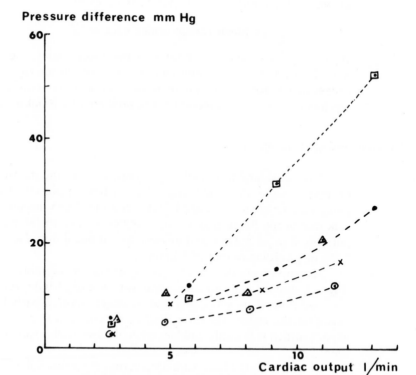

Figure 5. Results from dynamic tests of the mitral valves. The peak pressure differences across the mitral valves, Δ p (mm Hg) are plotted against cardiac output. (□ Beall, ⊙ Björk-Shiley, • Hancock, × Oxford, △ Starr-Edwards).

The Beall valve had a very high pressure drop across it, amounting to 52.5 mm Hg at the highest cardiac output (12.3 1/min). The Starr-Edwards and Hancock valves produced pressure differences about half those obtained with the Beall valve, and the Björk-Shiley and Oxford valves produced still lower values.

These peak-diastolic pressure differences can be estimated easily from Bernoulli's equation:

$$h + \frac{u^2}{2g} = \text{constant along a streamline}, \tag{3}$$

where h is the pressure, u the velocity, and g the acceleration due to gravity at a given point.

Continuity of mass flow implies that

$$u \, A = \text{constant} \tag{4}$$

where A is orifice area.

Combining equations (3) and (4),

$$\Delta h = \frac{u_o^2}{2g} \left\{ \left(\frac{A_o}{A_1} \right)^2 - 1 \right\} \tag{5}$$

where A_o is the area of the pipe entering the mitral valve, u_o the velocity in that pipe, A_1 the minimum orifice area of the mitral valve, and Δh the pressure drop across the valve. The smallest orifice of the Björk-Shiley valve was measured to be the area of the primary orifice (the area inside the sewing ring), less the cross-sectional area of the disc, multiplied by the sine of the opening angle. This area was found to be 2.83 cm² compared with a value of 5.07 cm² for A_o. The Beall valve had a primary orifice area 2.47 cm², and a smaller orifice, in which the flow was radial, of area 2.51 cm². However, the valve came close to the posterior wall of the ventricle, so some of the radial flow was deflected by the wall and the effective orifice was obviously less than the measured value.

The Hancock valve had a primary orifice of area 3.14 cm², but one cusp had a thickened muscular root which prevented that cusp from opening fully. This reduced the effective orifice area to 2.53 cm².

The Oxford valve had a primary orifice of area 2.27 cm². The Starr-Edwards valve had a primary orifice of area 2.27 cm², and a secondary annular orifice of area 2.87 cm², so the primary orifice was the determinant of pressure drop across the valve.

These effective orifice areas were substituted into equation (5). The calculated values of pressure drop across the valves for the two highest cardiac outputs are shown in Table 3. It is seen that quite good agreement

256

Table 3
Calculated values of peak pressure difference across the mitral valves (Δp) for two pulsatile flow-rates.

Pulse Rate /min	Flow Rate l/min	Calculated Peak Δp (mm Hg)				
		Beall	Björk-Shiley	Hancock	Oxford	Starr-Edwards
77	12.4	21.6	11.6	20.3	21.8	19.3
61	8.2	10.7	5.9	10.1	11.7	10.4

is obtained for all the valves except the Beall. The substantial underestimation for the Beall valve is attributed to the obstruction of the valve outlet by the posterior wall of the ventricle.

Flow Patterns Within the Ventricle

Strong vortices were formed in the ventricle for all the valves. The orientation of the Björk-Shiley valve determined the vortex direction; when inserted so that the disc opened like the anterior cusp of the natural mitral valve, the vortex rotated in the normal direction (Fig. 6). When the

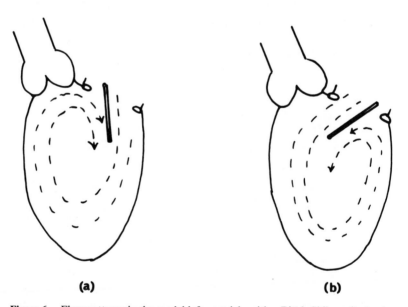

(a)   **(b)**

Figure 6. Flow patterns in the model left ventricle with a Björk-Shiley mitral valve with the disc opening (a) towards the outflow tract, (b) away from the outflow tract.

valve was turned by 180°, a vortex spinning in the opposite direction, but of equal strength, was established. The valve disc opened to its fullest extent and directed the flow, rather than being aligned by the flow, as happens in the natural mitral valve. In the latter part of diastole, however, the disc responded to decelerating flow through the mitral annulus and to the vortex behind the disc, and moved towards partial closure before the end of diastole.

The Hancock valve had one cusp with a thick muscular region at the base; this prevented that cusp from opening fully. The vortex in the ventricle was in the normal direction, and valve closure commenced before the end of diastole. The reversal of pressure difference across the valve during the latter part of diastole can be seen in Figure 7, when the pulse rate was 61/min and the cardiac output was 8.2 1/min. When the ventricular pressure exceeds the pressure at the mitral ring, the valve starts to close. The degree of diastolic closure depends both on the magnitude of the pressure difference and the length of time it is applied.

The Starr-Edwards valve also produced a vortex in the normal direction, although the asymmetry was not as marked as with the valves without central occluders. The Oxford valve produced a normal vortex also. The Beall valve produced a strong vortex in a direction opposite to normal, because the posterior wall obstructed part of its outflow region.

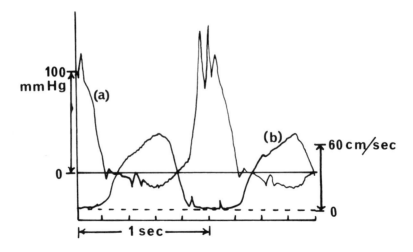

Figure 7. Measurements of (a) pressure difference across the Hancock mitral valve, and (b) velocity at the mitral ring. The pressure difference changes from a negative value at mid-diastole to a positive value towards the end of diastole, tending to close the mitral valve before the onset of systole.

DISCUSSION

The measurements of pressure drop across the mitral valves corre-lated well with calculations based on measured orifice areas. Although the three central-flow valves produced smaller energy losses than the centrally-occlusive valves (Beall and Starr-Edwards), this was a con-sequence of orifice area and not orifice shape. Wider opening of the Björk-Shiley valve would have permitted still smaller pressure differen-tials across it; had 90° opening been possible, the peak pressure differ-ence across it would have been reduced by 45% at all cardiac outputs. Full opening of the Hancock valve, possible if the muscular base of one cusp had been thinner, would have reduced the peak pressure difference across the valve by 25%. Obstruction of the outflow of the Beall valve by the posterior wall of the model ventricle is likely to be reproduced in vivo, and could be improved if the disc tilted as it opened, or if a smaller valve were used. The pressure drop across the Oxford valve could be reduced only by increasing the area of its orifice.

The very high leak rates of the three rigid valves, particularly the Björk-Shiley valve, and the high shear rates associated with that leakage, suggest that these valves may be hemolytic under unfavorable condi-tions. Measurements of the discharge coefficient C_D, given in equation (1) at low Reynolds numbers[6] justify the assumption that C_D is constant, and consequently, that the calculations of shear rate (derived from the experiments in water) are valid when applied to blood. Nevertheless, experimental confirmation is required, using blood as the test fluid.

$$\text{Reynolds number} = \frac{\text{mean velocity} \times \text{width of orifice}}{\text{kinematic viscosity of fluid}}$$

CONCLUSION

Five prosthetic mitral valves have been evaluated in both static leak tests and in a model left ventricle.

A very high leak rate was obtained in the static test of the Björk-Shiley valve (maximum 720 ml/min), and high leak rates were found in the Beall and Starr-Edwards valves (maximum 330 and 355 ml/min, respectively). Calculations of shear-rate showed that, under unfavorable conditions, leakage through these valves would be ex-pected to cause hemolysis. The two leaflet valves had smaller leak rates. The leak rate through the Hancock valve was at most 182 ml/min, and the maximum leak rate through the Oxford valve was only 23 ml/min.

Pressure drops across the mitral valves during diastole depended on velocity at the mitral ring and on orifice area, not shape. Except for the Beall valve, the orifice of which was obstructed by the posterior wall of the left ventricle, calculations of pressure drop agreed well with experiment. The maximum pressure drop across the Beall valve was 52.5 mm Hg at a cardiac output of 12.4 1/min. The Björk-Shiley valve had the largest orifice and the smallest pressure drop (maximum of 12.0 mm Hg at a cardiac output of 12.4 1/min). The Hancock valve had a thick muscular region at the base of one cusp which prevented that cusp from opening fully, with consequent stenosis even at the highest cardiac outputs. (Maximum pressure drop of 27.0 mm Hg at a cardiac output of 12.4 l/min.) The Starr-Edwards and Oxford valves produced maximum pressure drops of 21.0 and 16.5 mm Hg respectively, at cardiac outputs of 12.4 l/min. All valves permitted strong ventricular vortices to form in the normal direction, except for the Beall valve and the Björk-Shiley when it was hinged posteriorly, when, in both cases, the vortex rotated in the reverse direction. All five valves were competent, and the wide variations in leak rate had little effect on cardiac output.

REFERENCES

1. Bellhouse, B.J., Bellhouse, F.H. Fluid mechanics of the mitral valve. *Nature* 224:615, 1969.

2. Bellhouse, B.J. Fluid mechanics of a model mitral valve and left ventricle. *J. Cardiovascular Research* Vol. VI. 2:199, 1972.

3. Bellhouse, B.J., Bellhouse, F.H. Thin film gauges for the measurement of velocity or skin friction in air, water or blood. *J. Scientific Instruments* Series 2, 1:1211, 1968.

4. Massey, B.S. *Mechanics of Fluids*. 2nd edition. New York: Van Nostrand, 1970.

5. Blackshear, P.L. Mechanical hemolysis in flowing blood. Edited by Y.C. Fung, N. Perrone, N. Anliker. In *Biomechanics: Its Foundations and Objectives*. Englewood Cliffs: Prentice-Hall, 1970.

6. Liepmann, H.W. Gaskinetics and gasdynamics of orifice flow. *Journal of Fluid Mechanics* 10, Part 1, 65, 1961.

23 Velocity Profiles and Impedance of Prosthetic Mitral Valves*

D. E. M. Taylor, F.R.C.S.
Joan S. Whamond

Although there are many different designs of prosthetic mitral valve in current use, fluid dynamic studies in man show that they are notable more for their similarities in restricting diastolic filling than for their dissimilarities. The purpose of this chapter is to demonstrate how the hemodynamic performance characteristics of prosthetic mitral valves tend to resemble those of the diseased stenotic mitral valve rather than the normal valve. The reasons for this have not been fully elucidated, and it is, therefore, not possible to make other than tentative suggestions as to design criteria likely to lead to future improvements. The hemodynamic problems to be described are of only secondary clinical importance, as the major clinical difficulties with current prosthetic valves are concerned with thromboembolism

* Supported by grants from the Scottish Home and Health Department and the British Heart Foundation. The basic analog/hybrid computer used was provided by the Wellcome Trust.

and hemolysis rather than with minor degrees of valvular stenosis and incompetence. Improvement of the pressure/flow characteristics of prosthetic valves may well lead to a further reduction in post-implantation morbidity, for the major clinical complications have been ascribed to hemodynamic factors as well as to materials.

Studies have been carried out in the operating room at the time of valve implantation: the protheses studied were the Starr-Edwards caged ball, the Starr-Edwards caged disc, the Björk-Shiley tilting disc, the stented autologous fascia lata, and preliminary studies on the Hancock stented xenograft. Three groups of investigations have been carried out:

(1) Flow distribution and velocity profiles across the valve.

(2) Pressure drop and energy loss, and their dependence on cardiac output and heart rate.

(3) The contribution to transvalvular complex impedance of resistive and reactive components, and their dependence on flow and heart rate.

The methods used were those described previously in this book (see chapters 12 and 17).

FLOW PATTERNS AND VELOCITY PROFILES

Only two of the types of valves studied showed relatively stable flow patterns throughout most of diastolic filling; these were the two disc prostheses, the Starr-Edwards caged disc and the Björk-Shiley tilting disc (Fig. 1, b & c). The Starr-Edwards caged ball valve, and, somewhat surprisingly, the central channel fascia lata and Hancock xenograft valves, showed turbulence in the ventricle beyond the prosthesis for most of diastolic filling (Fig. 1a).

Starr-Edwards Caged Ball Prosthesis (Figs. 1a & 2a). At low rates of flow there were stable flow patterns on the upstream aspect of the prosthesis throughout diastole. When flow commenced, the occluder traveled the full excursion of the cage and an annular flat fronted velocity profile developed at the secondary orifice. Beyond this level there was an early attempt to form stable vortex systems in the ventricle, but flow separation with turbulence occurred on the downstream aspect of the occluder. As flow continued, the filling rate

Figure 1. Flow patterns in (A) early and (B) late diastole associated with (a) Starr-Edwards caged ball prosthesis, (b) Starr-Edwards caged disc prosthesis, (c) Björk-Shiley tilting disc prosthesis opening towards the ventricular outflow tract.

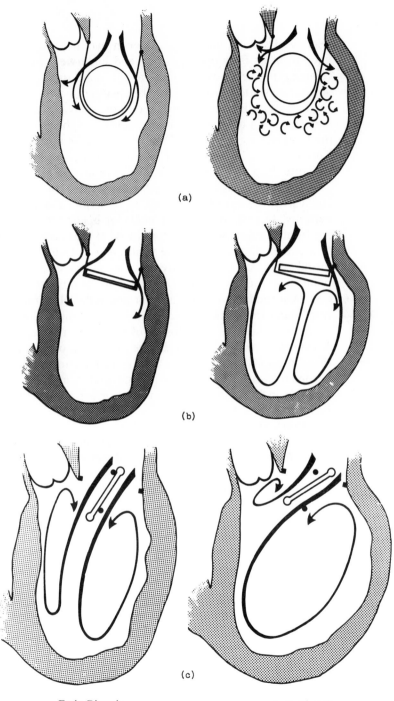

(a)

(b)

(c)

Early Diastole　　　　　　　　　　Late Diastole

263

decreased slowly, but the occluder in mid and late diastole moved back from its fully open position and underwent oscillations, thus reducing the secondary orifice; at the same time the level of flow separation shifted so as to lie on the upstream aspect of the equator of the ball. With increased cardiac output, such as was seen after the administration of isoprenaline to improve myocardial contractility, the level of flow separation jumped so as to lie upstream to the ball. This may have a significant bearing on the relationship between pressure drop and flow observed, where an inflexion occurs.

Starr-Edwards Caged Disc Prosthesis (Fig. 1b). Unlike the caged ball valve, the caged disc tends to be associated with stable flow patterns. In early diastole the occluder opens fully and an annular flat-fronted velocity profile is produced at the secondary orifice; this flow is then directed along the ventricular walls to form a stable and toroid vortex on the downstream aspect of the disc, with stagnation points near the apex of the heart, and on the downstream side of the disc. A secondary vortex is also formed in the left ventricular outflow tract under the aortic valve. As filling decelerates, the energy in the vortices causes a partial closure of the valve; in late diastole this is asymmetric, with a greater degree of closure occurring posteriorly than anteriorly. And so in a similar fashion to the ball valve, the secondary orifice dimensions are reduced in mid and late diastole. Changes in flow pattern have not been observed with this valve up to heart rates of 2.5 Hz.

Björk-Shiley Tilting Disc Prosthesis (Fig. 1c). This valve has been studied in detail only with the occluder opening towards the left ventricular outflow, as was the original method of insertion; complete studies have not been carried out on valves opening away from the aortic valve, as is now advocated.[2] Early in diastole the occluder opened to its full extent and stable vortices were generated in the left ventricle. Sometimes the line of the occluder separated two vortex systems with a stagnation point low down on the septum, but in some instances the level of separation was higher up the septum, with some of the flow through the major secondary orifice joining the vortex formed by the flow through the minor orifice. The latter was less common than the former, and this may be due to the tertiary orifice effect of the occluder against the septum proposed by Björk.[2] As flow decelerated, the occluder partially closed, and the vortex formed by flow through the smaller of the secondary orifices became predominant. In this valve also unstable flow patterns were not observed.

Stented Autologous Fascia Lata Prosthesis (Fig. 2b). The flow profile was flat and stable at the prosthesis, but, unlike the normal valve, ventricular vortex systems did not form. A jet was formed towards the apex of the ventricle, which broke up on reaching the ventricular wall, with turbulence in the ventricle apart from the region of the jet. A further point of difference from the normal valve was that the stagnation point did not move during diastolic filling, other than tracking movements of the seating ring. Because of the disturbed flow in the ventricle, estimates of jet dimension and flow-channel dimensions indicated that the valve 'cusps' did not open to their full extent, and it is likely that a fish-mouthed, rather than a circular, flow section was produced.

Hancock Stented Xenograft Prosthesis. Although only preliminary studies have been carried out on these prostheses, the indications are that the flow profiles and patterns produced are almost identical to those seen in the stented autologous fascia lata prosthesis.

PRESSURE DROP/FLOW RELATIONS

The different types of valves studied, despite their differing design and differing flow patterns and profiles, did not differ significantly in terms of pressure-drop/flow characteristics, the sole exception being the Starr-Edwards caged ball valve at high rates of flow. Therefore, only a single description will be given.

The pattern of diastolic filling showed that peak filling rate occurred early in diastole, but was considerably less than that encountered in the normal valve (Fig. 2); the deceleration during mid and late diastole was also less, so that, whereas in the normal valve the mean ratio of peak to mean Re was 3.1:1, for the prosthetic valve it was in the range 1.3–1.7:1, a figure similar to that for moderate to moderately severe mitral stenosis which was 1.3–1.6:1. In all valves closure was accompanied by backflow across the valve so that there was an early systolic incompetence of 3–8% of stroke volume (Fig. 2); this is not of great significance from the hemodynamic point of view.

The pressure drop and energy loss ($\int \Delta P * Q.dt$) varied from valve to valve, and for prostheses of equivalent annulus diameter, the rank ordering from least to most stenotic was Hancock xenograft, stented fascia lata, Björk-Shiley, Starr-Edward disc, and Starr Edward ball (see Chapter 23) (Fig. 3).

With changing cardiac output, all prostheses showed a power loss/cardiac output curve which approximated a square law (Fig. 3), but with the stented fascia lata having the steepest slope and, at heart rates below 2 Hz, the Starr-Edwards caged ball having the least. The latter, however, showed a sharp inflexion on the curve at a heart rate between 2 and 2.3 Hz, with a rapid increase in power loss above this rate (Fig. 3), a finding which has also been reported by Nolan (see chapter 25). This may correspond to the jump of flow separation from the ball equator to upstream of the primary orifice. For heart rates below 2 Hz the rank ordering of adaptation to changing cardiac output was from most to least adaptation: Starr-Edward ball, Björk-Shiley disc and Starr-Edward disc (equal), and stented fascia lata: there were insufficient data on the Hancock xenograft on this point. It will be seen that the order is the opposite of that for stenosis, and this should emphasize the inadvisability of basing opinions on the hemodynamic performance of a prosthesis on single criterion.

Overall, the prostheses would be clinically definable as mildly stenotic, and the associated diastolic filling curve and power law energy losses/cardiac output would confirm this assessment.

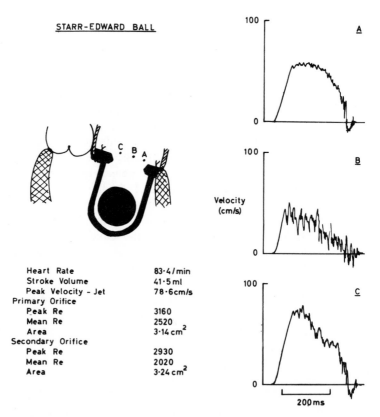

STARR-EDWARD BALL

Heart Rate	83·4 / min
Stroke Volume	41·5 ml
Peak Velocity – Jet	78·6 cm/s
Primary Orifice	
Peak Re	3160
Mean Re	2520
Area	3·14 cm^2
Secondary Orifice	
Peak Re	2930
Mean Re	2020
Area	3·24 cm^2

200 ms

Figure 2a. Velocity profiles at three points (A, B, C) on the primary orifice of a Starr-Edwards caged ball prosthesis. For discussion, see text and legend of Figure 2b.

IMPEDANCE, RESISTANCE, AND REACTANCE

As with the energy loss characteristics, all the types of prosthetic valve studied showed similar alterations in impedance, resistance, and reactance with changing cardiac output.

At resting heart rates, taking the division into resistive and reactive components, these were of the same order. This is similar both to the normal and to the stenotic valve, and would imply that the inertia of occluders plays an insignificant role in impedance at these rates. With raised cardiac output and heart rate, both the resistive and reactive components increased, following approximately the theoretical relationship to cardiac output and heart rate predicted by a rigid orifice analog.[3] This again is behavior similar to that seen in stenotic

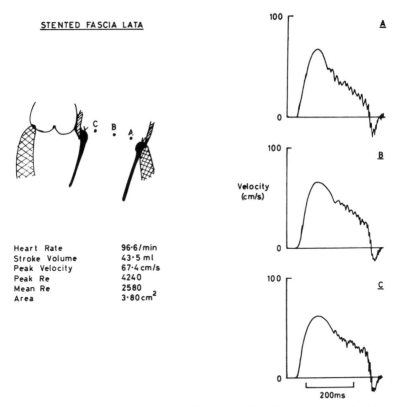

STENTED FASCIA LATA

Heart Rate	96·6/min
Stroke Volume	43·5 ml
Peak Velocity	67·4 cm/s
Peak Re	4240
Mean Re	2580
Area	3·80 cm^2

Velocity (cm/s)

200ms

Figure 2b. Velocity profiles for stented fascia lata. Note the central area of minimal and disturbed flow associated with a peripheral flow valve as compared to the more flat velocity profile of a central flow valve. Note also the backflow phase associated with closure of all prosthetic valves studied.

268

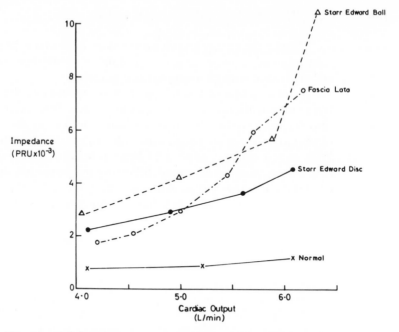

Figure 3. Relationship of impedance to cardiac output in different prosthetic valves. Note the relatively greater rate of increase of the autologous fascia lata leaflet prosthesis and also the inflection with the Starr-Edwards caged ball prosthesis.

valves[1,5] and unlike the adaptation of reactance which occurs in normal blood vessels[4] and across normal heart valves.[1,5]

Therefore, for the prosthetic valves studies, not only the dependence of energy loss, but also that of its resistive and reactive components to changing cardiac output, was similar to that of the stenotic mitral valve rather than the normal.

SUMMARY AND CONCLUSIONS

All the types of prosthetic valve studied, whether with a central or peripheral flow channel, were mildly stenotic and closed with minor but definite backflow. The change of energy loss across the valve with changing cardiac output and its resistive and reactive components was very similar to the stenotic mitral valve and did not show adaptions such as occurred with the normal valve.

These changes were qualitatively similar, although there were quantitative differences. The similarities in flow dynamics were associated with a wide variety of flow patterns from almost complete stability to complete turbulence.

At present the major morbidity and mortality of prosthetic heart valves is associated with factors such as thromboembolism, hemolysis, and structural failure: the degrees of stenosis and incompetence indicated by these studies are unlikely to be major factors in survival, although they may influence exercise tolerance. With the ability to adapt to the demands of increased cardiac output on exercise, and with improved materials, if the surgical problems are overcome, then improvement in valve hemodynamics, so as to produce a level of impedance more near to the normal valve, may well be required in order to improve the quality of life of our patients.

REFERENCES

1. Taylor, D.E.M., Whamond, J.S. Flow patterns and stability around normal, diseased and prosthetic mitral valves *in vivo*. *J. Bio Med. Eng.* In press, 1975.

2. Björk, V.O. Results of mitral valve replacements with the Björk-Shiley tilting-disc valve. This book, Chapter 38.

3. Eastell, R., Taylor, D.E.M., Whamond, J.S. Impedance change to differing heart rate and cardiac output across the acutely stenosed aortic valve. *J. Physiol.* 248:33, 1975.

4. Abel, S.L. Fourier analysis of left ventricular performance; evaluation of impedance matching. *Circulation Research* 28:119, 1971.

5. Carnie, N., Mukhtar, A.I., Pollock, C.G., Taylor, D.E.M., Whamond, J.S. Impedance spectra change across the aortic valve at different heart rates in the sheep. *J. Physiol.* 238:48, 1973.

24 Flow Dynamics in Prosthetic Valves—An Assessment of Hydrodynamic Performance*

J.T.M. Wright, Ph.D.

INTRODUCTION

The diseased mitral valve is usually replaced because it has become stenotic, incompetent, or both. It is, therefore, relevant to endeavor to measure the comparative pressure drops and incompetence levels of a range of mitral valve prostheses, for it is clearly desirable for the surgeon to be aware of the hemodynamic characteristics of prostheses to help make a valued judgment on the optimal type and size of valve to use in a particular patient. The hydraulic performances of some heart valve prostheses have been reported[1] using a special pulse duplicator.[2] Many of the prostheses then tested are no longer in clinical use, others have been further developed, and several new prostheses have become widely used. In this chapter,

* Supported in part with research grants from the British Heart Foundation and the American Heart Foundation.

Table 1
Prostheses Investigated

Type	Make	Model	Tissue Annulus Diameter mm
Pivoting	Björk-Shiley	MBP	25, 27, 29
Disc	Lillehei-Kaster	500	25.5, 27.5, 29.5, 32.5
Ball	Starr-Edwards	6400/32M	32
	Starr-Edwards	6320	30, 32
	Starr-Edwards	6120	30
	Smeloff-Cutter	856	27, 30, 32
Disc	Beall-Surgitool	106	30.5, 33, 35.5
	Cooley-Cutter	858	27, 30
	Starr-Edwards	6520	30
Tissue	Hancock	342	29, 31, 35

the results of recent tests undertaken on 23 currently used mitral valve prostheses (Table 1) are described.

Although the assessment is quantitative—measurements of mean diastolic pressure drop and incompetence—qualitative flow visualization studies have been carried out and are presented.

METHOD

Simple flow studies on two dimensional models of tilting disc valves carried out in this laboratory and elsewhere[3] demonstrated that strong vortices were produced in the model ventricular cavities. It was concluded that these vortices could affect the valve performance and that the closed cavity of the left ventricle was an essential feature in the design of a suitable test rig. A more refined pulse duplicator has therefore been developed, incorporating this closed ventricular chamber. The test rig is described briefly below. The general dimensions of the working sections were determined from a suitable casting made of a cadaver's left atrium, ventricle, and aorta.

The test rig is shown diagrammatically in Figure 1. The working

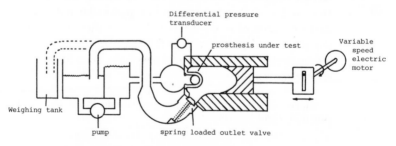

Figure 1. Circuit diagram of the pulse duplicator.

section of the test rig consisted of a flexible atrial chamber, a ventricular chamber, and an outflow tract. The atrial chamber was a thin-wall flexible container, approximately spherical in shape and of 60 mm diameter. The ventricular chamber consisted of a cylinder 52.5 mm in diameter containing a reciprocating piston shaped so as to represent the left ventricular apex. The piston moved back and forth 28 mm in a sinusoidal manner, being driven, via a Scotch yoke mechanism, by a variable speed electric motor. The volume displacement of the piston was 60.7 ml. The outflow tract, representing the aortic outflow tract, contained a spring-loaded output pressurising valve. The mitral valve prosthesis under test was mounted on a thin metal plate and sandwiched between the atrial and ventricular sections. The test liquid used was a water-glycerine mixture at 37°C of density 1.100 g/ml and viscosity approximately 3 cP. During the diastolic phase of the simulated cardiac cycle, liquid was drawn through the mitral valve prosthesis, and its mean diastolic pressure drop or gradient measured by a differential pressure transducer whose output was integrated over the diastolic period. During rig systole, the liquid was ejected through the pressurising valve. This caused the ventricular pressure to rise to about 120 mm Hg, thus subjecting the prosthesis to a near normal pressure cycle. The ejected liquid could be collected in a weighing tank for measurements of valve regurgitation. The difference between the volume collected per stroke and the volume displaced by the piston was due to mitral valve incompetence.

Flow visualization studies were made by photographing the flow patterns with a 35 mm single lens reflex camera. The shutter was actuated by a solenoid valve energized by a cam-operated micro switch. The flow was visualized by illumination of ion exchange resin beads (of diameter in the range 177-420 μ suspended in the water-glycerine mixture), with a thin sheet of light shone through the central axis of the model.[4] A series of photographs was taken at 1/15 second exposure at various phases of the cardiac cycle.

RESULTS

The pivoting disc valves were mounted so as to reproduce their recommended clinical orientation (i.e., the disc of the Björk-Shiley was directed away from the outflow tract while that of the Lillehei-Kaster was directed towards it). The mean diastolic pressure drop characteristics of the pivoting or tilting disc valves are shown in Figure 2. The vertical axis of the graph is mean diastolic pressure drop or gradient and the horizontal axis is pulse rate and equivalent pumped pulsatile flow (stroke volume × pulse rate). The largest valve, the Lillehei-Kaster 25 (the number designation of the Lillehei-Kaster refers to its orifice diameter, while in other prostheses, the number refers to the tissue annulus diameter) produced the lowest pressure drop. The much smaller Björk-Shiley 25 and Lillehei-Kaster 18 prostheses had much higher pressure drops.

The incompetence characteristics of this range of valves is shown in Figure 3. It may be seen that the regurgitation, expressed as a percentage of the stroke volume (60.7 ml), varied from 3% in the case of the smallest valve up to 14% for the Björk-Shiley 29. These results were taken with the ventricular test chamber horizontal and the outflow tract below it (as shown diagrammatically in Fig. 1). Under these conditions, gravitational forces aided the closure of the

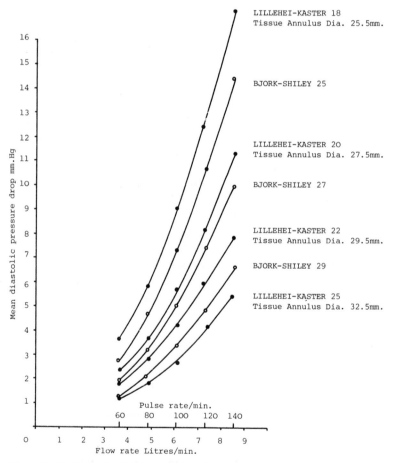

Figure 2. Pressure-drop characteristics of the tilting disc valves.

Lillehei-Kaster valves, but opposed closure of the Björk-Shiley prostheses. When the largest of these two types of prosthesis was tested with the ventricular section vertical and the prosthesis uppermost, then the incompetence level of the Lillehei-Kaster 25 rose to 16% at a pulse rate of 60, while that of the Björk-Shiley fell to a level of 11%. At the higer pulse rates the fluid dynamic forces dominated and, at a pulse rate of 140 per minute, incompetence was not influenced by orientation of the ventricle.

The pressure-drop characteristics of the disc valves are shown in Figure 4. Of particular interest is the Cooley-Cutter 30, which had a pressure drop only slightly greater than that of the much bigger Beall large valve. The incompetence levels of the disc valves are shown in Figure 5.

The pressure-drop characteristics of the ball valves are shown

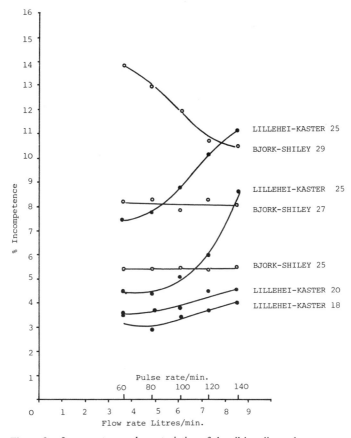

Figure 3. Incompetence characteristics of the tilting disc valves.

in Figure 6. In two cases the characteristics of two prostheses are virtually identical and are represented by single curves. The incompetence levels of these ball valves are shown in Figure 7. The highest regurgitation levels measured occurred in the three Smeloff-Cutter ball valve prostheses.

The hydraulic characteristics of the Hancock tissue valves are shown in Figures 8 and 9. It may be seen that the pressure drop at low flow rates is comparatively higher than those of mechanical valves and the curves are straighter. The latter implies that the valve acts as a variable area orifice, i.e., opens wider at higher flow rates. These valves, because of their nature, will probably show variation from sample to sample, although the valves supplied for test were selected as being typical. Note the very low incompetence levels of these prostheses, 3-5% for the Hancock 35, and 2-3% for the Hancock 29.

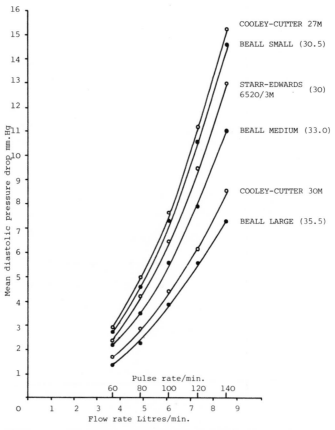

Figure 4. Pressure-drop characteristics of the disc valves.

FLOW VISUALIZATION STUDIES

Flow patterns produced by various prostheses are shown in Figures 10 to 14. In each photograph the prosthesis may be seen at the top of the ventricular cavity, and the blurred apex-shaped piston at the bottom. These photographs were taken near the end of the diastolic filling phase, while the piston was still moving, hence its blurring. The pulse rate was always 80 per minute. The superimposed arrows indicate the direction of movement of the particles. The length of a streak is directly proportional to the velocity of the particle.

Figure 10 shows the flow patterns produced by the Björk-Shiley valve. The flow entered passing either side of the tilted disc, and passed down the right hand side and up the left hand side of the ventricle to form a large vortex. This vortex continued to circulate

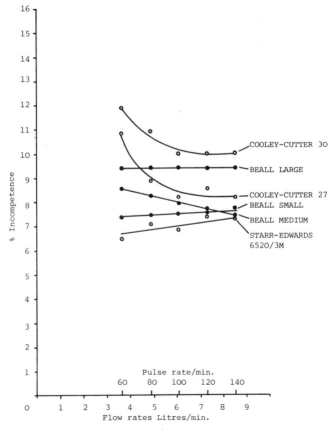

Figure 5. Incompetence characteristics of the disc valves.

after the cessation of diastolic filling and well into the systolic ejection period. As the angled disc lay directly in the path of the vortex, it is probable that its rapid closure at end diastole was aided by this vortex.

Figure 11 shows the patterns produced by the Lillehei-Kaster 22 prosthesis, oriented so that the disc opened towards the outflow tract. This prothesis also produced a strong intraventricular vortex, and again this vortex probably aided valve closure at end diastole.

The flow patterns produced by the Beall small valve prosthesis are shown in Figure 12. The flow entered the valve orifice, then bifurcated to flow close to the disc and down the wall of the ventricle. An annular vortex was set up distal to the valve such that a central stream of fluid (of velocity 30-40 cm/sec) was directed up the central axis of the ventricle towards the rear of the valve poppet. Thus the

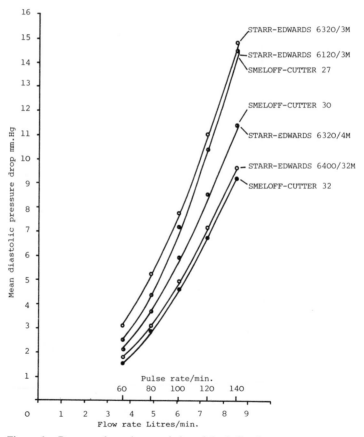

Figure 6. Pressure-drop characteristics of the ball valves.

disc valve was also subjected to a vortex which could have aided valve closure at end diastole. A small secondary annular vortex circulated in the area between the sewing ring and ventricular wall adjacent to the mitral orifice ring position.

Figure 13 shows similar patterns for a Starr-Edwards ball valve prosthesis. Again major and minor annular vortices were produced. By contrast Figure 14 shows the patterns produced by the Hancock porcine xenograft. The central flow characteristics of the valve are easily seen. This flow set up two main annular vortices and a minor (unmarked) vortex adjacent to the valve sewing ring and ventricular wall junction.

DISCUSSION

In general, the valves (of a particular type) with the largest tissue annulus diameters produced the lowest pressure drops. Exceptions

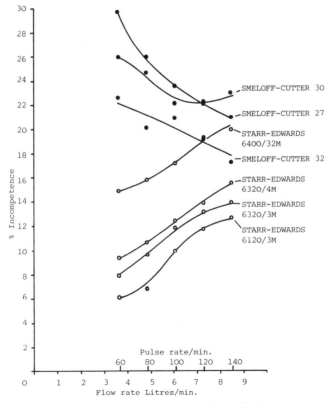

Figure 7. Incompetence characteristics of the ball valves.

were the Beall medium and Beall small, which had pressure drops greater than the smaller Cooley-Cutter 30. All the mechanical prostheses produced square-law pressured drop curves, implying that they behaved as turbulent orifices. The straighter pressure drop curves of the tissue valves implied that they behaved as variable area orifices. The incompetence levels of many of the prostheses with a closed leakage path were comparatively higher at low pulse rates than at higher rates. This was due to the longer period in which systolic leakage could occur. The valves that came into this category were the Björk-Shiley pivoting disc valves, the Cooley-Cutter disc valves, and the Smeloff-Cutter ball valves.

Some prostheses had poppets with densities quite different from

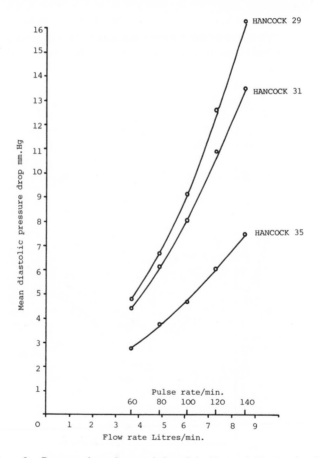

Figure 8. Pressure-drop characteristics of the Hancock Xenograft valves.

blood. The incompetence levels of this group of valves was affected by valve orientation at low pulse rates.

The flow visualization studies demonstrated that significant vortices are produced in a closed ventricular type cavity distal to the prosthesis. In the mechanical prostheses, the vortices probably aided early valve closure at end diastole, thus minimizing incompetence.

Clinically significant incompetence has been classified by Kennedy et al.[5] as being less than 20%. Only the Smeloff-Cutter valves exceeded this value. In spite of the large orifice diameters and low pressure drop characteristics of the largest pivoting and tilting disc valves, their incompetence levels were well within acceptable limits. In clinical use, the likely effect of an incompetent valve will be to cause the heart to increase its stroke volume or pulse rate so as to achieve the net output flow required to meet metabolic requirements of the body. The extra volume of blood which has to be pumped by the heart will increase the pressure drop across the incompetent valve. To take account of this effect, Table 2 has been drawn up listing valves in order of their hydraulic merit. Pressure drops are shown at

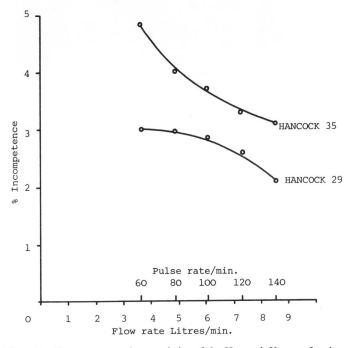

Figure 9. Incompetence characteristics of the Hancock Xenograft valves.

282

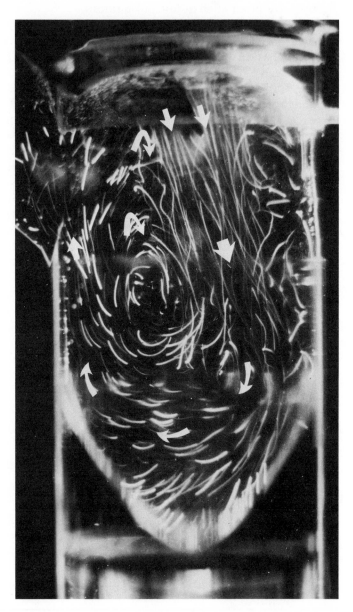

Figure 10. Flow patterns produced by the Björk-Shiley 27 tilting disc valve.

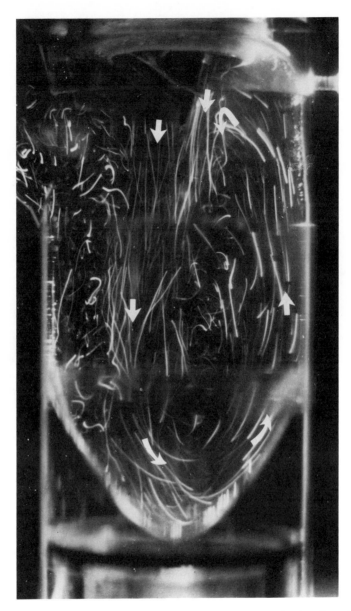

Figure 11. Flow patterns produced by the Lillehei-Kaster 22 pivoting disc valve.

284

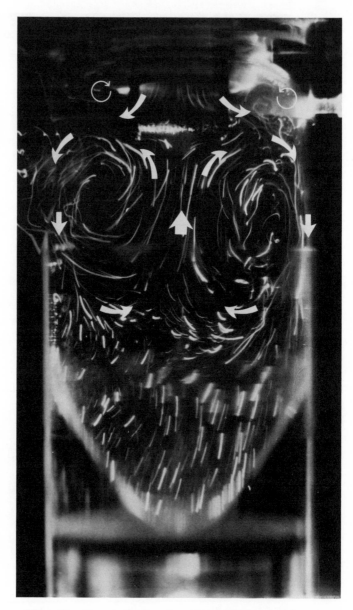

Figure 12. Flow patterns produced by the Beall-Small disc valve.

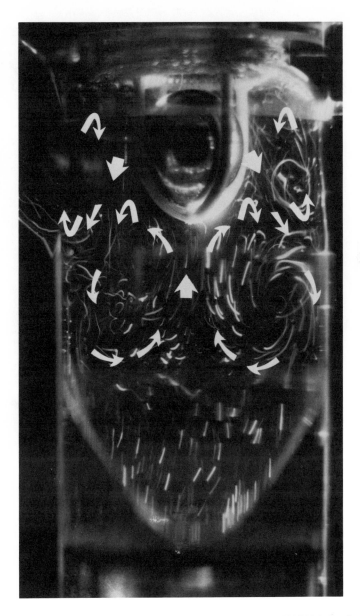

Figure 13. Flow patterns produced by the Starr-Edwards 6320/3M ball valve.

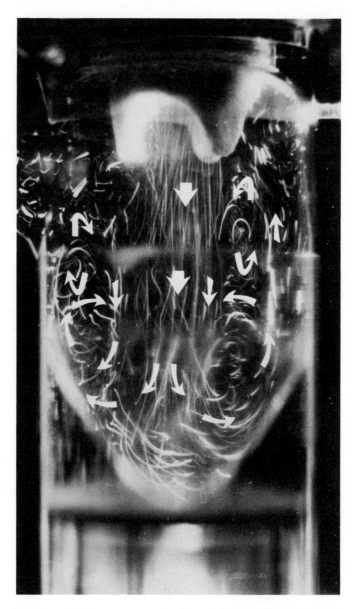

Figure 14. Flow patterns produced by the Hancock 29 Xenograft valve.

simulated cardiac outputs of 4.5 liters/min (representing cardiac resting) and at 8.5 liters/min (representing exercise conditions). Table 2 shows the order of hydraulic merit of valves with a tissue annulus or mounting diameter of 31 mm or greater. Note the great difference between the pivoting disc valves and the ball valves. Table 2 also shows the order of hydraulic merit of valves in the range 29-31 mm. The list is now headed by the Björk-Shiley pivoting disc valves, followed by the Lillehei-Kaster. The next three are the disc valves, then the tissue valve, and last the three ball valves. The exact position of the Hancock tissue valves is open to discussion as it has a higher pressure drop at cardiac resting but a lower pressure drop under exercise conditions compared to some mechanical valves.

Finally the order of hydraulic merit of the smaller valves (with tissue annulus diameters in the range 27-29 mm) is also shown in Table 2. Although the smaller sizes of tissue valve and Edwards ball valves

Table 2
Order of Hydraulic Merit

Make	Model	Pressure drop mm Hg at cardiac output of 4.5 l/min	Pressure drop mm Hg at cardiac output of 8.5 l/min
Tissue Annulus Diameter ≥ 31 mm			
Lillehei-Kaster	25	1.9	6.4
Björk-Shiley	31	2.3	7.9
(BS29 with large sewing ring)			
Beall-Surgitool	Large	2.3	8.3
Hancock	342/35	3.5	7.6
Beall-Surgitool	Medium	3.5	12.4
Smeloff-Cutter	M8	3.6	12.7
Starr-Edwards	6400/32M	3.6	13.7
Starr-Edwards	6320/4M	3.8	14.0
Tissue Annulus Diameter ≥ 29 mm < 31 mm			
Björk-Shiley	29	2.3	7.9
Lillehei-Kaster	22	2.7	8.9
Cooley-Cutter	30	3.1	9.8
Starr-Edwards	6520/3M	4.1	14.4
Beall-Surgitool	Small	4.5	16.5
Hancock	342/29	6.3	15.0
Starr-Edwards	6120/3M	4.3	18.7
Smeloff-Cutter	M7	4.9	18.5
Starr-Edwards	6320/3M	5.4	18.5
Tissue Annulus Diameter ≥ 27 mm < 29 mm			
Björk-Shiley	27	3.3	10.3
Lillehei-Kaster	18	3.4	12.4
Cooley-Cutter	27	5.2	17.5
Smeloff-Cutter	M6	5.2	20.5

were not tested, there is no obvious reason to believe that they would have changed the order of merit.

CONCLUSIONS

These tests showed that from a hydrodynamic point of view the preferred valve replacement is the pivoting or tilting disc type of prosthesis, followed by the disc and tissue valves. The ball valve comes last. Except in the largest size, the Björk-Shiley valves proved to be hydrodynamically slightly superior to the Lillehei-Kaster valves. Apart from the Smeloff-Cutter ball valves, all the prostheses produced clinically insignificant regurgitation. However, it is also clear that only the largest of the prostheses came close to providing clinically insignificant stenosis. While it is recognized that this method of test does not necessarily provide results identical to those found in clinical practice, it is put forward as a fair method of measuring the relative performance of prostheses.

Finally, it must be emphasized that mitral valve replacement is a compromise. The levels of pressure drops of a prosthesis are important, but other characteristics are also important. These include the relative thromboembolic incidence, freedom from the use of anticoagulants, sizes of the prosthesis in relation to that of the left ventricular cavity, and the age and physical condition of the patient.

A mitral valve replacement could be considered, figuratively speaking, as a crutch to support the patient. It cannot strictly be thought of as a device which allows him to return to physiological normality.

SUMMARY

The pressure drop and incompetence levels of a range of mitral valve prostheses have been measured under pulsatile flow conditions. Pivoting or tilting disc valves were found to be hydraulically superior to disc, xenograft, or ball valve prostheses. Flow visualization studies showed that the mechanical prostheses examined produced strong vortices which could aid poppet closure at end diastole.

REFERENCES

1. Wright, J.T.M., Temple, L.J. Relationship between the physical size, incompetence, and stenosis of prosthetic mitral valves. *Thorax* 27:287, 1972.

2. Wright, J.T.M., Temple, L.J. An improved method for determining the flow characteristics of prosthetic mitral heart valves. *Thorax* 26:81, 1971.

3. Naumann, A., Kramer, C. Flow investigations on artificial heart valves. *AGARD Conference Proceedings No. 65,* AGARD-CP-65-70, 4-1, 1970.

4. Wieting, D.W. Dynamic flow characteristics of heart valves. Ph.D. Thesis, University of Texas at Austin, 1969.

5. Kennedy, J.W., Yarnall, S.R., Murray, J.A. et al. Quantitative angiocardiography. *Circulation* 41:817, 1970.

25 Flow Characteristics of Mitral Valvular Prostheses: Ball, Disc, and Xenograft

Stanton P. Nolan, M.D.

INTRODUCTION

The dynamic characteristics of devices for mitral valve replacement are of great importance in determining the relative merit of each prosthesis. In vitro studies, using pulse duplicators, may provide the starting point for such evaluation; however, it is ultimately necessary to determine the instantaneous flow occurring across the valve and the simultaneous pressure gradient in vivo during periods of varied heart rate and cardiac output.

A series of experiments was performed to determine the intracardiac flows and pressures in calves whose mitral valves had been replaced by ball, disc, or xenograft devices.

METHODS

An electromagnetic flow transducer was incorporated into the base of the device to be studied. The hydraulic characteristics of the two valves were similar. At a steady state flow of 7 liters per minute, the pressure drop across the 2 M valve was 1.6 centimeters of water, and across the flowprobe prosthesis, it was 1.8 centimeters of water. The sensitivity of the transducer was linear, with flow from 1,000 to 20,000 ml per minute.

The experiments were performed in calves under halothane anesthesia. Using cardiopulmonary bypass, the mitral valve was excised and replaced with the flowprobe prosthesis. An extravascular flow transducer was placed on the ascending aorta, and pressure was measured in the left atrium, left ventricle, and aortic root. The following data were recorded simultaneously: 1) lead 2 electrocardiogram; 2) instantaneous ascending aortic blood flow; 3) instantaneous mitral valve blood flow; and 4) pulsatile, aortic, left ventricular, and left atrial pressures.

The heart rate was varied by atrial pacing, and cardiac output was controlled by the infusion or withdrawal of blood through a cannula in the right atrium. The studies were carried out during periods of constant heart rate and stable pressure. This allowed assessment of valvular function at heart rates of 75 to 300 per minute and cardiac output rates of 800 to 5,000 ml per minute.

RESULTS

Figure 1 is a recording obtained from one animal with a ball valve and a heart rate of 110 per minute. During systole, there was no flow through the mitral valve, and the recorded pressure events were normal. In diastole, there is a striking loss of the Phase I period of flow noted in the normal mitral valve, and there is a consistent 30 to 50 msec time lag from reversal of the atrioventricular pressure gradient to the onset of mitral valve flow. Mitral flow accelerates rapidly and, at heart rates below 130 to 140 per minute, a secondary acceleration of flow due to atrial contraction is evident. With reversal of the atrioventricular pressure gradient, there is a rapid deceleration of flow and finally, a brief period of regurgitation that always occurs during initial ventricular contraction. However, the normal Phase V flow that should follow the period of regurgitation is lost with these prostheses and xenografts.

The effects of a 2 M mitral ball valve prosthesis on pressure and flow were analyzed and the following summary observations were made: When heart rate was increased in steps from 100 to 300 per minute, 1) stroke volume decreased; 2) mean mitral flow rate fell from 190 to 54 ml per diastolic second; 3) cardiac output fell from 3600 to 1400 ml per minute; 4) the duration of forward flow through the mitral valve decreased; 5) with the same increase in heart rate, left ventricular end-diastolic pressure rose from 6 to 12 ml of mercury; 6) mean left atrial pressure increased from 14 to 30 ml of mercury; and 7) the antrioventricular pressure gradient increased from 9 to 18 ml of mercury.

In all animals with ball and disc valves, there was mitral regurgitation just prior to valve closure. When regurgitation was present, its volume varied from 1.3 to 3.6 ml. With the xenograft, however, there was no detectable regurgitation.

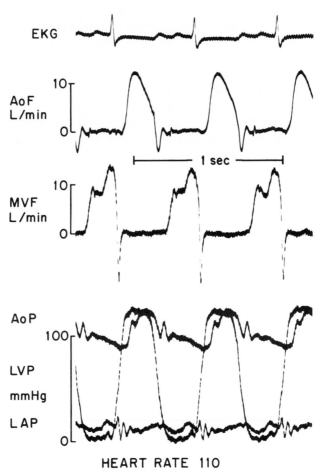

Figure 1. Simultaneous recordings of the electrocardiogram (EKG), ascending aortic blood flow (AoF), instantaneous blood flow across a ball valve in the mitral position (MVF), and the pressures in the aorta (AoP), left ventricle (LVP), and left atrium (LAP). Heart rate 110 per minute.

In Figure 2, the transvalvular stroke power loss in milliwatts is plotted against the mitral forward stroke volume in ml. Power loss defines the rate at which energy must be expended to achieve flow. Each line represents the relationship at a different heart rate. At a heart rate of 80, a stroke power loss of 25 milliwatts is required to achieve a stroke volume of 15 ml. If the stroke volume is doubled to 30 ml, the power loss rises to 60 milliwatts, for an increase of 140%. In general, above a heart rate of 100, a twofold increase in stroke volume causes a fourfold increase in power loss. Also, at a constant stroke volume, power loss increases with any rise in heart rate.

In Figure 3, the minute valvular energy loss in joules is plotted against cardiac output in ml per minute. This defines the cost in terms of pressure work needed to achieve a given cardiac output. Again, each line represents the relationship at a different heart rate. At each heart rate, from 80 to 180 per minute, the relationship appears to be linear up to the point marked here with an arrow. Above this point there is a marked increase in the energy loss for any increase in cardiac output. Thus, at a heart rate of 80, there is a linear relationship up to the cardiac output rates of 2700 to 3000 ml per minute. Above

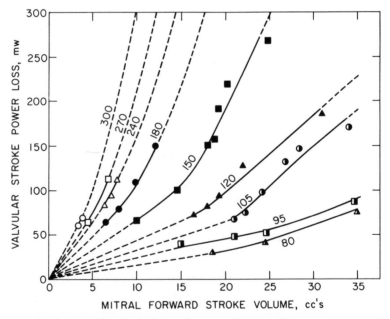

Figure 2. Relationship of valvular stroke power loss in milliwatts to mitral stroke volume in cubic centimeters, plotted at several heart rates. The experimental data are drawn in solid lines and the extrapolated points indicated by dashes. At all heart rates an increase in stroke volume results in an increase in power loss.

this level, the energy loss increases in a ratio of 4 to 1 for any increase in cardiac output. Also, at any level of cardiac output, the minute energy loss increases with a rising heart rate.

The increase in stroke power loss with increasing heart rate, at a constant stroke volume, was predictable from the decreased duration of flow. However, the cause of the disproportionate increase in minute energy loss above a critical cardiac output at a constant heart rate is less obvious. One of three factors might be involved: 1) there could be a decrease in the effective orifice area of the valve; 2) the physical design of the valve may be such that, above a given flow rate, turbulence or disturbed flow develops; or, 3) there might be an alteration in the kinematic viscoscity of the blood, due to an increased velocity of flow.

The data presented indicate that the adverse characteristics of the 2 M mitral ball valve are: 1) inertance of the poppet decreases the effective orifice area and shortens the duration of flow; 2) the duration of flow decreases significantly above a heart rate of 90; 3) the transvalvular power loss increases above a heart rate of 100; 4) early

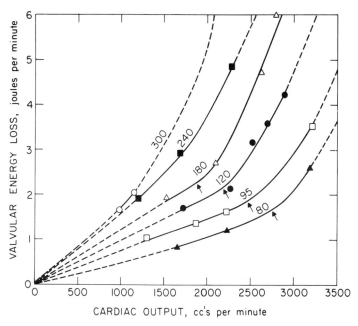

Figure 3. The relationship of valvular energy loss in joules per minute to cardiac output plotted at several heart rates. The experimental data are drawn in solid lines and the extrapolated points indicated by dashes. At heart rates from 80 to 180 per minute there is a change in the slope of the line indicated by an arrow. Above this point there is a disproportionate increase in energy loss for any increase in cardiac output.

systolic regurgitation decreases the net stroke volume and the left ventricular end-diastolic volume; and 5) transvalvular energy loss increases with heart rate if cardiac output is held constant, and, at a constant heart rate, energy loss increases disproportionately above a critical level of cardiac output.

The conditions under which optimal function of a 2 M ball valve prosthesis may be achieved are: 1) with heart rate maintained between 80 and 100 per minute, power loss will be minimized while producing an adequate duration of flow; 2) at this heart rate, cardiac output should be maintained between 2500 and 3000 ml per minute, which will minimize regurgitation and energy losses; and 3) if it is necessary to obtain a cardiac output greater than 3000 ml per minute, there will be no change in the percentage of regurgitation and a disproportionate increase in the energy loss. However, an increased cardiac output will always be achieved more efficiently by increasing the stroke volume rather than the heart rate.

Similar studies were carried out using a Kay-Shiley disc prosthesis (size #6) with a primary orifice comparable to the 2 M ball valve. This prosthesis functioned in a manner similar to the ball valve prosthesis at cardiac outputs of less than 2500 ml per minute and heart rates less than 150 per minute. However, the disc valve operated with a 30% lower power loss at cardiac outputs between 2500 and 3000 ml per minute, and at heart rates above 150 per minute. Both of these prostheses were less efficient than the normal mitral valve, and required an estimated two- to four-fold increase in the power output of the left atrium.

Stent-mounted xenograft aortic valves were inserted in the mitral position. The orifices of these valves were much larger than the ball and disc prostheses studied. The patterns of mitral valve flow across the xenograft were essentially the same as those of the normal mitral valve, with the exception of the loss of oscillations associated with papillary muscle contraction: that is, Phases I and V of normal mitral valve flow. It was also observed that there was no regurgitation across the xenograft, absence of Phase IV flow, and only a slight increase in the pressure gradient above that of the normal mitral valve.

SELECTED READING

1. Nolan, S.P., Stewart, S., Fogarty, T.J., Dixon, S.H., Morrow, A.G. *In vivo* studies of instantaneous blood flow across mitral ball-valve prostheses: effects of cardiac output and heart rate on transvalvular energy loss. *Annals of Surgery* 169:551, 1969.

2. Gelbert, D.B., Nolan, S.P., Stewart, S., Fogarty, T.J., Harris, E.K. An *in vivo* study of energy losses of ball and disc valves in the mitral position. *Journal of Applied Physiology* 28:282, 1970.

3. Rawitscher, R.E., Botero, L.M., Lee, R.J., Nolan, S.P. Hemodynamic characteristics of heterograft valves in the mitral position (abstract). *Circulation* (Supplement III), 51:90, 1970.

DISCUSSION: PART V

Dr. Somerville: All the valves demonstrated were used with a ventricle of fixed dimensions which never changed regardless of heart rate, filling pressure, or other factors. This never happens in life. Human valves are replaced when the ventricle is to a greater or lesser extent diseased, and abnormal compliance is the rule. Valve closure, too, resulting from flow vortices as shown in Dr. Taylor's beautiful models, depends on ventricular size. It seems unlikely that the secondary vortices would behave in exactly the same way as shown if, as in human situation, the ventricular cavity were larger, as it would be in diseased states.

Dr. Yellin: These comments are all quite in order and very relevant. What we have been examining are hemodynamic relations: the pressure-flow energy losses. None of the authors can really discuss long-term effects or other complications, and it is clear that quite a bit remains to be done in terms of the influence of the shape of the ventricle into which the valve goes, and in terms of the shape of the driving pressures.

Dr. Reid: I would like to congratulate Drs. Wright, Bellhouse, and Taylor on the precision of their experiments and the clarity of their conclusions. However, the conclusion that only minor modifications of a central occluding valve would produce a clinically acceptable valve needs qualification and seems optimistic to me for one important reason. One aspect of the discussion which has not so far been considered is, if you like, the nonvalvular function of the mitral valve, namely, ventricular filling. The left ventricle consists of a prefixed organization of muscle fibers and sarcomeres, and if they are to be optimally distended at the end of diastole, the filling pattern is all important. In 1970, I introduced the concept of diastolic dyskinesis as an explanation of poor postoperative cardiac performance, an area subject to much speculation.[1] This original concept was based on cineangiographic studies of diastolic cardiac silhouettes after ball, disc, and homograft valve replacement. Each particular valve type has a very characteristic end-diastolic silhouette. In the case of the disc and ball valves, the normal filling pattern of the ventricle is entirely reversed. Very abnormal, dyskinetic movement of the ventricular wall is observed, and this observation is further substantiated by echocardiography when paradoxical movement of the septum is confirmed. This observation now forms the basis of a routine preoperative assessment where mitral valve dehiscence is suspected when paradoxical septal movement is usually abolished. Where central flow homograft valves are concerned, the end-diastolic configuration is improved although it remains abnormal, and optimal distension of sarcomeres, at the end of diastole, remains markedly compromised.[2]

Dr. Beall: In his study, Dr. Bellhouse has illustrated something that many of us have been trying to stress for a number of years, and that I think is of considerable importance. It is that the prostheses must be sized to the ventricle rather than to the annulus. In an attempt to get low gradients, a prosthesis that is too large may be put in, and this produces obstruction, not in the primary or secondary orifice, but in the tertiary orifice. Whether you are using ball or disc valves, if the ball or disc is too large and is not allowed to open completely by the ventricular wall, this will produce stenosis. I think Dr. Bellhouse demonstrated this very well. If the prosthesis doesn't open completely, there will be stenosis; this demonstrates the importance of size to the ventricle and not to the annulus.

Dr. Kaster: I would like to talk for a moment about the central flow prosthetic disc valve. Relative to the plane of the base, the disc of the Lillehei-Kaster Pivoting Disc (LKPD) prosthesis is inclined 18° in the closed position and 80° in the full open position (Fig. 1). The disc is contained in a free-floating relationship within the valve housing. During the opening phase, the disc moves out of the orifice approximately 1 mm in the downstream direction. This allows blood to flow freely through the pivot areas during each stroke.

An echocardiographic examination of patients with the LKPD mitral prosthesis shows the opening and closing events of the disc to be both rapid and spontaneous.[3] The closing event of the LKPD prosthesis is characterized by two event sounds. The first closing sound occurs when the disc regresses approximately 1 mm into the orifice and engages the wall of the valve housing. The second part of the closing sound occurs when the disc comes to rest on the disc stop, closing off the orifice. The closing time of the disc is extremely short when compared with the duration of ventricular systole (Figure 3 of Reference 3).

The valve closes in response to a combination of two forces acting upon the disc. Blood flowing back through the large orifice passes from a larger area distal to the valve into a smaller area bounded by the orifice and the anterior surface of the disc. In this narrower region, the blood flow velocity increases, causing the pressure to decrease. As a result, the disc is drawn into the closed position. The second force that acts to close the valve is caused by a substantial blockage of the regressing blood behind the disc. The resultant force acts to push the disc closed. The combination of these two forces acting on the disc—the pulling force on the anterior surface plus the pushing force on the posterior surface—act in concert to accelerate the closing event of the central flow disc prosthesis.

Dr. Frater: I'd like to make comments on both Dr. Bellhouse's and Dr. Wright's presentations. Both suggested that, concerning distinctly artificial ventricles, central occluder prosthetic valves tend to move towards closure, towards the end of diastole. However, if these valves are mounted in a beating natural ventricle as we have done, with synchronized simultaneous ciné, pressure, and flow studies, they may bounce during diastole. They do not start closing until systole starts, which is in complete contrast to the natural valve. We have data (Fig. 2) for an eccentrically opening valve, showing the amount of obligatory insufficiency that occurs during closure of this valve (and which occurs with all central occluder prostheses). Forward flow is on the left, and regurgitant flow in closure on the right. The amount of fluid that must flow backwards into the atrium, past the occluder, in order to pull it closed is the same whether the rate is 80 or whether the rate is 180. But since with reduced filling time at rapid rates the forward flow is reduced, the effective stroke volume is disproportionately reduced at the rapid rate because a greater proportion of the blood that flowed through the valve during diastole must

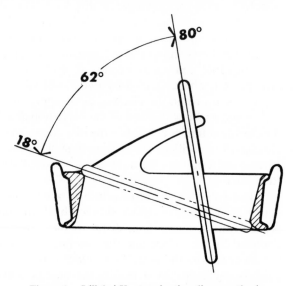

Figure 1. Lillehei-Kaster pivoting disc prosthesis.

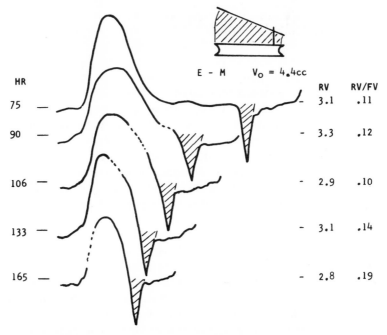

Figure 2. Graphic representation of data for an eccentrically opening valve. See text for discussion.

flow back through it at the end of diastole in order to close it. And this is one of the reasons why the effective orifice area of a central occluder valve at the rate of 180 is less in calculation than the effective orifice area at the rate of 80.

Dr. Bellhouse: Only by undertaking frame-by-frame analysis of my ciné film of valve action could I say whether or not the ball valve started to close before the end of diastole, and I have not yet undertaken this analysis. It was clear that some reversed flow was necessary to complete the closure movements of the valve.

REFERENCES

1. Reid, K.G. Design criteria for a prosthetic orthoptic heart and mitral valve. *Guys Hospital Reports* Vol. 119, No. 3 (1970).

2. Reid, K.G. Cited in *Year Book of Cardiovascular Medicine*, ed. J.W. Kirklin. Year Book Publishers: 1971.

3. Gibson, T.C., et al. Echocardiographic and phonocardiographic characteristics of the Lillehei-Kaster mitral valve prosthesis. *Circulation* 49:434, 1974.

SUMMARY: PART V

J.T.M. Wright, Ph.D.

The hemodynamic characteristics of the Björk-Shiley pivoting disc valve were discussed by Dr. Viking Björk, who emphasized that the prosthesis had a greater ratio of the orifice diameter to mounting diameter than other valves, and hence produced minimal pressure drop for a given size of valve. Measurements made of pressure drop at various steady flow rates indicated that an opening angle of 60° was optimal. Dr. Björk also compared in vitro tests in which the hemolysis produced by the Björk-Shiley valve was lower than that produced by a Likllehei-Kaster. This was thought to be due to the nonoverlapping nature of the closed disc.

Dr. Brian Bellhouse described pulsatile flow studies carried out on Beall, Starr-Edwards ball, Hancock, and Björk-Shiley prostheses, and a three cusp prosthesis with sinuses constructed in his laboratory. A short ciné film was used to illustrate vortices produced by these valves. The lowest pressure drop occurred with the Björk-Shiley, and the highest with the Beall large. However, with this valve the disc was proximal to the posterior part of the flexible ventricular cavity, thus forming a restriction to flow. A leakage flow study under a steady pressure head showed that the Björk-Shiley had a high closed leakage path compared to other valves, and calculations of shear rates indicated the probability of red cell destruction.

The pressure drop and incompetence levels of a range of valve prostheses, under pulsatile flow conditions, were presented by Dr. John Wright. The tests were carried out using a mechanical model of the left ventricle over a range of pulse rates of 60-140 per minute at a stroke volume of 60 milliliters. The prostheses tested were listed in order of hydraulic merit: pivoting and tilting disc valves, disc valves, tissue valves, and ball valves. A series of flow visualization studies for each valve type was shown.

Dr. David Taylor described fluid dynamic studies, carried out at the time of implantation, using needle pitot techniques. The valves investigated were the Starr-Edwards ball and disc valves, the Björk-Shiley, stented fascia lata, and the Hancock tissue valve. With both types of disc valves, stable flow patterns appeared to be established, and in the case of the tilting disc valve a toroidal swirl appeared to be established in the ventricle. This could cause partial valve closure after early diastole. The rank ordering for least resistance were fascia lata, Björk-Shiley, Starr-Edwards disc, and Starr-Edwards ball valve.

302

Dr. Stanton Nolan described his findings on the flow characteristics of ball, disc, and xenograft valves. Electromagnetic flow transducers were incorporated into the base of the valve prostheses which were implanted into calves. One finding was that the disc valve operated at 30% less power loss than the ball valve, but both types produced a two-to-four-fold increase in the power output of the left atrium. By contrast, the mounted heterograft produced only a slight increase in the pressure drop above the normal mitral valve, there was no regurgitation, and the patterns of mitral valve flow were essentially the same as the normal valve.

A feature of the session was that the different workers, using different techniques, produced results which showed general agreement in the flow patterns, pressure drops, and order of hydraulic merit for the prostheses.

PART SIX

NEW TRENDS IN NONINVASIVE ULTRASONIC DIAGNOSIS OF MITRAL VALVE DISEASE

26 Contribution of Ultrasonic Echography to the Diagnosis of Mitral Valve Disease

J. Pernod, M.D.
J. Kermarec, M.D.
D. Richard, M.D.
M. Terdjman, M.D.

This chapter schematically presents the information that can be given by ultrasonic echography in mitral cardiopathies.

METHOD

The echographic examination is performed with a commercial echograph* and a transducer (2.5 megahertz). The patients are examined in the recumbent position, and the transducer is placed in the third or fourth intercostal space along the left sternal border. The transducer is directed posteriorly and slightly medially so that the anterior mitral-valve echo may be observed. The posterior leaflet is recorded by directing the transducer slightly more inferiorly and laterally. Signals are visualized either on an oscilloscope or on a recorder.

---

* Hewlett Packard

STUDY OF THE MITRAL VALVE
Mitral Stenosis

A full study of the mitral lesions must be undertaken on the anterior mitral leaflet, the posterior mitral valve, and the subvalvular system.

Anterior Mitral Leaflet[1] The characteristic appearance of the graph is seen in Figure 1 a. During diastole, the normal double-peaked aspect (the peaks corresponding respectively to the maximum aperture of the mitral valve and the auricular contraction) is replaced by a slightly inclined plateau (as shown by the low value of the angle indicated in the figure) which immediately suggests the diagnosis of a mitral stenosis.

Measurement of the speed of the diastolic plateau can be made on graphic recordings such as the one shown in figure 1 a, by checking amplitude and knowing the unwinding speed of the recorder. The speed of the plateau here is 8 millimeters per second. The mean values are 88.9 for the normal subjects (standard deviation = 19.1) and 20.6 for the subjects with mitral cardiopathies (standard deviation = 12.0). A correlation between a great number of patients, 140 of whom had tight and operated stenosis[2] allows the following conclusions:

1. There is an obvious difference between loose and tight operable stenoses. The speed of a tight stenosis is always less than 25 and in most cases may even be less than 20 millimeters per second. Therefore, a speed greater than 30 mm per second indicates that the stenosis is not very tight.

2. However, in tight stenoses, the speeds are always so diminished that it is useless to look for a straight parallel between the ostium surface and the echographic speed. The speed of the valve is in fact influenced not only by the degree of the stenosis, but also by the degree of the valvular anatomical lesion.

To determine the speed of the opening of the mitral valve, two parameters may be measured. The first one is the B2-OM delay time between the second noise of the phonocardiogram and the maximum aperture point on the echographic curve. Its measurement is identical to the measurement of the interval B2-CO of the phonocardiogram, the point OM being contemporaneous with the opening snap of the mitral valve and with the declivous point O of the apexogram. The

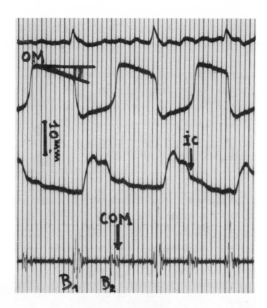

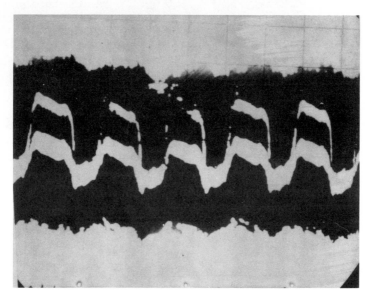

Figure 1. Mitral Stenosis. (Top) The simultaneous recording from bottom to top of the phonocardiogram (with the opening snap of the mitral valve, COM), of the carotidian pulse, of the echographic curve of the anterior mitral valve with a slow moving plateau contour (8 mm per second), and of the electrocardiogram (complete arrythmia). (Bottom) Visualization of the two mitral valves: the small valve, like the large one, moves forward. The respective thickness of the curves show that there is no predominance of the anatomic lesion in either of the two valves.

interval B2-OM has an advantage over the interval B2-CO, because it is always measurable, whereas there is not always an opening snap.

The second parameter is the time taken by the mitral valve to open, i.e., the delay time between the foot of the echographic curve and the maximum opening point, OM. This interval is weak, so it is not usually measured; yet it is possible to do so accurately by using a digital-analogical converter. As shown in Figures 2 a and 2 b, the curve is transformed automatically into a series of points separated by the expected interval of time (0.01 second in Figure 2 a, two milliseconds in Figure 2 b). A minicomputer carries out the measurements given in Table 1.

The average speed of opening expressed in hundredths of a second is 6.83 in the normal subject. It is slightly emphasized in cardiopathies without mitral disease (7.43), and greatly emphasized (more than 40 percent) in cardiopathies with mitral disease (10.45).

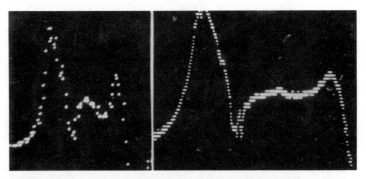

Figure 2. Analogical-digital conversion of the curve of the movement of the mitral valve depending on the time. Each point is separated from the following by 0.01 second on the left side of the diagram, and by 0.002 second on the right side. A very precise measurement of the opening time of the mitral valve can be made.

Table 1
Speed of Opening of the Mitral Valve (expressed in hundredths of second)

	Normal Subjects	Cardiopathies Without Mitral Disease	Cardiopathies With Mitral Disease
Number of subjects	23	23	33
Average	6.83	7.43	10.45
Average interval of trust (at 5%)	±0.34	±0.41	±0.32
Standard deviation	0.78	0.94	0.94
Degree of meaning in relation to the normal subjects	/	$p < 0.05$	$p < 0.000\ 001$

There is a correlation between the speed of the opening of the mitral valve and the speed of the diastolic plateau (on 79 pairs of values r = 0.835 corresponding to p < 0.0001). The two parameters discussed above probably do not depend equally on the two factors likely to influence the speed of opening: pressure gradient and pliancy of the valve.

The amplitude is a less reliable parameter than the speed because it is less reproductive. A long time ago, Edler[3] showed that the amplitudes are altered only in highly pathological valves—in particular, those that are calcified.

The study of the character and timing of the echo as shown on the graph is important; it allows one to evaluate the degree of anatomic disease of the valve.[4]

Posterior Mitral Valve[5] After the anterior mitral leaflet has been located, it is enough to modify the placement of the transducer slightly to get the data for the posterior mitral valve. Figure 1b shows that, in the case of mitral stenosis, the posterior mitral valve moves in the same way that the anterior mitral leaflet does, as opposed to the normal case. The distance between the plotting of the two valves gives an approximate idea of the surface of the opening. We have confirmed this paradoxical movement of the small valve during surgical procedures in the office of Dr. Servelle; the small valve is located, and the transducer is placed on the heart directly in front of the posterior valve.

The diagram of the posterior valve looks like a plateau, and one can measure the speed, amplitude, and thickness as it is done for the anterior leaflet. The comparison of the morphology of the two valves is very instructive: for example, in the case of Figure 1 b, it is evident that they are already damaged by the pathologic process, because the thicknesses of the corresponding lines are identical.

Subvalvular System The examination should also include the subvalvular system. The presence of thick echos is important evidence of its impairment. The surgeon must then be careful if a comissurotomy is to be performed.

Mitral Insufficiency

Mitral insufficiency theoretically leads to modifications opposite to those made by stenosis: large amplitude and great speed. But this is true only for pure mitral insufficiencies with pliable valves. Actually, one cannot diagnose mitral insufficiency solely on the basis of echography, because it is too unreliable. Nevertheless, it has a considerable value in revealing some mechanisms of mitral insufficiency, particularly ruptured chordae tendineae and mitral valve prolapse syndrome.[6,7] Figure 3 a is of a patient suffering from a mitral insufficiency, with signs of irreducible cardiac insufficiency. The diagnosis of ruptured chordae tendineae is confirmed by echography: the plotting indeed shows that the large and small valves have entirely independent movements, and are not coupled at any time. Anatomic testing actually showed that the posterior valve had lost all connections, and that several chordae of the anterior leaflet were broken.

Figure 3 b is of a patient with a telesystolic murmur. From echography, we note the posterior valve is not, as normally, coupled with the anterior valve for the duration of systole; during telesystole, it moves down, thus showing the mechanism of this mitral insufficiency: mitral valve prolapse.

Mitral Disorder

As a general rule in case of mitral disorder, the symptoms of stenosis predominate over those of insufficiency. Therefore, one cannot rely on echography either to detect an unimportant leak associated with a mitral stenosis or to evaluate the respective importance of the two processes of stenosis and insufficiency.

On the other hand, if in the course of a mitral disorder a fast diastolic speed of the mitral valve is noted, one can assert that insufficiency is large.

MEASURING THE SIZE OF THE LEFT ATRIUM[8]

In order to measure the size of the left atrium, the anterior mitral leaflet is first located and then the orientation of the transducer is modified to be progressively higher and more medial. The anterior mitral leaflet extends by the posterior wall of the aorta, which is at the same time the anterior wall of the left atrium, whereas the posterior wall of the left ventricle extends by the posterior wall of the atrium. The diameter can be measured in this way. The measurements are very reproducible: there are only slight differences between the measurements made by several operators in the same day; the same is true for those made by the same operator during a long time. The sizes are emphasized in the case of mitral stenosis, as is shown in Table 2, which is based on 163 subjects.

The average is between 27 and 30 mm for normal subjects or cardiopathies without mitral disease, and it is 46.2 mm for mitral

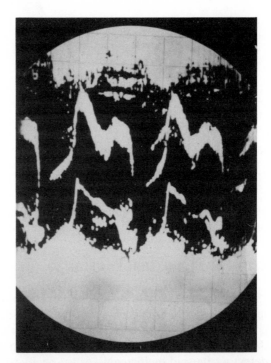

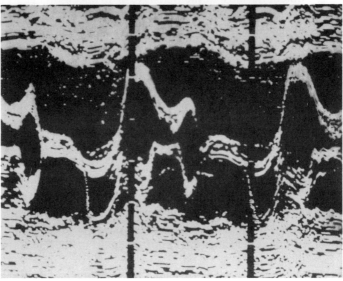

Figure 3. Mitral Insufficiencies. (Top) Break in the chordae: the movement of the two valves is totally independent. (Bottom) Mitral valve prolapse syndrome: in telesystole there is a backward movement of the small valve, which separates itself from the large one.

Table 2
Size of the Left Atrium

	Number of Subjects	Average (in mm)	Interval of Trust at 5% of the Average	Standard Deviation
Mitral Disease	77	46.2	± 3.0	13.4
Cardiopathies without Mitral Disease	51	29.6	± 1.5	5.6
Normal subjects	35	27.3	± 1.2	3.5
Total	163			

cardiopathies. The difference between this last group and the two previous ones is significant statistically at more than 1 for 10,000.

EXAMINATION OF THE OTHER VALVES

With a mitral cardiopathy the examination should consist of investigating the tricuspid echo and studying the aortic sigmoid echoes. It is more difficult to show the movements of the tricuspid than those of the mitral valve. The examination is often unable to detect a tricuspid inefficiency, or to specify its degree. It can, however, enable one to detect a stenosis[9] with a characteristic plateau aspect, and it can give an idea of the degree of anatomic damage of the valve, based on the loudness of the echo.

It is easier to show aortic sigmoids. Here again the most valuable information is supplied by the thickness of the echoes obtained, which will give an indication of the level of their bearing; however, in most cases they do not enable one to specify the extent of a stenosis or leakage.

MYOCARDIAL CONTRACTILITY

In the case of all cardiopathies to be operated on, it is essential to have an idea of the myocardial contractility. Karliner[10] and others have shown that a sufficiently reliable parameter is the VCF (velocity of circumferential fiber shortening), a method used in cineangiocardiography.

In echography, the speed of shortening of the diameter of the left ventricle is measured during systole. This is proportional to the VCF, and has an advantage over the latter, since it can be measured directly without any hypothesis on the geometry of the ventricle.

On a recording of the cavity made by an optical-fibers recorder or an electronic reprograph, the distance between the echo of the left side of the septum and that of the posterior endocardium of the ventricle is measured. The measuring of the diastolic and systolic diameters enables one to calculate the average speed of shortening of the diameter, bearing in mind the duration of the systole.

A greater precision can be obtained by selecting the echoes through a system of electronic gates, and by sending them into a small computer. After the analogic-digital conversion shown in Figure 4 a (with a sample length of 0.01 second) the minicomputer automatically plots the variation in diameter depending on the time (Figure 4 b, top) and the standardized derivative (Figure 4 b, bottom); the maximum value gives the highest speed of shortening expressed in diameter per second, which is a more precise parameter than the average speed.[11] In addition to the graphical plotting, the computer prints a list of all numerical values, thus freeing the operator from all measuring and calculation.

CONCLUSIONS

Ultrasonic echography is a rich source of information in establishing a diagnosis and a preoperatory balance in mitral cardiopathies. In the course of mitral stenosis the anatomic balance of the mitral system can be seen by checking three types of information:

1. The speed of the large valve during the diastolic plateau. As it has been shown by correlation with surgical findings, this speed is not only dependent on the degree of stenosis, but also on the anatomic condition of the valve.

2. The duration of aperture of the large valve. This measurement can be done precisely using a digital-analogic transformation. It depends on the same factors as the diastolic speed but not to the same degree.

3. The respective thicknesses of the echoes of the anterior and posterior valve enables one to check whether the condition involves or prevails in only one of the two valves. The examination is done in such way to show up a possible disease of the subvalvular system.

Echography has only limited use in the positive diagnosis of mitral insufficiency; it is, however, of great interest in supporting

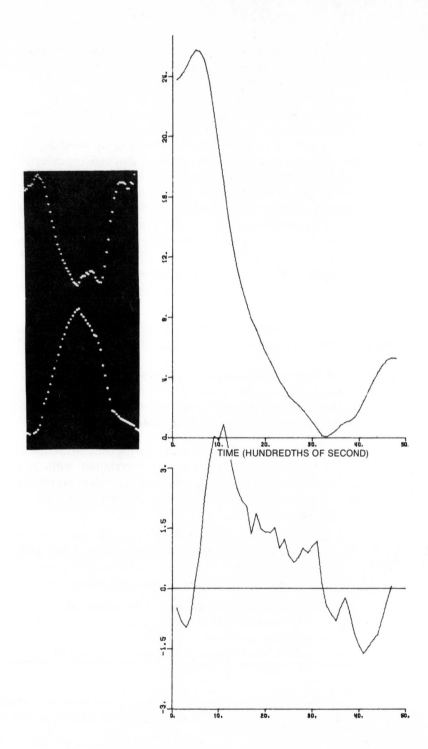

TIME (HUNDREDTHS OF SECOND)

some of its mechanisms, such as ruptured chordae tendineae or mitral valve prolapse.

In addition to the examination of the mitral valve, echography will inform about the size of the left atrium, as well as the degree of anatomic disease of the aortal sigmoïds and possibly of the tricuspid valve.

Finally, the determination of the myocardial contractility is as important as the study of the valves themselves in the evaluation of an indication or an operative technique. A good indication of contractility might be available by determining the average and maximal speeds of shortening of the transverse diameter of the left ventricle. This determination can be done manually or better with a minicomputer after digital-analogical transformation.

REFERENCES

1. Effert, S. Pre and postoperative evaluation of mitral stenosis by ultrasound. *Amer. J. Cardiol.* 19:59, 1967.

2. Pernod, J., Servelle, M., Haguenauer, G., and Kermarec, J. Corrélations entre échographie par ultrasons et constatations anatomo-chirurgicales dans les cardiopathies mitrales (à propos de 140 corrélations). *Arch. Mal. Coeur.* 66:333, 1973.

3. Edler, I. Ultrasound cardiography in mitral valve stenosis. *Amer. J. Cardiol.* 19:18, 1967.

4. Castillo-Fenoy, A., Houeix, J.M., Veber, G., and Tricot, R. Appréciation de l'état valvulaire mitral par l'échographie. *Gazette Médicale de France* 81:2281, 1974.

5. Duchak, J.M., Chang, S., and Feigenbaum, H. The posterior mitral valve echo and the echocardiographic. *Amer. J. Cardiol.* 29:628, 1972.

6. Sweatman, T., Selzer, A., Kamagi, M., and Cohn, K. Echocardiographic diagnosis of mitral regurgitation due to ruptured chordae tendineae. *Circulation* 46:580, 1972.

7. Popp, R.L., Brown, O.R., Silverman, J.F., Harrison,

Figure 4. Definition of the speed of shortening of the diameter of the left ventricle by a mini-computer. (Left) Analogical-digital-transformation of the movements of the left side of the septum (top) and of the posterior endocardium (bottom). Two successive points are separated by 0.01 second. (Right) A minicomputer automatically plots the variations in diameter, taking account of the time (top) and the standardized derivative (bottom), showing the maximum speed expressed in diameters per second.

D.C.   Echographic abnormalities in the mitral valve prolapse syndrome. *Circulation* 49:428, 1974.

8. Hirata, T., Wolfe, S.B., Popp, R.L., Helmen, C.H., Feigenbaum, H.   Estimation of left atrial size using ultrasound. *Amer. Heart J.* 78:43, 1969.

9. Joyner, C.R., Hey, E.B., Johnson, J., and Reid, J.M.   Reflected ultrasound in the diagnosis of tricuspid stenosis. *Amer. J. Cardiol.* 19:66, 1967.

10. Karliner, J.S., Gault, J.H., Eckberg, D., Mullins, C.B., and Ross, J.   Mean velocity of fiber shortening. A simplified measure of left ventricular myocardial contractility. *Circulation* 44:323, 1971.

11. Pernod, J., Kermarec, J., Richard, D., and Chenille, E.   Determination de la contractilité myocardique par échographie ultrasonique. *Nouvelle Presse Medicale* 4:1113, 1975.

27 Special Features and New Data in Mitral Valve Echocardiography*

Richard L. Popp, M.D.

Echocardiography allows us to observe mitral valvular motion non-invasively. I would like to point out some of the strengths and weaknesses of the technique, since most clinicians now realize its vast diagnostic ability. In the past we have been studying the method, and such critical analyses must continue. But now we have begun to use the method to study pathologic states. As examples I will concentrate on recent work regarding the mitral valve prolapse syndrome and also idiopathic hypertrophic subaortic stenosis.

I would point out our reference system for all echocardiographic studies is a transducer fixed at the chest wall and tilted to encounter cardiac structures. This is distinguished from internal reference systems used by other techniques. We know the normal systolic echocardiographic mitral valvular motion is toward the transducer on the chest wall. This is due to ejection of the ventricular blood which lies between the closed mitral valve and the chest wall. Thus the mitral echo inscribes a positive motion above the horizontal in our

* Supported in part by a Research Career Development Award No. K04-HL-704-39, and a grant from the Bay Area Heart Research Association.

320

strip chart recordings (Fig. 1). The patient with mitral valve prolapse (MVP) has this ventricular ejection bringing the valvular ring towards the anterior chest wall, but also has motion of the valvular leaflets toward the posterior left atrial wall. Hence we see the resultant net motion by echocardiography. The classic echocardiographic pattern shows abrupt midsystolic posterior motion of the closed valve echoes, after initial anterior, horizontal, or posterior motion.[1,2] In such records it is common to see multiple discrete echoes from the mitral valve region. These echoes are seen less strikingly in normal valves, and represent echo production by multiple areas of both the anterior and posterior leaflet, rather than separation of these two leaflets. Therefore it is not possible to diagnose mitral regurgitation on the echocardiogram, as "separation" of the leaflets cannot be recognized.

In addition to the abrupt mid-systolic motion of the leaflet echoes towards the left atrium in MVP, we have seen another pattern which corresponds with the clinical and angiographic picture of MVP. In these cases the posterior motion begins with systole (the "C" point) and inscribes a smooth "U" shaped contour.[3] The patients with

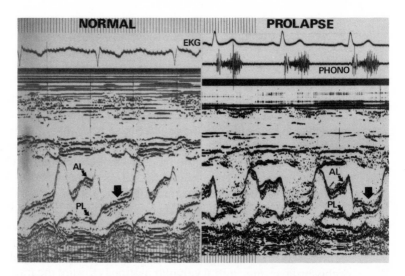

Figure 1. Left: Echocardiogram of the mitral valve in a normal subject. During systole there is gradual migration of the closed valve toward the transducer on the chest wall (black arrow). Right: Mitral valve in a patient with mitral valve prolapse. During systole the valve echoes move away from the transducer and toward the left atrium (black arrow). A late systolic murmur is recorded in the phonocardiogram. AL = anterior leaflet; PL = posterior leaflet. EKG = electrocardiogram.

midsystolic or early systolic posterior valve motion are exactly similar on angiography and probably represent nothing more than recording from different areas of the mitral valve, and/or more early cancellation of the anterior annulus motion by posterior motion of the leaflets in the latter form. This suggestion is supported by recent work by Dr. David Sahn of the University of Arizona.[4] We have found that the position of the transducer on the chest wall and the angulation of the transducer in the sagittal plane affect the echocardiographic pattern. In a study done in our laboratory with Dr. Walter Markiewicz, we found that transducer placement high on the chest wall (second interspace) uniformly gives a smooth posterior mitral echo similar to the "U" shaped or holosystolic prolapse. This is due to shortening of the apex-base cardiac dimension, which is registered by high transducer placement, but not registered by the sound beam perpendicular to this motion when the transducer is perpendicular to the chest wall. Even in the case of patients with a pattern of MVP recorded with this lower transducer position, angulation in the horizontal plane may give both typical and atypical patterns in the same patient. One may record a false negative pattern if the transducer is low on the chest wall as well. In this study we called in 100 apparently normal women aged 18-35 for clinical history, physical exam, EKG, phonocardiogram, echocardiogram, exercise treadmill, and Holter EKG testing. Depending on the criteria used to label these subjects as having evidence of MVP (on at least two types of exam), we found 4 to 10% of these apparently healthy women to have MVP. This is interesting in light of our prior study showing patterns of MVP by echocardiogram and angiocardiogram without auscultatory findings such as clicks or murmurs.[3]

Thus we have used the echocardiogram to identify subjects with "silent" forms of MVP, and have made a first attempt to learn the prevalence of this condition in a preclinical state. We have also used this tool to explore the dynamics of MVP under physiologic and pharmacologic interventions. Work done in conjunction with Dr. Roger Winkle of our laboratory has shown a clear association of auscultatory findings, when present, and the timing of abrupt valve motion during systole. However, discrete clicks or onset of a murmur fail to coincide with either apparent onset or maximum degrees of posterior valve motion. These studies show congruous translocation of clicks, or onset of murmur and onset of posterior echographic motion of the valve, but either the area of the valve causing clicks is not visualized in any of our studies or the sounds are not related to abrupt valve motion.[5]

Another area of exploration of the MVP syndrome has related to the coexistence of infective endocarditis and this valvular condition. Dr. Denton Corrigall has analyzed all the cases of endocarditis indexed in the medical records of our hospital since 1972. When one chooses cases of clear mitral valve involvement, two facts emerge. First, 20 to 30% of patients with isolated mitral valve endocarditis had echocardiographic, angiographic, or pathologic evidence of MVP; and second, the murmur in these patients was often holosystolic and indistinguishable from that of patients with rheumatic mitral disease. We found many echocardiograms with "fluffy" echoes in the area of the mitral valve which are consistent with masses of vegetations in these patients. These findings may be absent despite positive blood cultures, and a murmur of mitral regurgitation (false negative) and echoes similar to the pattern associated with valvular vegetations may be seen in pure MVP without any evidence for current or past endocarditis (false positive).

These examples of our use of echocardiography show our concern with establishment of echocardiographic patterns associated with disease, and our use of this method to search out groups of patients with this condition for further study. Through these investigations we hope to learn more of the syndrome in general and the natural history in particular.

We have used a similar approach to investigate patients with idiopathic hypertrophic subaortic stenosis (IHSS). Concentrating only on our impressions regarding the motion of the mitral valve in this condition, we can make several statements. Combination of echocardiography and phonocardiography shows a close correlation of the contour of the systolic murmur and the contour of the left ventricular outflow tract, defined as the area between the left endocardium of the interventricular septum and the mitral valve echo (Fig. 2). This suggests an important role for the abnormal systolic anterior motion of the mitral valve in the production of an outflow obstruction in this condition. Dr. Walter Henry and his colleagues at the National Heart and Lung Institute in the United States have shown an inverse relationship between the calculated echocardiographic outflow tract area and the magnitude of the outflow tract gradient.[6] While this concept is generally correct, the localized sampling of the outflow tract available by ultrasound may not be representative of this three-dimensional orifice in each case.[7] Thus we believe we may follow patients serially with echocardiography after establishment of the relation between the echocardiographic outflow tract and the catheterization-recorded gradient on a beat-to-beat basis. Thus echocardiography has great strength for assessment of therapy

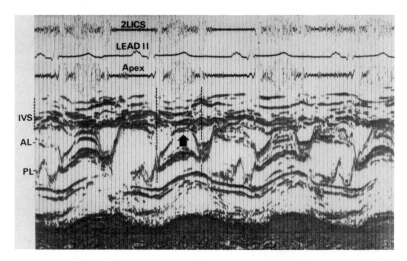

Figure 2. Echocardiogram in a patient with hypertrophic obstructive cardiomyopathy (IHSS). The systolic anterior motion of the mitral valve (arrow) is coincident with the murmur recorded on the phonocardiogram. Systole is indicated by the dashed lines. 2LICS = second left intercostal space; LEAD II = electrocardiogram; IVS = interventricular septum; AL = anterior mitral leaflet; PL = posterior mitral leaflet.

in this condition, as well as diagnosis, if one recognizes the limitations of the technique.

From the observations mentioned here I conclude that echocardiography is an excellent tool to study the motion of cardiac structures in humans. It enables us to get direct dynamic information. But an understanding of the physical basis and limitations of the technique is critical in placing significance on any recorded signals.

REFERENCES

1. Kerber, R.E., Isaeff, D.M., Hancock, E.W. Echocardiographic patterns in patients with the syndrome of systolic click and late systolic murmur. *NEJM* 284:691, 1971.

2. Dillon, J.C., Haine, C., Chang, S., Feigenbaum, H. Use of echocardiography in patients with prolapsed mitral valve. *Circulation* 43:503, 1971.

3. Popp, R.L., Brown, O.R., Silverman, J.F., Harrison, D.C. Echocardiographic abnormalities in the mitral valve prolapse syndrome. *Circulation* 49:428, 1974.

4. Sahn, D.J., Friedman, W.F. Cross-sectional echocardio-

graphic evaluation of mitral valve prolapse in children. *Amer. J. Cardiol.* 35:179, 1975.

5. Winkle, R.A., Goodman, D.J., Popp, R.L. Simultaneous echocardiographic-phonocardiographic recordings at rest and during amyl nitrite administration in patients with mitral valve prolapse. *Circulation* 51:522, 1975.

6. Henry, W.L., Clard, C.E., Glancy, D.L., Epstein, S.E. Echocardiographic measurement of left ventricular outflow gradient in idiopathic hypertrophic subaortic stenosis. *NEJM* 288:989, 1973.

7. Rossen, R.M., Goodman, D.J., Ingham, R.E., Popp, R.L. Echocardiographic criteria in the diagnosis of idiopathic hypertrophic subaortic stenosis. *Circulation* 50:747, 1974.

28 Echocardiographic Assessment of Prosthetic Mitral Valves*

Richard L. Popp, M.D.

Despite continued improvements in engineering, manufacturing, and techniques of implantation of prosthetic mitral valves, some patients experience malfunction of these prostheses. There are not a large number of patients with true prosthesis malfunction, but enough of these patients are seen to bring this possibility to mind continually when dealing with postoperative patients experiencing heart failure. We have been impressed with the finding that continued myocardial disease, rather than prosthesis malfunction, is the cause of heart failure in a great many of these patients.

The caged-ball prostheses are made of materials which produce very intense echoes on the echocardiogram. When the transducer is placed between the apex and lower left sternal border in patients with prosthetic mitral valves, it is possible to align the sound beam with the path of ball travel within the cage and consistently track ball motion (Fig. 1). Proper alignment of the transducer is indicated by maximum excursion of the ball when comparing echocardiographic recordings

* Supported in part by a Research Career Development Award No. K04-HL-704-39, and a grant from the Bay Area Heart Research Association.

325

from several transducer positions in this general area of the chest. When properly recorded, echoes from the apex of the cage and the sewing ring may be identified. These two echoes move identically and have a general sinusoidal wave form. They move towards the transducer during systole and away from the transducer during diastole.

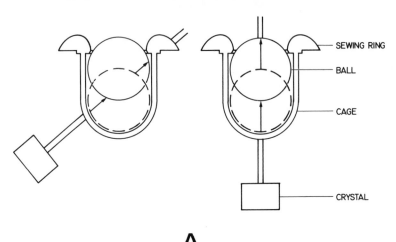

A

Figure 1A. Diagram of the effect of alignment of the sound beam (from the transducer crystal) and the path of ball travel within the prosthesis. When the paths are parallel, maximum ball motion will be recorded. Transducer drawn with placement near the cardiac apex. Opening is recorded toward the transducer.

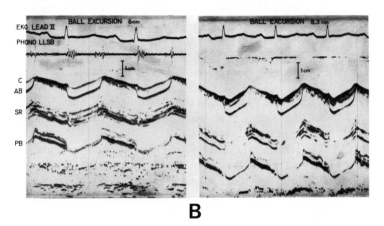

B

Figure 1B. Two echocardiograms from the same patient using different transducer locations. The left panel shows 6 mm excursion vs. 8.5 mm on the right. The latter indicates close alignment of the sound beam and ball path. Here the transducer reference would be presented at the top of the paper, so opening is recorded toward the EKG.

Between these two echoes one records the ball moving toward the apex of the cage at the onset of diastole and away from the cage toward the sewing ring at the onset of systole. The posterior portion of the ball, i.e., the interface between the posterior ball and blood, is recorded as if it were behind the sewing ring with the ball appearing approximately twice its actual size. This effect is due to calibration of the ultrasonic instruments, which measure distances by measuring the time taken for sound to travel a given distance, assuming that sound travels at a speed of 1540 m/sec (the average speed of sound through soft tissue). However, the silastic material conducts sound at 960 m/sec, so it takes approximately twice as much time for sound to travel through the ball as it would take for sound to travel through a comparable thickness of soft tissue. For this reason the ultrasonic instrument presents the ball as if it were twice its actual size.[1] This presents some advantage in interpretation since the posterior ball echo is presented in bold relief, allowing study of its movement without nearby echoes.

When the valve opens, the ball moves towards the apex of the cage, and the point of contact of these two structures is exactly coincident with recording of the opening click on the phonocardiogram. The ball generally remains at the apex of the cage during ventricular filling. Full excursion closure of the valve with the onset of systole is coincident with a high-intensity closing click. Occasionally during a long diastole the ball may drift towards the sewing ring, and then completed closure is associated with a low intensity closing click.[2] Prosthetics "S3" or "S4" are associated respectively with an initial bounce of the ball during opening, or full re-opening of the ball by atrial systole after some drift of the ball away from the cage in mid-diastole. Ball bounce on opening is most striking in low output states, but may be seen normally. One may recognize full immobilization of the ball by thrombus when seeing lack of independent ball motion with respect to the cage.[3] This is verified by the posterior ball echo being presented independent of the cage and sewing ring echoes, but having identical motion as the valve structure. An example of this situation is shown in Figure 2. If the prosthesis has enough thrombus around it to cause intermittent sticking of the ball, one may recognize this both by wide beat-to-beat variations of the interval between the aortic component of the second sound and the opening click, and by an unusual pattern on the echocardiogram.[3,4] The ball should open at the same point on the sinusoidal curve of cage motion with each cycle. The mitral ball should move to the apex of the cage at the point of maximum anterior cage position. If ball motion is delayed beyond this point, and especially if ball motion is delayed irregularly, one can be

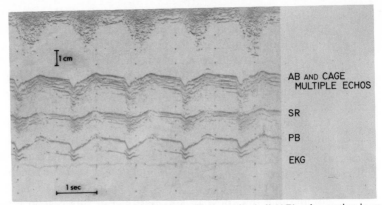

Figure 2. Thrombosed mitral prosthesis: The anterior ball (AB) echo motion is not seen independent of the cage and sewing ring (SR). The posterior ball (PB) echo recorded separate from, but moving with, the sewing ring indicates the sound beam is passed through the prosthesis in the proper way.

confident of the diagnosis (Fig. 3). In studies done by Dr. Theodore Berndt in our laboratory, it was found that maximum beat-to-beat variation in the A2 opening click interval should be no greater than 20 msec in the presence of normal sinus rhythm and no more than 30 msec in the presence of atrial fibrillation.[2]

In patients presenting with very soft or inaudible valve sounds

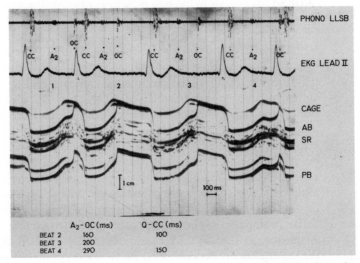

Figure 3. Sticking prosthetic ball: The cage and sewing ring (SR) echoes show a consistent sinusoidal wave form. The anterior (AB) and posterior ball (PB) echoes show irregular patterns of opening motion relative to the cage. The phonocardiogram shows wide variation in the A2-opening click (OC) interval.

the echocardiogram is of help, since a totally thrombosed valve may be recognized as described above. Full-excursion ball motion will be seen in the presence of other causes of decreased valve sounds. We have often recorded normal excursion of these prosthetic balls in the aortic and mitral position in the presence of severely depressed ventricular function resulting in soft valve sounds (Fig. 4). One should be able to make this differentiation in patients with mitral prostheses, since over 90% of these prostheses may be successfully recorded with echocardiography. Only approximately 50% of patients with aortic prostheses yield adequate recordings of the valve for assessment, and several patients with aortic valve malfunction have shown no recognizable echocardiographic abnormality. Therefore these comments are restricted to mitral prosthetic valves.

A common type of valve malfunction occurs because of partial detachment of the sewing ring from the mitral annulus. In the presence of major detachments of this type there is sufficient rocking of the valve cage to prevent continuous alignment of the ultrasonic beam and the axis of ball travel. Consequently one records abrupt motion of the cage at the onset of both diastole and systole. In this situation, experienced investigators cannot continuously record the usual waveform of the cage and sewing ring as well as the anterior and posterior ball echoes.[3]

By combining echocardiography and phonocardiography, one is able to determine the origin of valve sounds in patients with multiple

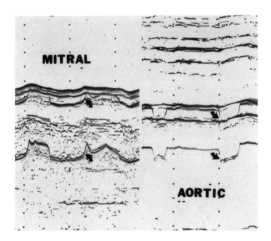

Figure 4. Normal ball motion with severely depressed ventricular function. The mitral and aortic prosthetic balls move well within their respective cages. Marked bounce of the balls after each opening is seen. Opening indicated by the arrows. This patient had virtually inaudible valve sounds.

prosthetic valves in place.[3] This is especially important in patients with mitral and tricuspid prostheses. Recognition of an extremely short A2-opening click interval may not be possible in such patients unless the echocardiogram is recorded simultaneously to identify the components of the phonocardiogram associated with opening and closure of each valve.

We also have studied the echocardiographic pattern associated with stent-mounted homograft and porcine heterograft valves placed in the mitral position. In vitro experiments have allowed us to recognize the origin of valve echoes.[5] With extremely low flow rates, only one cusp of the porcine heterograft valve opens while the small cusp and the cusp originally containing muscle seem to resist opening. In high flow situations, all three cusps open fully. These valves may be recorded with the sound beam traversing both sides of the valve ring and recording up to two cusps moving toward and away from the transducer. This is usually best achieved from the left sternal border. Dr. Michael Horowitz in our laboratory has demonstrated the optimal technique for recording such valves through a conventional M-mode sector scan of the left ventricle.[5] An example of this type of record is shown in Figure 5.

Our studies may be summarized as follows. The early diastolic slope or rate of motion of the stent may be taken to represent the rate of right and left ventricular filling. If this slope is below 19 mm/sec,

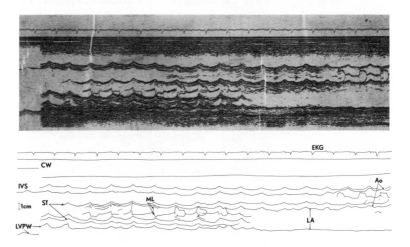

Figure 5. Strip chart record and corresponding diagram of a patient with a mitral bioprosthesis. The similarity of the aortic valve (AO) and the mitral prosthesis (MV) are shown; however, the EKG reference shows diastolic opening of the mitral valve.

decreased mitral valve flow is expected.[6] An echocardiogram of the left ventricle may indicate very poor myocardial contractility and low stroke volume, in which case the low diastolic slope may be directly attributable to this low output state. However, the presence of this finding with good left ventricular motion suggests inflow occlusion of the mitral valve. If this diastolic slope is greater than 33 mm/sec, we may suspect increased mitral valve flow often associated with valvular regurgitation. One may expect the valve leaflets to have an excursion greater than 10 mm, and if the leaflet excursion is not greater than 55% of the total stent diameter, one may suspect possible thrombus or other material preventing leaflet opening.[6] In this situation again, one must check for high or low flow states, since a low flow state itself may cause incomplete valve opening. The leaflet echoes should be of less intensity than the stent echoes. If the leaflet echoes do not appear delicate and if they are of equal intensity with the stent, calcification of the leaflets may be suspected.[6] An example of a homograft valve which deteriorated with calcification and subsequent thrombus formation is shown in Figure 6 with the associated echocardiogram.

The vast majority of patients that we study with echocardiography do not have a pattern diagnostic of valve malfunction. However, confirmation of ball motion and the occasional diagnosis of frank malfunction stimulates us to continue studying patients with prosthetic valves. Echocardiography, especially when combined with phonocardiography, may develop into a major tool for the diagnosis of mitral prosthesis malfunction. Only further studies and experience in many laboratories can establish the sensitivity and specificity of the patterns found by us and mentioned in this report.

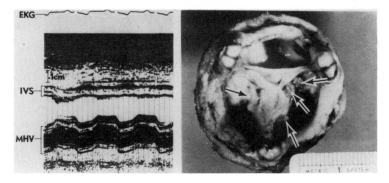

Figure 6. Calcified homograft bioprosthesis removed at surgery on right. Corresponding echocardiogram on left. MHV = mitral homograft valve; IVS = interventricular septum.

REFERENCES

1. Johnson, M.L., Paton, B.C., Holmes, J.H. Ultrasonic evaluation of prosthetic valve motion. *Circulation* 42 (Suppl II): II-3, 1970.

2. Berndt, T.B., Goodman, D.J., Popp, R.L. Echocardio-graphic-phonocardiographic studies of normally functioning caged ball valve prostheses. (Submitted for publication.)

3. Berndt, T.B., Goodman, D.J., Popp, R.L. Echocardio-graphic-phonocardiographic evaluation of suspected caged mitral valve malfunctions. (Submitted for publication.)

4. Pfeifer, J., Goldschlager, W., Sweatman, T., Gerbode, F., Selzer, A. Malfunction of mitral ball valve prosthesis due to thrombus. *Amer. J. Cardiol.* 29:95, 1972.

5. Horowitz, M.S., Tecklenberg, P.L., Goodman, D.J., Harrison, D.C., Popp, R.L. Echocardiographic evaluation of the stent mounted aortic heterograft valve in mitral position: *in vitro and in vivo* studies. (Submitted for publication.)

6. Horowitz, M.S., Goodman, D.J., Hancock, E.W., Popp, R.L. Non-invasive diagnosis of complications of the mitral bioprosthesis. (Submitted for publication.)

29 Ultrasonic Two-dimensional Analysis of the Mitral Valve

J. Roelandt, M.D.
F.J. ten Cate, M.D.
W.G. van Dorp, B.S.
C.M. Ligtvoet, M.Sc.
C.T. Lancée, M.Sc.

Dynamic two-dimensional cardiac imaging is a recent development in diagnostic ultrasound and is rapidly coming into clinical use. The electronic scanning instruments in particular create a lot of enthusiasm because they non-invasively provide images of the heart similar to those obtained with cine-angiocardiography.[1-4] However, we must realize that there are no echo data present in two-dimensional cardiac images that cannot be recorded with conventional echocardiography. Indeed, the basic unit of information, the echo signal which indicates presence and location in depth of an interface (i.e. a cardiac structure) in the direction of the sound beam, is the same for both techniques. The fundamental difference between the techniques is the manner in which the echo data are manipulated and displayed. These different representations provide additional information, but may each have some disadvantages for purposeful applications. However, in general, one can say that they complement each other, so that the clinical possibilities are extended when they are used in combination. To make this clear, one has to fully understand how two-dimensional imaging of the heart is realized. Since the mitral valve is the subject of this book, this contribution will focus on the relative role of both techniques in the recognition of the mitral valve structures.

ONE-DIMENSIONAL VERSUS TWO-DIMENSIONAL DISPLAY OF THE MITRAL VALVE

A thorough understanding of the cross-sectional anatomy of the heart is necessary in order to understand its three-dimensional anatomic relationships. This is only achieved by the study of cardiac anatomy, physiology, and angiocardiograms, and not the least after extensive experience with clinical ultrasound. The cross section of the heart that yields most of the useful diagnostic echo information follows a sagittal plane through the long axis of the left ventricle. Therefore, we shall confine ourselves to this cross section. In Figure 1, the anatomic relationships are depicted. The anterior mitral valve leaflet is in anatomic continuity with the posterior wall of the aorta and extends downwards to the apex of the heart. The leaflet is connected to the papillary muscles of the left ventricle by the chordae tendineae. As a consequence, the anterior leaflet divides the basilar portion of the left ventricle into an anterior outflow tract and a posterior inflow tract. It is of interest to realize that the plane of the anterior mitral leaflet in its neutral or midposition is parallel to the anterior chest wall. Behind the inflow tract is the posterior mitral valve leaflet, which is a much smaller structure.

In Figure 1, a single element transducer is placed at the appropriate position to study the mitral valve. The sound beam traverses from anterior to posterior: the anterior heart wall, the right ventricular cavity, the interventricular septum, the left ventricular cavity, the free edges of both anterior and posterior mitral valve leaflets, and the left ventricular posterior wall. The echoes of these structures can be represented in three types of oscilloscope display, referred to as A, B, and M-mode. The B-mode is the intermediate step where the A-mode or amplitude-modulated echoes are converted to dots, their relative intensity being indicated by their brightness. The M-mode is then realized by moving the B-mode at a constant speed over the screen. When recorded with a stripchart recorder, the depth of the echo signal on the vertical axis is displayed as a function of time, yielding a graphic representation of the change in range of any particular echo. In this manner a detailed and specific analysis of the characteristic motion pattern of that part of the mitral valve "insonified" by the sound beam becomes possible. With a narrow sound beam, this information is therefore in principle one-dimensional.

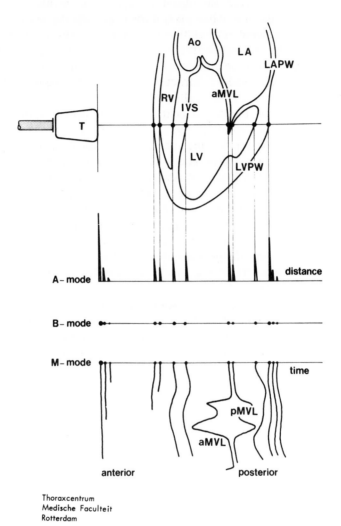

Thoraxcentrum
Medische Faculteit
Rotterdam

Figure 1. Schematic cross section of the heart from the base towards the apex with cardiac structures included. The single element transducer (T) in front is aimed so that the sound beam traverses from anterior to posterior: the anterior heart wall, right ventricle (RV), septum (IVS), left ventricular cavity (LV), the tips of the mitral valve leaflets, and the left ventricular posterior wall (LVPW). The echoes which originate from these boundaries are classically represented in three types of oscilloscope display and are referred to as the "A," "B," and "M-mode." (Ao = aorta; aMVL and pMVL = anterior and posterior mitral valve leaflets; LA = left atrium; LAPW = left atrial posterior wall).

336

However, the mitral valve is a complicated three-dimensional structure and what we aim for is at least the knowledge of its two-dimensional interrelationships in the investigated cross section. This can be realized with conventional echocardiography by comparing depth with the direction of the sound beam, and by anatomical continuity of specific structures recorded in sequence by angling the transducer. This is called the M-mode sector scan, and is achieved by sweeping the sound beam from the aorta towards the apex while recording continuously. The sequential directions of the sound beam from aorta to the apex are diagrammatically shown in Figure 2. The resulting M-mode record, obtained from a normal individual, is represented in Figure 3. As one can see, the echoes from the anterior mitral valve are in continuity with the posterior aortic root, and terminate in the region of the posterior papillary muscles, as do the chords of the posterior papillary muscle. Thus, the anatomic relationships of the mitral valve can be appreciated on such a record. However, some distortion is always introduced, as a wedge-shaped sector of the heart (see Fig. 2) is represented in a rectangular format on this M-mode display.

The examination technique requires skill and experience, since the resulting M-mode display is not simply related to the true cardiac anatomy, i.e. the cross section as seen in Figure 2. For this reason, a two-dimensional pictorial representation of the entire cardiac cross

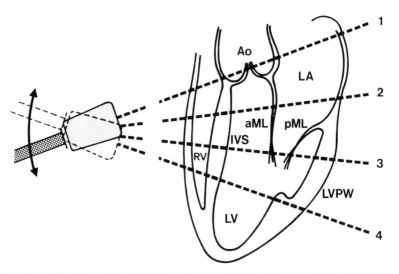

Figure 2. Same schematic cross section of the heart as shown in Figure 1, demonstrating the manner in which the transducer is swept from the aorta (direction 1) towards the apex (direction 4) to perform a sector scan (for abbreviations see Figure 1).

section with its true anatomic relationships is attractive. This has been achieved with the use of a multi-element transducer array.[1] Twenty elements incorporated in one transducer are placed in front of the cardiac cross section under exploration. Starting at the top, each element in sequence is used to produce a single sound beam. The echoes from the underlying cardiac structures are displayed in the B-mode (Fig. 1). While the sound beam is being scanned across the transducer probe, an image is simultaneously being created on the display oscilloscope screen, and the horizontal lines are traced in the same relative position as each sound beam arising from the transducer. Very rapid electronic switching permits instantaneous visualization of the cross section under observation.

Resulting images obtained from a normal individual are shown in Figure 4. The right end edges of the simultaneously recorded ECG indicates the timing of the image within the cardiac cycle. In these images the effects of motion are eliminated but the echo signals are displayed in "correct anatomic orientation" at that particular moment. As a consequence, this stop-action image directly resembles the anatomic appearance of the whole cross section under study at that particular moment, while the M-mode echocardiogram does not. Carrying the development one step further, the two-dimensional system displays the motion of all echo signals in their correct anatomic orientation when time is introduced. Thus, real-time two-dimensional images yield morphologic, anatomic, and functional information simultaneously, whereas the M-mode sector scan only yields dynamic information of selected parts of structures. For these

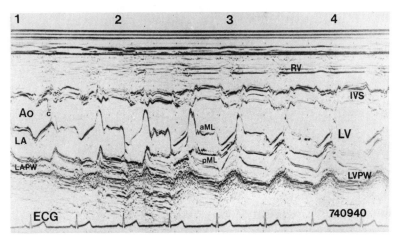

Figure 3. M-mode scan of the heart. The directions of the sound beam labelled 1 to 4 on the diagram of figure 2 correspond to the areas labelled 1 to 4 on this record.

338

reasons, an M-mode recording is more likely to demonstrate functional and physiologic abnormalities, while two-dimensional techniques are more able to visualize gross anatomic and structural abnormalities. As a result, the techniques are complementary and mutually supportive in the applications where anatomy and function overlap.

Any individual element of the multi-element transducer array can be selected, and the echo information, being in the B-mode on its display axis, can be recorded in the M-mode. This combines the

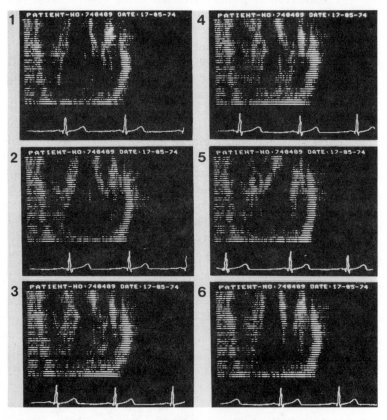

Figure 4. Six long-axis cross sections demonstrating the dynamic events of the normal mitral valve. For orientation see diagram of Figure 1. The right end of the electrocardiogram in each frame indicates the timing of the cross section within the cardiac cycle. At end-diastole (frame 1), the anterior mitral valve leaflet closes in a superior and posterior direction and remains in that position throughout systole (frames 2 to 4). At end-systole, the left ventricle is markedly smaller. In early diastole (frame 5) the anterior mitral valve leaflet opens and moves anteriorly towards the septum. In mid-diastole (frame 6) it is in its neutral position in the prolongation of the posterior aortic wall.

two-dimensional orientation facility with the detailed analysis of cardiac structures. In Figure 5, the example is shown where a crystal whose sound beam passes the mitral valve is selected. The situation is comparable to the diagram of Figure 1. The echo information received by the crystal is displayed in the B-mode on the cross sectional image. Hardly any information is present on that isolated axis, whereas the actual position of the entire mitral valve is visualized on the image. Thus, at any moment, much more data (i.e., a complete section of the heart) are present on the cross-sectional display. However, when time is added to the scanty information present on the selected line, the

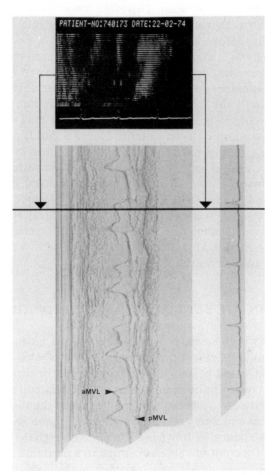

Figure 5. End-diastolic stop-action image obtained from a normal individual. A single crystal of the transducer is selected and its echo information, being in the B-mode on the two-dimensional image, is represented as a function of time on the tracing below. The motion pattern of the mitral valve is nicely tracked.

motion pattern of that part of the valve hit by the sound beam is nicely tracked (Fig. 5). The advantage is that the ultrasonic beam path is now identified, and distortions can be accounted for. Thus, more accurate dimensional measurements should be possible, as one knows exactly how the sound beam intersects the structures. This example also strikingly demonstrates that basically the same echo information is used for two apparently different types of display.

Real-time visualization of an entire cardiac cross section results in images which look directly familiar to those with some previous knowledge of cardiac anatomy. This can hardly be said from an M-mode sector scan. Therefore, two-dimensional echocardiography is attractive and explains the increasing interest in echo techniques today. However, it also poses more serious problems for recording, analysis, and interpretation. Indeed, at each instant, much more data are present on one single frame as compared to the M-mode record. This makes instantaneous analysis extremely difficult. The problem is exactly the same as encountered in quantitative angiocardiography, where the analysis of videolines rather than the complete image is now accepted as an easier and more accurate process.[5] Echocardiography actually started with a single-element recording, and quantitative analysis of, for example, the motion pattern of the mitral valve, remains easier on such a one-dimensional display recorded on a handy paper strip. Furthermore, the M-mode record obtained from any selected crystal of the multicrystal array is completely analogous to videotechniques, where the data of a selected videoline are represented as a function of time to track motion patterns of the LV wall or cardiac valves (Fig. 5).

PITFALLS IN THE ULTRASONIC ANALYSIS OF THE MITRAL VALVE

With an ideal "pencil-like" sound beam, the recorded echoes should represent the correct position of each reflecting structure in that sound beam axis. Unfortunately, the ultrasound beam spreads out over a finite angle, which limits the lateral resolution of presently used echo systems. This may result in the display of off-axis structures and thus problems in interpreting the record.[6] This problem is schematically shown in Figure 6. Although the labeled parts 1, 2, and 3 of the mitral valve are struck in a predominantly vertical manner, they are seen behind each other on the display axis. On the M-mode record, they will be recorded as multiple parallel echoes. A clinical example obtained from a patient with an atrial septal defect of the secundum type is shown in Figure 7. The valve was found to be

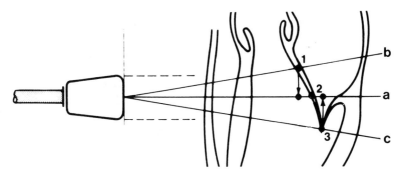

Figure 6. Diagrammatic representation of the mitral valve with a single element transducer in front. The main beam (a) passes through the valve at position 2. However, due to the finite beam width, part of the energy along the directions b and c will also encounter the valve at positions 1 and 3. Thus, different parts of the valve which are side by side will be displayed behind each other, resulting in spurious parallel moving echoes on the M-mode display.

completely normal during open heart surgery, although the multiple mitral valve echoes during systole could suggest mitral valve disease. Thus, the echographic separation of structures does not necessarily mean anatomic separation, and all echoes seen on the display do not necessarily correspond to an anatomical structure. On a two-dimensional display, the off-axis echoes may result in some distortion

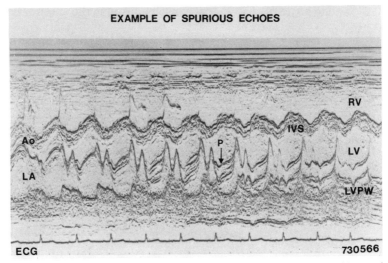

EXAMPLE OF SPURIOUS ECHOES

Figure 7. Example of spurious echoes (P) of the mitral valve in a patient with an atrial septal defect (type secundum). The valve was found to be normal during open heart surgery. (Ao = aorta; IVS = interventricular septum; LA = left atrium; LV = left ventricle; LVPW = left ventricular posterior wall; RV = right ventricle).

of structures, and thus of the mitral valve as well. With each single element, multiple adjacent parts of the same valve leaflet are displayed as if they are behind each other. The effect shown in Figure 6 is thus multiplied and a "verticalization-effect" results on cross sectional images. This is demonstrated on the stop frame of Figure 8, which was obtained from a normal individual in end-diastole. Note the peculiar display of the mitral valve seen as multiple vertical rows of echoes. The valve seems to be distorted and appears much thicker than the thin structure it really is. Viewing the moving images alleviates some of these problems, since the eye-brain system is unsurpassed in integration.

CROSS SECTIONAL STUDY OF THE MITRAL VALVE

The Normal Mitral Valve

The normal anterior mitral valve leaflet appears as a freely moving structure which opens anteriorly towards the septum in early diastole. It closes partially to its neutral position (i.e., in the prolongation of the posterior aortic root and parallel with the chest wall), and reopens during atrial systole. After ventricular activation, it closes primarily in early systole by a posterior and superior movement against the posterior leaflet which serves as a baffle. The movement of the posterior valve, less conspicuous than the anterior leaflet, varies

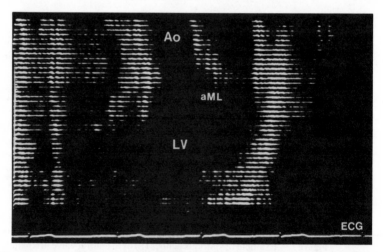

Figure 8. The summation of the spurious echoes on the display axis of each single crystal results in a "verticalization pattern" of the mitral valve. As a consequence, it appears on a two-dimensional display as a much thicker structure than it is in reality.

considerably between individuals, but always has a lesser amplitude, as it is a much smaller structure. When seen, it moves in the opposite direction to the anterior leaflet. It is impossible to define the free edges of the valve leaflets, and they appear as continuous structures with the papillary muscles, including the chordae tendineae. The dynamic events of the normal mitral valve are demonstrated on the six frames of Figure 4.

Mitral Stenosis

In mild mitral stenosis, valve motion becomes jerky or stiff, with decreased amplitude. This is most marked in its midportion, which normally shows the largest amplitude of motion. This part bulges anteriorly throughout diastole in this condition.[4] Other abnormalities, consistent with and as a result of mitral stenosis such as the dilatation of the left atrial and right ventricular cavities, are directly appreciated. The latter is of course only seen in cases with severe mitral stenosis. Here the leaflets move as a unit and appear often as dense, thickened echoes as a consequence of fibrosis and/or calcification. In these cases, the slow filling rate of the left ventricle can be appreciated when one watches the left ventricular walls during diastole. In a recent study, it has been reported that one could directly measure the mitral valve orifice from cross sectional images.[7] Up to now we have not been able to confirm this experience.

Left Atrial Myxoma

The characteristic appearance of an atrial myxoma is that of a mass of echoes behind the mitral valve in diastole when the tumor prolapses through the valve. The resultant obstruction to left atrial emptying produces a motion pattern of the valve similar to that seen with mitral stenosis. Cross sectional study is very helpful for the diagnosis, as the tumor can be followed throughout the cardiac cycle; often this is not possible with the single-element technique.

Dilated Cardiomyopathy

It seems from multiscan observation that mitral valve mechanics are altered because of the stretched valve apparatus by left ventricular dilatation in congestive cardiomyopathy. The reduced, vibrating motion pattern of the mitral valve, of which both leaflets are nearly

344

always distinguishable, is striking, and it appears as if the valve cannot close in systole. Ring dilatation seems an unlikely explanation of the mitral regurgitation in these patients. Furthermore, the left ventricular shape in this condition becomes globular, with reduced motion amplitude of the walls (low ejection fraction). It should be emphasized that appreciation of left ventricular shape is a unique capability of a two-dimensional system.[4]

Asymmetric Septal Hypertrophy

Most of the typical features of this asymmetric type of hypertrophic cardiomyopathy are easily demonstrated using a two-dimensional system. The disease manifests with and without outflow obstruction (idiopathic hypertrophic subaortic stenosis), and the difference lies chiefly in a functional and not an anatomic abnormality, although some structural differences have been reported recently.[8] In patients with idiopathic hypertrophic subaortic stenosis, there is pathognomonic abnormal systolic anterior movement of the anterior mitral valve leaflet, which narrows the outflow tract of the

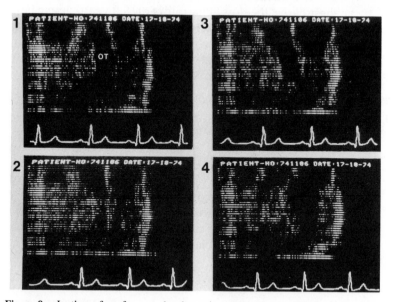

Figure 9. In these four frames, the dynamic events of the mitral valve are demonstrated in a case of asymmetric septal hypertrophy with outflow obstruction (idiopathic hypertrophic subaortic stenosis). In early systole (frame 1), the anterior mitral leaflet is in its closed position and the outflow tract (OT) wide open. In midsystole (frame 2), the valve is in an anterior position, close to the septum. This causes narrowing of the outflow tract. The valve returns to its closed position in late systole (frame 3) to open again normally in early diastole (frame 4).

left ventricle and impedes the ejection of blood. This is demonstrated by the cross sectional images obtained from a patient with idiopathic hypertrophic subaortic stenosis in Figure 9. In early systole, the valve is closed in a posterior and superior position. However, it reopens in mid-systole and is in apposition to the septum, which bulges into the left ventricular cavity, giving it its abnormal shape.[4] The outflow tract becomes narrowed, and a pressure gradient results. In late systole, the valve recloses for a short time, and opens normally in early diastole. In Figure 10, stop frame images of a patient with asymmetric septal hypertrophy without outflow obstruction are shown. In this condition the mitral valve remains closed throughout systole, and the outflow tract stays wide open.

Prolapsing Mitral Valve

A prolapsing anterior mitral valve exhibits a flailing exaggeration of the normal diastolic movement, and in some cases actual prolapse of the anterior leaflet past the posterior leaflet is seen during systole. This pendular motion is so typical that the diagnosis is easy. Assessment of the posterior mitral valve leaflet has been found very difficult in this condition.

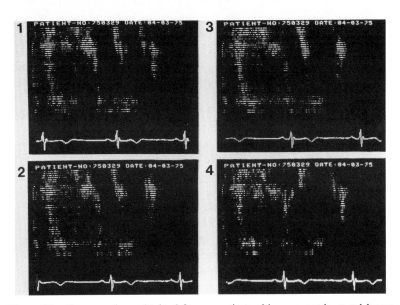

Figure 10. Cross sections obtained from a patient with asymmetric septal hypertrophy without obstruction of the outflow tract. The anterior mitral valve leaflet remains closed throughout systole and the outflow tract wide open (frames 1 to 3). The valve opens normally in early diastole and touches the septum (frame 4).

CONCLUSION

Because of its non-invasive nature and highly favorable benefit-to-risk ratio, ultrasonic two-dimensional imaging of the heart may eventually become the principal method for visualization of intracardiac structures and for studying their function. Multiple element echocardiography is a valuable extension of the single element technique. The additional information it provides relates to the dimensional relationships in time, although at present, for a quantitative study of the motion patterns, analysis of a single dimension will undoubtedly remain the best approach.

REFERENCES

1. Bom, N., Lancee, C.T., van Zwieten, G., Kloster, F.E., Roelandt, J. Multiscan echocardiography. I. Technical description. *Circulation* 48:1066, 1973.

2. Kloster, F.E., Roelandt, J., ten Cate, F.J., Bom, N., Hugenholtz, P. Multiscan Echocardiography. II. Technique and Initial clinical results. *Circulation* 48:1075, 1973.

3. Roelandt, J., Kloster, F.E., ten Cate, F.J., Bom, N., Lancée, C.T., Hugenholtz, P.G. Multiscan echocardiography. Description of the system and initial results in 100 patients. *Heart Bull.* 4:51, 1973.

4. Roelandt, J., Kloster, F.E., ten Cate, F.J., van Dorp, W.G., Honkoop, J., Bom, N., Hugenholtz, P.G. Multidimensional echocardiography. An Appraisal of its clinical usefulness. *Brit. Heart J.* 36:29, 1974.

5. Schelbert, H.R., Kreuzer, H., Dittrich, J., Schmiel, F.K., Loogen, F. A videotechnique for recording continuously left ventricular wall motion and changes in wall thickness. *Am. Heart J.* 87:597, 1974.

6. Roelandt, J., van Dorp, W.G., Bom, N., Laird, J.D., Hugenholtz, P.G. Resolution problems in echocardiology. A source of interpretation of errors. *Am. J. Cardiol.*, in press.

7. Henry, W.L., Griffith, J.M., Michaelis, L.L., McIntosh, C.L., Morrow, A.G., Epstein, S.E. Measurement of mitral orifice area in patients with mitral valve disease by real-time, two-dimensional echocardiography. *Circulation* 51:827, 1975.

8. Henry, W.L., Clark, C.E., Griffith, J.M., Epstein, S.E. Mechanism of left ventricular outflow obstruction in patients with obstructive asymmetric septal hypertrophy (idiopathic hypertrophic subaortic stenosis). *Amer. J. Cardiol.* 35:337-345, 1975.

30 Diagnosis of Mitral Valve Disease Using Doppler Echocardiography*

Donald W. Baker, BSEE
Steve L. Johnson, M.D.

INTRODUCTION

A new ultrasonic device is being developed which promises to provide new insight into the performance of the normal and diseased mitral valve. This new device, called a pulsed ultrasonic Doppler,[1,2] processes signals which are present in any pulse echo machine but which have not been previously analyzed.

The physical characteristics of the mitral valve can be described in terms of two components. The first relates to the physical structure of the valve apparatus and the motion of the leaflets. The second component of the valve performance, previously neglected, is the detection and analysis of blood flow traveling through the valve orifice, during either mitral systole or mitral diastole for the evaluation of stenosis or regurgitation. Pulsed echo techniques have been thoroughly described in the literature for assessing the motion of the mitral valve leaflet during a variety of clinical circumstances.[3] A

* Supported by NIH Grants HL-07293-14, HL-13517-04.

catalog of valve motions has been developed and serves as a reference for the detection of abnormal valve displacements. In certain clinical situations the data produced by pulsed echo techniques represent nearly an optimal measurement of the valve performance, bordering on what might be called a gold standard. The apparent success of this approach does not necessarily mean this is the best method to evaluate all of the mitral valve characteristics.

Doppler techniques are another approach which may allow more direct measurement of important clinical or physical variables and which will provide additional insight into the performance of the valve. Blood flow through the mitral valve orifice certainly should be a very direct indicator of mitral valve performance, since it is the purpose of the valve to allow flow with low pressure drop into the left ventricle during diastole and to prevent backflow into the left atrium during systole. While mitral stenosis may be easily evaluated using pulsed echo techniques, mitral regurgitation is relatively difficult to detect. The assessment of mitral valve disease using conventional auscultatory techniques can often be misleading in the presence of aortic insufficiency, tricuspid stenosis, or pulmonic stenosis; the timing of these sounds in the cardiac cycle can coincide with the sounds of mitral stenosis or mitral regurgitation. It would be very convenient to be able to differentiate between these various valve dysfunctions.

The flow patterns through the mitral valve are very complex, since they are a function of both time and of space. These flow signals are further complicated by a wide range of characteristics, ranging from smooth, ''well-behaved'' laminar-type flow to turbulent or ''disturbed'' flows. The signal patterns produced by this variety of flow patterns require special equipment to detect, and will require some period of time to evaluate and understand clinically.

DOPPLER PRINCIPLES

The pulsed ultrasonic Doppler device is a new development which is significantly different from a conventional pulse echo machine. Its functional characteristics can be easily compared to pulse echo methods. In Figure 1 an example is shown with the pulsed Doppler transducer pointed in the direction of a blood vessel. Immediately below the transducer is the raw echo pattern that might be seen on the oscilloscope trace. Notice that there are echo artifacts which occur at the instant of the transmit time, and that there are large echoes produced by the walls of the vessel. If the device is equipped for echo detection, then the signal processing serves to outline the envelope of the raw echo pattern on the right side of the illustration. The smoothed wave form corresponding to the echo envelope is called the video signal. The position of the wall echo is readily apparent. This simple detection process provides information mainly

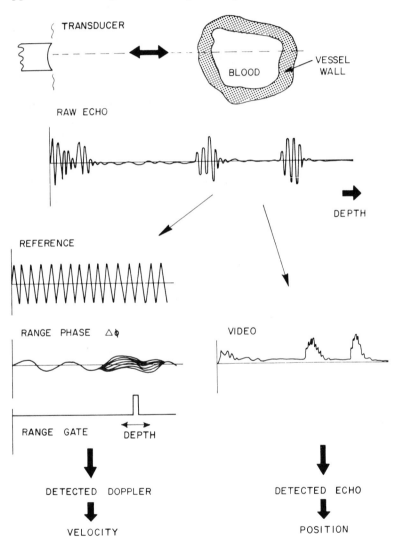

Figure 1. The raw echo signal from tissue structures can be analyzed simultaneously for both the position and velocity of an interface.

about the position of interfaces. Pulse echo systems designed for evaluation of valve motion show the echo video signal on a TM or time-motion type display. On this display, shown in Figure 2, interface depth is presented on the vertical axis, time on the horizontal axis, and the amplitude of the echo on the Z or intensity axis. As the valve leaflet moves through its normal cycle, the distance from the interface to the transducer will vary, shifting the timing of the echo. Recording the displacement of this echo as a function of time will produce a record of the motion or displacement of the valve leaflet. Using this recording method makes it very easy to study mitral valve leaflet motion. The clinical diagnosis in this case is based on the particular motion characteristics of the valve.

The Doppler detection of flow can be derived from the same raw echo signal. When the echo is compared to a reference signal corresponding to the original transmitted frequency, it is possible to detect the velocity of the interface at a selected depth along the sound beam. This is done by detecting the amount that the echo frequency is shifted from the transmitted frequency due to the interface motion. This comparison is accomplished in a phased detector. The output of the phased detector produces a signal called the range phase, shown on the left, Figure 1. If there is motion, i.e., velocity, then the range phase will be modulated according to the velocity. A range gate is set to sample the range phase signal at a particular depth corresponding to the time delay for the transmitted burst to travel to the interface and return. This rate of travel corresponds to 13 μsec of delay per cm of depth. The fluctuation frequency of the range phase corresponds to the Doppler difference frequency. This sampled output is then filtered

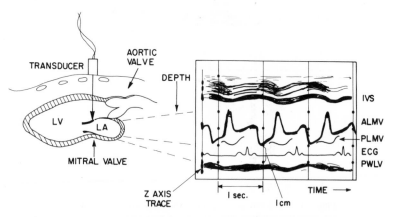

Figure 2. The motion of the mitral valve is mapped out using a Time Motion "TM" display.

and is called the detected Doppler signal. The frequency of this signal corresponds to the velocity of the interface. It is apparent that the original raw echo signal can be processed in two ways. The simplest or echo method gives us the position information, and the more complex frequency comparison scheme leads to the detection of the Doppler shift corresponding to the velocity.

In the pulsed Doppler device being described in this chapter, we are concerned with the detection of the Doppler shift due to the movement of blood flow through the mitral valve orifice. While it would be highly desirable to quantitate the flow velocity and the volume flow rates through the valve orifice both for stenosis and regurgitation, this goal is still beyond our present knowledge. Less quantitative but equally useful applications have been found for this technique based on the use of our hearing and mental processes to evaluate the Doppler signal. Fortunately velocities in the range of 0 to 100 cm per second will produce Doppler shifts in the range of 0 to about 5 kHz for a 3 mHz carrier. These frequencies are audible and can be utilized to evaluate the temporal and spatial characteristics of the flow signals. In Figure 3 we can see an example of how these flow signals might vary as we shift the depth of the Doppler sample volume (sensing point) through a flow constriction. On the left of the illustration in the region where the flow is accelerating due to the Venturi effect, we would find that the Doppler spectrum would be relatively

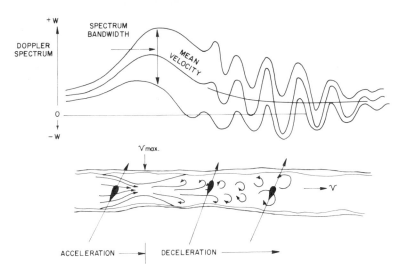

Figure 3. The Doppler spectrum is a very sensitive indicator of the characteristics of blood flow within the tear-drop sample volume. The more disturbed the flow, the wider the spectrum.

narrow due to the small velocity gradient that would be present within the teardrop-shaped sample volume region. As the streamlines proceed through the orifice, a point of maximum velocity is reached, producing a broad Doppler spectrum as turbulence develops. Downstream, distal from the occlusion, flow begins to decelerate and vortices or eddies will be formed. These will start small and gradually increase in size while translating downstream. These vortices and eddies will produce velocity components within the sample volume which are both toward and away from the transducer at the same time. This produces two effects. One, the spectrum bandwidth increases, and two, as the vortices become larger they will actually rotate through the sample volume so there will be an apparent flow reversal, shown by the oscillating pattern in the upper half of the illustration. These flow characteristics form the basis for the current clinical application of pulsed Doppler techniques.

PRINCIPLES OF CURRENT CLINICAL APPLICATION

Quantitation of blood flow through the valve orifices will require the measurement of the flow stream cross-sectional area, the instantaneous average velocity over the flow lumen, and the angle between the sound beam axis and the flow velocity vector.[4] The measurement of all these variables is well beyond the capability of present instrumentation. Techniques are in development to accomplish these measurements; however, other useful clinical applications have been found short of achieving these long-term developments. From the previous example we can see that smooth, well-behaved flow will produce a smooth, tonal-like Doppler signal of relatively narrow spectral width, whereas disturbed or turbulent flow associated with vortices and eddies produces a wide range of velocities and a corresponding broadening of the Doppler spectrum. The presence of "turbulence" has the effect of adding a harsh sound to the Doppler signal. This harsh, white-noise type characteristic is readily distinguishable from the smooth tonal quality of the signal for so-called normal flows. Because this distinction is easy to make with the ear, this leads to several practical applications of the listen-only output from the Doppler device. These simple analytic procedures have led to a number of significant clinical findings.

The method that has been used in the evaluation of mitral valve disease is relatively straightforward.[5] The pulse Doppler sample volume is positioned within the left atrium close to the mitral valve orifice. The characteristic normal flow signal has a systolic component due to left atrial inflow from the pulmonary veins, and a dyastolic flow signal that peaks early in diastole due to rapid left atrial emptying. It may also peak in late diastole due to the "A" wave. These normal flow signals have a tone-like quality with a narrow frequency bandwidth, indicating a relative lack of turbulence. In mitral regurgitation the harsh, wide frequency band with the systolic signal can be detected. If the regurgitation is minimal, this abnormal jet is well localized and of low intensity. In moderate to severe regurgitation the abnormal jet can be detected over a much larger region of the left atrium, and is often heard in the left atrium posterior to the aortic valve. In addition to this spatial dispersion, the intensity of the signal is also proportional to the severity of the mitral regurgitation.

A preliminary investigation of the accuracy of pulsed Doppler detection of mitral regurgitation has been completed involving 86 patients who were studied by echo and Doppler procedures preceding the cardiac catheterization. There were 9 true positives and 29 true negatives, with a significant number of false positives and false negatives. Four of the 7 false positives had a very faint, well-localized jet of mitral regurgitation, and it is possible that they could have been missed with cardiac catheterization. There were 11 false negatives; 4 of these 11 patients were described as having faint, well-localized "whiffs" of mitral regurgitation that were present only with premature ventricular contractions. In another 2 patients there was disagreement as to the presence or absence of regurgitation in the angiograms. The remaining 5 patients all had mitral stenosis, and we have since learned that the minimal or mild regurgitation often present in these patients is difficult to detect without a thorough pulse Doppler examination. While the preliminary study was performed with the original cardiac pulsed Doppler unit, a new model is now being used with improved signal-to-noise ratio and improved penetration, so we now obtain a much higher quality signal from the left atrium. Our current impression is that the pulsed Doppler is far more accurate in the detection of mitral regurgitation than the above study would indicate, and we are in the process of repeating this study. Even with the original study, all of the false negative results were in patients described as having minimal (9 patients) or mild (2 patients) regurgitation. The principal difficulty of this clinical approach is in the fact that the analysis of the signal is almost an art. There is no hard-copy graphical record made which can be passed on to other physicians for their interpretation and for inclusion into the patient's records. It would be very desirable to have a hard-copy record to document the procedure in a fashion which is possible with the pulse echo devices.

HARD-COPY GRAPHICAL RECORDINGS OF MITRAL VALVE SIGNALS

The record format which many have become accustomed to in interpreting the pulse echo exam would be a good example to follow for the development of a graphical record from the pulsed Doppler device. An example of a new readout scheme for recording these signals is shown in Figure 4. This is another new development which has not been completely evaluated, but will serve to show examples of mitral valve flow wave forms as we are currently able to record them. The validity of the flow waveforms has not been established, and they are presented as examples only. It should be possible to recognize similarities in the mitral valve flow waveforms to those previously recorded from experimental animal preparations using electromagnetic flowmeters. The top half of the record is devoted to a Doppler TM type of display which is essentially identical to the echo TM display. The display has centimeter calibration markers for depth, and half-second time markers. The path of motion of the mitral valve echo is shown, and the heavy line at the depth of the mitral valve orifice indicates the location of the Doppler sample volume. The TM portion of the record is helpful in identifying the flow detection site.

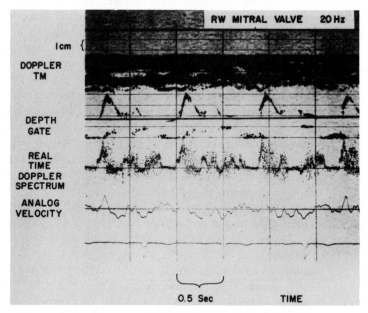

Figure 4. A new recording format for the pulse Doppler shows both the echo type TM display plus the flow signals detected at the location of the depth gate.

Immediately below the TM record in the figure is a plot showing the real-time Doppler spectrum. The spectrum analyzer[4] measures and analyzes the time interval between each zero crossing of the raw Doppler signal. Because of the complex nature of the raw Doppler signal, the interval of the zero crossing will vary in a fashion which corresponds to the frequency spectrum of the Doppler signal. Therefore, a recording of the spectrum of the zero crossing intervals will be analogous to the Doppler spectrum derived from using more rigorous analytical methods, for example the Fast Fourier Transform (FFT). In the real-time Doppler spectrum examples, the display consists of a dot pattern in which each dot corresponds to an actual zero crossing event. The vertical axis corresponds to the Doppler shift, the horizontal axis corresponds to the time base, and the dark pattern corresponds to the spectral distribution of the signal as a function of time. Narrow-band or tonal-like signals produce a narrow dot pattern. Noisy, broad-band signals associated with stenosis produce a broad dot pattern as shown in Figure 5 for pulmonic stenosis. The next lower tracing of the illustration shows the analog velocity. This waveform corresponds to the mean frequency of the instantaneous spectrum and is analogous to the conventional zero crossing analog output available on most continuous wave Doppler devices. In the

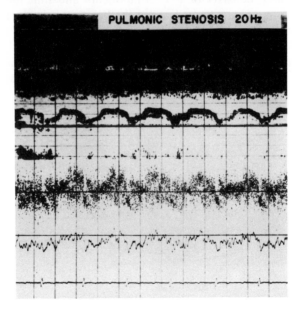

Figure 5. Pulmonic stenosis produces a flow jet which causes a wide-band Doppler signal as indicated by the broad dot pattern.

examples to be presented we will be concerned with both of these signals. The real-time Doppler spectrum will show the spectral broadening due to the detection of turbulence, and the analog velocity will show the general trend in velocity as well as motion effects of the cardiac structures.

Figure 6 shows another example of the Doppler TM record in which the various components of the display are associated with the physical structure of the heart, the location of the sound beam, and the pulse Doppler apparatus. If one looks closely at the analog velocity waveforms one will notice that there is a low frequency periodic motion of a sinusoidal character in the signal. This low frequency periodic motion is attributed to the motion of the mitral valve apparatus throughout the cardiac cycle. The lower trace of Figure 6 shows the electrocardiogram for a timing reference. We can see that the mitral valve flow tract moves anterior in systole and posterior in diastole. We will also notice that the flow through the mitral valve occurs during the period in which the mitral valve outflow tract is moving posteriorly. There are two components to the flow wave form as recorded transcutaneously, the initial ejection followed by a brief delay, and then the waveform associated with the atrial kick. Yellin[6] and others have shown that the flow waveform through the mitral valve consists of two components and that the spacing of these components depends upon the heart rate. In the example, the heart rate is approximately 60 beats per minute, which results in an appreciable gap between the two flow components. Had the heart rate been higher, one might have anticipated that the atrial kick component would have fused with the initial mitral ejection pattern. No examples

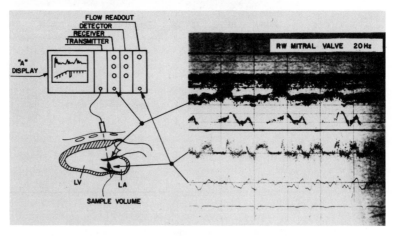

Figure 6. Functional relationship between pulse Doppler, heart, and display.

of these circumstances have been recorded to date. Many examples will have to be recorded and analyzed before the true mitral valve flow patterns for transcutaneous measurement will be known.

A particular problem of this measurement technique is that the system is sensitive to the total velocity of blood with respect to the transducer which is located on the chest wall. This means that motion of the heart is added to the flow velocity components. This is very apparent in the real-time spectral plot in Figure 7, where one can observe the low frequency motion component superimposed on the flow component.

Close examination of the real-time spectral pattern in the graphic recording reveals variations in spectral broadening which may be associated with disturbed flow. In following the real-time spectral pattern along its time course in Figure 7, we see that the dot pattern broadens significantly in the interval between the initial mitral valve ejection and the atrial kick. It is conceivable that there are backflow eddies in the valve orifice or around the leaflets of the valves at this instant which are detected by the Doppler device. These are shown as a spread in the Doppler spectrum. We also notice in ventricular systole that there is a broadening of the spectral pattern in the left

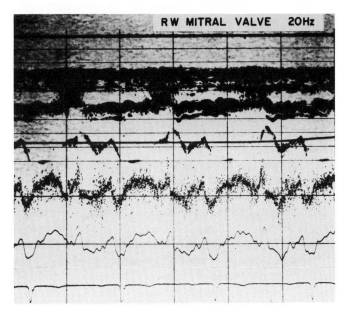

Figure 7. Doppler readout for mitral valve flow signals with superimposed cardiac AP motion. Slight spectral broadening occurs between initial ventricular filling and atrial kick.

ventricular outflow track near the mitral valve apparatus. The implications of these findings are not clearly understood.

DIFFERENTIAL DIAGNOSIS OF OTHER MIMICKING SIGNALS

Conventional auscultatory examination of the heart for mitral disease can, on occasion, lead to an erroneous conclusion. This is particularly true in cases of mitral stenosis when there may be a possibility of aortic insufficiency or tricuspid stenosis. Similarly, in evaluation of mitral regurgitation, incidences of pulmonic stenosis may also obscure the desired signal. Severe cases of emphysema or altered pulmonary function may produce passageway sounds which can mask the mitral valve signals. The pulse Doppler device is particularly useful in differentiating mitral valve disease from these other clinically common situations. The sample volume of the pulse Doppler device measures approximately 2 × 4 mm and is an extremely sensitive point sensor. With experience it can be positioned directly in the outflow track or in the backflow region of any of the valves of the heart. The echo pattern and its motion are helpful in assuring the physician that the sound beam is in fact aimed at the structure he believes it to be. Examples of these echo patterns are shown in Figure 8a, b, and c. These are sequentially (a) the echo pattern for the aortic valve apparatus, for the detection of aortic stenosis, (b) the evaluation of aortic valve insufficiency, and (c) mitral regurgitation. It is quite apparent in these examples that the pattern for the aortic valve apparatus is quite different from that of the mitral valve apparatus. In the example, Figure 8c, the sample volume is located in the left atrium for the purpose of detecting mitral regurgitation. The echo pattern, along with the unique and readily distinguishable Doppler flow signal, makes the signature for mitral regurgitation clearly different from the signature for aortic stenosis or aortic insufficiency. In addition, the flow waveforms that can be recorded at these various sites are also quite different. Based on these data, it is relatively easy to rule out aortic insufficiency and tricuspid stenosis in the presence of mitral stenosis, or pulmonic stenosis in the presence of mitral regurgitation.

These are preliminary findings on the application of pulsed Doppler techniques in cardiology for the evaluation of mitral valve disease. A great deal of work needs to be done to optimize the approach and eventually to lead to some form of quantitation of the signals detected.

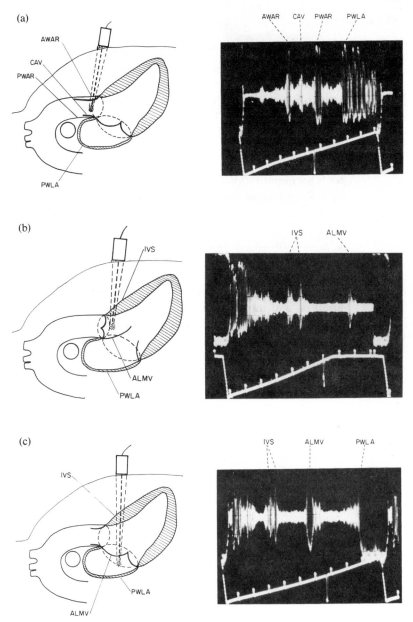

Figure 8. Typical echo patterns from three different flow sites. (a) aortic valve, AS, (b) Left ventricular outflow tract, AI, (c) left atrium, MR.

360

REFERENCES

1. Baker, D.W. Pulsed ultrasonic doppler blood flow sensing. IEEE Trans. on sonics and ultrasonics, Vol. SU-17, 3:170, 1970.

2. Peronneau, P., Hinglais, J., Pellet, M., and Leger, F. Velocitmetre sanguin par effet Doppler à emission ultrasonore pulsée. *L'onde Electrique* 50:369, 1970.

3. Feigenbaum, H. *Echocardiography*. Philadelphia: Lea and Febiger, 1973.

4. Baker, D.W., Johnson, S.L., and Strandness, E.E. Prospects for quantitation of transcutaneous pulsed Doppler techniques in cardiology and peripheral vascular disease. *Cardiovascular Applications of Ultrasound*. Amsterdam: North Holland Publishing Company, 1974.

5. Johnson, S.L., Baker, D.W., and Lute, R.A. Doppler echo cardiography: the localization of cardiac murmurs. *Circulation* 47:810, 1973.

6. Yellin, E.L., Laniado, S., Peskin, C., and Frater, R. Analysis and interpretation of the normal mitral valve flow curve: inertiance, resistance and compliance. International Symposium on the Mitral Valve, Paris, 1975.

DISCUSSION: PART VI

Dr. Tsakiris: A question to Dr. Popp. Recent information seems to indicate that mitral leaflet motion recorded by echocardiography may be delayed compared to the true time-motion of the leaflets, and that this delay may be unpredictable. Do you have any comments?

Dr. Popp: Yes, I believe the studies that we have done and that others have done prove that the signal that one receives from the echocardiograph is without delay from the event one is recording. However, the event that makes a sound, or makes some other correlated recording, may not be from the area we are visualizing with the sound beam. This is the point I was making: If one sees two leaflets come together on the echocardiogram we are only recording the element of motion which is within the sound beam, so if the leaflets come together and then move towards the atrium, and this is perpendicular to the sound beam, we have no way of recording that with a single element echocardiogram.

Dr. Tsakiris: And would you, then, record for instance the opening or the closing of the mitral valve several milliseconds later than it really happened?

Dr. Popp: If we are talking about an event stopping, then one part of the valve may start or stop before another part, and we could miss that slightly. This is why we try to see all areas of the valve with strip chart recording rather than look at one specific area and try to make comment.

Dr. Barlow: Dr. Popp has raised the possibility of silent prolapse being common. I am not sure that I really believe that. There is little doubt that for many years we all missed a lot of clicks, but when one gets more oriented to listening for them specifically, then one does hear more and more. I have a large number of patients referred to me for elucidation of abnormal electrocardiograms and of symptoms such as palpitations, chest pain, syncope, or anxiety, and it is our experience that if these patients are auscultated very carefully, and often with change in their posture such as standing, squatting, and lying in the left lateral position, then very many do, in fact, have clicks. I submit that a true silent prolapse is extremely rare.

Dr. Popp also made the interesting observation that, following an answer to a newspaper advertisement, he detected prolapse on echocardiography in 4 to 10% of 138 subjects. However, I doubt whether these numbers give an indication of the true prevalence in a normal population. I would have thought that his 138 subjects might well include some who did not disclose to him that they have had chest pain, are anxious, or have been aware of palpitations. I don't think anyone yet knows the true prevalence of the billowing mitral leaflet syndrome in a so-called normal population. Rizzon in Bari, Italy, auscultated several hundred young student girls and found an incidence of 0.33%. We have auscultated over 12,000 so-called normal Black school children on the outskirts of Johannesburg and found that the incidence of non-ejection clicks and late systolic murmurs was about 1.4%. These results, however, are probably affected by the fact that there is a high incidence of rheumatic heart disease in urban Blacks, and many of the children may have had rheumatic heart disease rather than the specific billowing leaflet syndrome.

Dr. Fawzi: I would like to ask Dr. Popp how many of his patients who have silent prolapse on echocardiography have evidence of prolapse on left ventricular angiography?

Dr. Popp: In the original series there were 20 patients, and 2 of the 20 had silent prolapse. All 20 had angiographic correlation. If one gives the majority of patients with clinically silent prolapse amyl nitrite one can develop some clicks or murmurs, but there are definitely some in whom this is not possible at any one time, yet they have anatomic prolapse by angiography.

Dr. Somerville: Dr. Popp, you can see the lively interest in silent prolapse. Of those who answered your advertisement, 4 percent had silent prolapse. However, you omitted the age. The importance of age was emphasized yesterday by a number of speakers, in that with increasing age, the left atrial floor approximates to the apex in systole, the chordae become lax, and mitral prolapse may occur.

Dr. Popp: The advertisement was in the campus newspapers at Stanford University, and we limited the applicants to females between the ages of 18 and 35. All of the patients were given a questionnaire on their health, and any who had previous heart disease of any type were excluded. All of the records were taken; examinations and recordings were done by one group; the phonocardiograms, electrocardiograms, echocardiograms were each read blind by a different group.

Dr. Thiron: I would like to put a question to Dr. Popp. Did you ever demonstrate any abnormal movement of the mitral valve leaflet under the effect of methoxamine? This mid-systolic click rarely occurs alone, and it is very common to notice the presence of a systolic murmur following the click by increasing the systolic blood pressure for example from 120 to 150 mm/hg using methoxamin. Did you have an opportunity to carry out echograms under isoproterenol or amyl nitrite, and did you see dyskinesia of the septum or of the left ventricular wall?

Dr. Popp: In answer to the first part of the question, we used hand grip as the afterload stimulus and studied the incidence of development of clicks, but we did not give isoproterenol or a drug of that type. In every patient that we have, the echocardiographic pattern of prolapse is the same at rest and whatever intervention we used. If it is there anatomically, it seems to be recorded echocardiographically. The purpose of our studies is to try to figure out what the valve is doing during all of these maneuvers. We have some results which do not fit into a nice pocket so far, and so we continue the analysis.

Dr. Carpentier: As a surgeon, I would like to make three points. First, regarding Dr. Roeland and Dr. Popp's papers. There may be a discrepancy between the interpretation of the echocardiogram and the findings at surgery. We must be careful in making correlations between findings at surgery and the echocardiogram, because during open heart surgery, the surgeon is faced with nonphysiological conditions which make the assessment of mitral regurgitation difficult.

Second, I would like to offer a possible explanation for the discrepancy sometimes found between the echocardiogram denoting a prolapse of the mitral valve and the angiogram which shows no evidence of mitral regurgitation. This may be due to a confusion between two different lesions which give a similar echocardiographic appearance: one is the *valve prolapse* of the mitral valve leaflet due either to elongation or rupture of the chordae which give mitral regurgitation. The other is the *valve ballooning* of the mitral valve due to excess valvular tissue with grossly normal chordae without regurgitation.

Third, I would like to end by saying that we, as surgeons, expect a great deal from the various methods of investigation because they should help us understand more fully the exact pathophysiological mechanisms involved in mitral valve disease, thereby leading us to develop better techniques for valvular reconstruction.

Dr. Hugenholtz: As Dr. Carpentier just said, surgeons, who are peculiar beings as we all know, do seem to like ultrasound very much.

Dr. Popp: Dr. Shumway and his colleagues are sometimes my most severe critics, but I think we are beginning to win them over.

And I totally agree that the diagnosis of mitral regurgitation is not something that can be made with the echocardiogram alone. One needs to use other techniques—as well as his own ears—to diagnose this. I think this is recognized as much by echocardiographers as by anyone else.

Dr. Sonnenblick: Perhaps Dr. Popp and Dr. Roelandt might comment on the use of echocardiography to follow up patients with mitral insufficiency regarding their ventricular function over a certain period.

Dr. J. Roelandt: Since the application of ultrasound is a safe and noninvasive procedure, it can be applied to the critically ill as well as to the ambulatory patient. The examination can be easily repeated and thus used to study patients with valvular heart disease (e.g., mitral insufficiency) postoperatively on a daily basis or over an extended time to follow the severity of the disease. However, two-dimensional real-time systems currently allow only a qualitative assessment of LV function from its size, shape, and wall motion. The assessment of LV shape is especially unique for the two-dimensional system. For a quantitative analysis, the conventional single element technique is still the method of choice because of its higher resolution and the fact that a hard copy is readily available.

Dr. Popp: There is some recent information from Dr. Henry's group at NIH in the United States that one can see serial changes in ventricular VCF, or ventricular change in dimensions within 5 to 10%, as a trend. But I don't think that anyone has done the study to see how sensitive this is to a deterioration in patients with valvular disease.

SUMMARY: PART VI

R.L. Popp, M.D.

The initial paper of this session by Dr. Pernod was a review of the wave form of the mitral valve in health and in several diseased states. This review gives a taste of the multiple uses of ultrasound in the recognition and quantitation of mitral valve disease as the primary diagnosis. In addition, the sampling of abnormal mitral valve diagnostic patterns in a great many cardiac pathologic states was nicely reviewed. The third paper gave examples of the extension of pulsed reflected ultrasound to study various pathophysiologic aspects of disease states, rather than simply recognizing the presence of the conditions. The exciting technique of Dr. Roelandt and associates has the great advantage of presenting pictures of the heart which are extremely recognizable to any cardiologist. As Dr. Roelandt mentioned, there are still some problems to be worked out regarding the resolution of the technique and the ability of clinicians to obtain quantitative information from records of this type.

Just as Dr. Roelandt's paper extends conventional pulsed reflected ultrasound to give added information above the normal echocardiogram, so Dr. Baker has added a new dimension to our diagnostic abilities. The addition of gated Doppler signals to echocardiography is extremely exciting. Obviously, further experience and refinement of the technique is indicated but one can certainly envision a great many patients in whom the diagnosis of mitral stenosis can be made with certainty using conventional techniques, and the presence and degree of mitral regurgitation could be quantitated using Doppler methods. In many such patients early diagnostic cardiac catheterization can be eliminated.

The paper on diagnosis of mitral prosthetic valve function demonstrates the use of echocardiography to supply information which is extremely hard to get by any other technique. However, because of the limitations of ultrasound in this area, the clinical impression, the phonocardiogram, and other objective tests are used best when integrated for the patient's benefit.

It is important to keep these papers in proper perspective; one must understand that the use of ultrasound is in its infancy in general, and that the presentations here give only a glimpse of what may be developed for patients and physicians over the next few years. The rapid growth of echocardiography as a diagnostic tool for mitral valve disease shows the enthusiasm with which clinicians accept noninvasive methods. It is almost certain that this attraction, coupled with the improvements of existing instruments made by sophisticated engineering techniques, will result in an ever increasing clinical demand for the family of diagnostic and investigative procedures that were presented in this session.

PART SEVEN

ASSESSMENT OF MITRAL VALVE DISEASE AND OF ASSOCIATED MYOCARDIAL FUNCTION

31 The Dynamic Determinants of Experimental Mitral Insufficiency

The Influence of Left
Ventricular Size, Shape,
and Contractility*

Edmund H. Sonnenblick, M.D.
David M. Borkenhagen, M.D.
Juan Serur, M.D.
Douglass Adams, M.D.
Richard Gorlin, M.D.

In mitral insufficiency, the mitral regurgitant flow or volume (MRV) is dependent on three identifiable factors: the area of the mitral regurgitant orifice (MRA), which is generally thought to be fixed in a given lesion at a given time, the systolic pressure gradient between the left ventricle and the left atrium (MRG), and the ventricular ejection period or interval (VSI). These variables have been expressed by the Gorlin formula as:

$$MRV = k \times MRA \times VSI \times \sqrt{MRG} \quad \text{where k is } 36^1$$

Were the MRG to be the only variable which changes significantly, MRF should be reasonably constant. However, we have been impressed with the fact that the clinical course followed by patients with rupture of a chordae tendineae accompanied by acute mitral regurgitation is quite variable, and seemingly massive early regurgitation may subsequently be reasonably well tolerated. Further in the clinical

* These studies were supported in part by NHLI Grant HL11306.

369

course of chronic mitral regurgitation secondary to chronic rheumatic valvular disease, ventricular shape and contractility may affect the ultimate clinical course which may be followed.[2]

Earlier approaches to the study of experimental mitral regurgitation have generally employed mechanical shunts across the mitral valve[3] or external shunts between the left ventricle and left atrium.[4,5] These studies have demonstrated that left ventricular performance can be well maintained in the face of very substantial amounts of mitral regurgitant flow, so long as left ventricular contractility is adequate. Furthermore, the decompression of the left ventricular flow into the low pressure outlet of the left atrium in early systole leads to a rapid reduction of ventricular size and hence wall tension, which produces a converse increase in velocity of wall motion and further enhanced ventricular emptying. This may be viewed as a positive feedback which helps sustain adequate ventricular function.[4] The experimental design of these studies, however, did not permit analysis of the contribution of ventricular size and shape to regurgitant orifice area and flow.

METHODS

In the present study, acute mitral regurgitation was induced in twelve anesthetized mongrel dogs (wt 20 to 31 kg) by passing a valvulectome (KIFA, Sweden) on a wire-guided catheter from the external jugular vein across the interatrial septum into the region of the mitral valve, excising a portion of the free edge of the leaflet and associated chordae. A semiquantitative estimate of the degree of regurgitation was made angiographically, and then studied by hemodynamic and cineangiographic methods. Although the dog's chest was closed, respiration was assisted and heart rate controlled by a pacing catheter in the coronary sinus.

Catheters were placed into the central aorta and left ventricle for the injection of angiographic dye and the measurement of aortic and left ventricular pressures. Left atrial and pulmonary artery pressures were also measured. Effective forward stroke volume was determined by the dye dilution method; 0.7 ml of indocyanine green was injected into the coronary sinus, while density changes in the pulmonary artery were measured with a Gilson densitometer.

Mean pressure gradient (MRG) in mm Hg across the mitral regurgitant orifice during ventricular systole was taken as the difference between mean systolic pressure in the left ventricle and left atrium. The ventricular systolic interval (VSI) in msec was measured from the onset systolic ventricular pressure to the decrotic notch on the aortic pressure curve.

Biplane left ventricular cineangiograms were performed in the 60° right anterior oblique and 30° left anterior oblique positions at 100 frames per second (Siemens Corp.). Ventricular volumes were calculated by the method of Dodge,[6] using the biplane diameters and the ventricular length in the right anterior oblique position. Mitral regurgitant volume (MRV) was calculated as the difference between total angiographic stroke volume and effective forward stroke volume. In 16 experiments, left ventricular forward stroke volume calculated from angiograms exceeded effective stroke volume determined from the right ventricle by dye dilution methods by 5.5%.

The mean area of the regurgitant orifice during systole (MRA) was calculated from the formula[1]:

$$\overline{MRA} = \frac{MRV}{VSI \cdot k \sqrt{MRG}}$$

where k equals the constant 36. Direct measurements of subvalvular diameter of the mitral valve were made extending from the superior margin of the left ventricular outflow tract to the inferior wall of the left ventricle near the inferior margin of the mitral annulus. The mitral annular diameter was measured from the insertion point superiorly of the anterior mitral leaflet into the fibrous skeleton of the heart to the insertion point inferiorly of the posterior leaflet into the annulus itself.

RESULTS

With the production of acute mitral regurgitation, the regurgitant volume (22 ± 2 ml/beat) was actually greater than the forward stroke volume (18 ± 2 ml/beat) with a calculated mitral regurgitant orifice area (MRA) of 0.41 ± 0.04 cm². Both in controlled mitral regurgitation and during the interventions to be described, the calculated $\overline{MRA}$ and its changes correlated well with directedly measured values of subvalvular diameters and mitral annular areas from cineangiograms. Nevertheless, this massive mitral regurgitation was well tolerated, with left ventricular end-diastolic pressure (LVEDP) remaining normal (< 13 mm Hg) in 11 of 12 animals, and left atrial mean pressure and atrial V waves averaging 8 ± 1 mm Hg and 13 ± 2 mm Hg respectively.

With the infusion of dextran to increase diastolic ventricular volume (Fig. 1), LVEDP increased from 5 ± 1 to 12 ± 2 mm Hg, while LV end-diastolic volume increased from 60 ± 7 to 88 ± 9 ml. Total ejection fraction was not altered significantly (0.63 vs. 0.65), although both forward stroke volume and MRV increased substantially from 18 ± 2 to 26 ± 5, and from 19 ± 2 to 35 ± 5 respectively. Left artrial pressure rose 160%, while MRG only rose an insignificant 6.5%. The 68% increase in regurgitant volume (MRV) was 4 times greater than the 17% increase predicted by the hydraulic formula for regurgitant flow were MRA to remain constant. Alternatively, MRA increased 44% from 0.34 ± 0.03 to 0.49 ± 0.08 cm², while mitral annular diameter measured from angiograms increased from 2.48 ± 0.17 to 2.96 ± 0.25 cm.

Angiotensin was infused to increase left ventricular systolic pressure (Fig. 2). Aortic pressure rose 23%, left ventricular peak pressure, 20%, and the MRG, 20%, from 114 ± 5 to 137 ± 2 mm Hg. The LVEDP rose from 9 ± 2 to 12 ± 3, while LV diastolic volume increased slightly from 68 ± to 79 ± 13 ml. Total ejection fraction rose insignificantly from 0.52 ± 0.05 to 0.63 ± 0.03, although effective forward stroke volume fell from 18 ± 3 to 14 ± 3, while MRV rose substantially from 18 ± 4 to 31 ± 3. The ventricular systolic time interval (VSI) decreased 14%, while left atrial pressure rose from 8 ± 2 to 11 ± 3 mm Hg. The 72% increase in MRV was several times larger than the increment predicted from the increase in MRG. The calculated MRA, however, increased 64% from 0.39 ± 0.08 to 0.64 ± 0.04

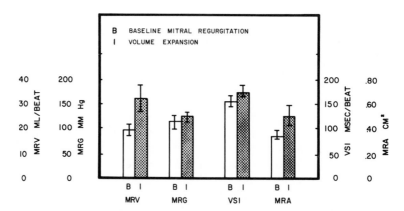

Figure 1. The effects of volume expansion on mitral regurgitation. The clear bar-graft illustrates the control state (B), while the hatched bar (I) shows the same values after the increment in ventricular volume induced by dextran administration. MRV = mitral regurgitant volume; MRG=mitral regurgitant gradient in systole; VSI=ventricular systolic interval; and MRA=calculated mitral regurgitant area. Volume expansion produced a substantial increase in MRV and MRA with trivial changes in MRG or VSI.

cm², while the measured annular diameter increased from 2.60 ± 0.20 to 2.97 ± 0.10 cm.

During inotropic stimulation with either epinephrine or calcium (Fig. 3), mean aortic pressure, left ventricular peak pressure, or the MRG did not change significantly. The LVEDP fell from 12 ± 3 to 8 ± 2, while the total ejection fraction rose slightly. However, the forward stroke volume rose from 18 ± 3 to 20 ± 5, while the MRV fell substantially from 29 ± 3 to 17 ± 2 ml. The VSI fell from 150 ± 10 to 140 ± 5 msec. The 41% decrease in MRV was decreased by 35% from 0.49 ± 0.06 to 0.32 ± 0.5 cm², while the measured mitral annular diameter was decreased from 2.62 ± 0.14 to 2.16 ± 0.08 cm.

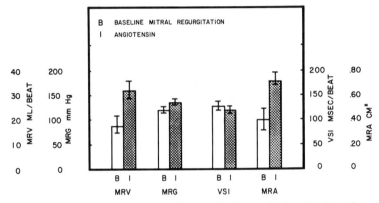

Figure 2. Effects of angiotensin infusion on mitral regurgitation. Angiotensin produced a small increase in MRG but induced a very large increase in MRV, which correlated with the increment in MRA.

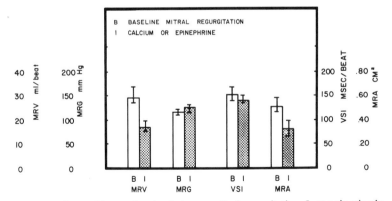

Figure 3. Effects of inotropic stimulation on mitral regurgitation. Inotropic stimulation produced a large decrease in MRV despite the fact that MRG rose. This decrease in MRV was only partly explained by a decrease in VSI, but was largely due to the decrease in MRA.

Assessment of relative ventricular shape in terms of eccentricity[2] indicated that both volume infusion and angiotensin administration made the ventricle assume a more globular or spherical form, while during inotropic stimulation the ventricle assumed a more eccentric or cylindrical shape.

DISCUSSION

We have found that acute mitral regurgitation produced experimentally in the dog is well tolerated, with trivial increments in left-sided filling pressures. This tolerance of massive regurgitation occurs so long as ventricular contractility is well maintained. These findings agree with prior studies where fixed amounts of regurgitation were produced in the open-chested dog.[4] Further, the unloading of volume into the atrium helps to reduce wall tension and hence facilitates further wall shortening.

We have also found that the amount of mitral regurgitation (MRV) is not fixed for a given lesion, but is increased by volume or pressure loading, and decreased by positive inotropic ventricular stimulation. To our surprise, these changes in MRV were not explained by changes in the mitral regurgitant gradient (MRG) or the ventricular systolic interval (VSI); however, they correlated well with changes in the mitral regurgitant area (MRA), which has been calculated from measured regurgitant volumes and pressures, or with alterations in sub-mitral valve diameter measured directly from bi-plane angiograms. Angiotensin, which increases the MRG, also produces a secondary increase in ventricular diastolic volume and hence MRA, and it appears that this increase in diastolic volume is vastly more important than the change in the gradient in augmenting MRF. The minor influence of MRG on the MRV also reflects the fact that the MRV is proportional to the square root of the gradient, but directly proportional to the MRA.[1]

These induced changes in MRA also correlate with changes in eccentricity of the ventricle, and it has long been held that ventricular dilatation itself may induce or worsen mitral regurgitation. We would suggest that the effective orifice for regurgitation includes the sub-mitral portion of the ventricular muscle,[7] so that decreasing ventricular volume by whatever means should tend to reduce MRF. Such a hypothesis would help to explain the salutary effects of reducing ventricular volume in acute mitral regurgitation such as occurs with ruptured chordae tendineae in humans. The reduction in ventricular size consequent to therapy may help to reduce the extent of regurgitation, while also reflecting an improved tolerance of the regurgitation.

Alternatively, an enlarging left ventricle may not only reflect a decrease in ventricular contractility for a given lesion, but also may serve to further increase the amount of regurgitation and place an added burden on an already compromised ventricle. Accordingly, ventricular dilatation generates further mitral regurgitation leading to further dilatation, while reduction in ventricular size, whether from inotropic stimulation or reduced volume or pressure load, will reduce the MRV, largely independent of mitral pressure gradients. Whether these principles are directly applicable to mitral regurgitation in humans has yet to be demonstrated, although we have shown that progressive increments in ventricular diastolic volume, a decreased ejection fraction, and globularity reflect a poor course in a given patient.

SUMMARY

Acute mitral regurgitation (MR) was produced in 12 closed-chest dogs by partial valvulectomy to determine the relative effects of MR pressure gradient (MRG), orifice area (MRA), and ventricular contractility on MR flow (MRF). Aortic, left ventricular, and left atrial pressures, bi-plane left ventricular (LV) angiography, forward flow (FF), and MRF were obtained following acute MR, during an angiotensin infusion to increase diastolic ventricular volume, and during calcium or epinephrine infusion to increase contractility.

Angiotensin increased the MRG substantially, but could only account for 20% of the observed increase in MRF, while MRF was highly correlated with LV end-diastolic (ed) basilar diameter, ed mitral annular diameter, and LV ed volume. The influence of LV morphology was also demonstrated by dextran infusion, which augmented LV ed volume and increased MRF substantially with a trivial change in MFG; augmentation of LV contractility increased the MRG, while reducing MRF concommitant with a reduction in sub-mitral valve dimensions.

It has been concluded that LV size and shape importantly effect MRF independent of MRG by changing MRA. These observations may help to explain the labile clinical picture observed in ruptured chordae tendineae in humans and the salutary effects of reducing ventricular end-diastolic volume as a result of vigorous therapy.

REFERENCES

1. Gorlin, R., and Dexter, L. Hydraulic formula for the calculation of the cross-sectional area of the mitral valve during regurgitation. *Am. Heart J.* 43: 188, 1952.

2. Vokonas, P.S., Gorlin, R., Cohn, P.F., Herman, M.V., and Sonnenblick, E.H. Dynamic geometry of the left ventricle in mitral regurgitation. *Circulation* 48: 786, 1973.

3. Braunwald, E., Welch, G., and Sarnoff, S. Hemodynamic effects of quantitatively varied experimental mitral regurgitation. *Circulation Research* 5: 539, 1957.

4. Urschel, C.W., Covell, S.W., Sonnenblick, E.H., Ross, J., Jr., Braunwald, E. Myocardial mechanics in aortic and mitral valvular regurgitation: The concept of instantaneous impedance as a determinant of the performance of the intact heart. *J. Clin. Invest.* 47: 867, 1968.

5. Urschel, C.W., Covell, J.W., Graham, T.P., Clancy, R.L., Ross, J. Jr., Sonnenblick, E.H. and Braunwald, E. Effects of acute valvular regurgitation on oxygen consumption of canine heart. *Circulation Research* 23: 33, 1968.

6. Dodge, H.T., Sandler, H., Baxley, W.A., Hawley, R.R. Usefulness and limitations of radiographic methods for determining left ventricular volume. *Am. J. Cardiol.* 18: 10, 1966.

7. Tsakaris, A.G., Sturm, R.E., and Wood, E.H. Experimental studies on the mechanisms of closure of cardiac valves with use of Roentgen videodensitometry. *Am. J. Cardiology* 32: 136, 1973.

32

Assessment of Mitral Regurgitation Using Indicator Dilution, Especially Roentgen-Densitometry

W. Rutishauser, M.D.
R. Simon, M.D.
A. Kléber, M.D.
J. Wellauer, M.D.

Upstream sampling methods are the most sensitive indicator-dilution techniques for assessment and quantitation of mitral regurgitation.[6,9] The fundamental relationship—flow × concentration × time = mass of indicator—can be used to derive mitral regurgitant flow. Indicator is injected downstream of the incompetent valve; the ratio of the areas of the resultant indicator-dilution curves inscribed in the upstream and downstream chambers is equal to the regurgitation fraction, which is defined as regurgitant flow in relation to total flow.[5,2] Total flow is equal to the sum of regurgitant and net forward flow. The mitral regurgitant fraction therefore equals the ratio of the areas of the left atrial and left ventricular (or aortic) indicator dilution curves.

The thermal dilution method—infusing cold saline into the left ventricle and sensing temperature with thermistors in the left atrium and in the aorta—is a typical upstream sampling technique for calculation of mitral incompetence. However, until recently we had not been able to check the accuracy of this method. From experience, we know that if sampling is confined to a point in the left atrium, the position of the sampling catheter is critical, since the indicator and blood do not mix completely. If the left atrial thermistor catheter is repositioned away from the mitral valve, the area of the left atrial curve may vary considerably.

Roentgen-cine-densitometry and roentgen-video-densitometry can also be used to quantitate mitral regurgitation. Fundamental to both roentgendensitometric methods is that they provide the mass, and not the concentration, of the contrast medium. In cine-densitometry, calibration of the amount of contrast medium is mandatory in every single case; it can be achieved by pulling a contrast wedge over the area of interest, and leaving a water layer during the injection of contrast medium. By this procedure the changes in light intensity during the projection of the film in the areas of interest can be converted into the amount of contrast medium in the field of interest.[7] In video-densitometry, since there is no film-developing process, a calibration with a contrast wedge is not regularly necessary, provided the conditions during recording are standardized.

Earlier attempts for assessment of mitral regurgitation in our laboratory and other centers using roentgen-cine-densitometry and video-densitometry have been based on measurements using relatively small circular or rectangular sampling areas on both sides of the valve.[1,7, 12-14] In a series of experiments in which the goal was to study the mechanism of closure of the mitral valve, these windows were positioned over the silhouette of the left ventricle about 3 mm downstream to the mitral valve ring, and over the left atrium at a similar distance upstream to the maximal excursion of the valve cusps. The windows were made equisensitive, and in order to have an empiric measure of the degree of regurgitant flow, the area under the left atrial curve, expressed as the percentage of the area of the left ventricular curve, was termed the regurgitant index. Although this method proved to be very sensitive for small regurgitations, exact quantitation was not possible. The same holds true for cine-densitometric measurements. As shown in Figure 1, the densitometric method with small windows allows one mainly to study the temporal relationship of forward or backward flow at the mitral valve. In this example of a 59 year old woman with 3 degree AV-block, the phenomenon of so called "atriogenic reflux"[8,14] can be demonstrated. Three small areas over the aorta, the left ventricle, and the left atrium are sampled during the injection of contrast medium into the left ventricle. While the oblique arrows point to the rapid inflow of undyed blood from the left atrium into the left ventricle in early diastole, an atrial contraction wave which was not followed in normal sequence by a ventricular contraction led to a regurgitation of contrast medium from the left ventricle to the left atrium during atrial relaxation, as indicated by the vertical arrow. An attempt to quantitate this atriogenic reflux in humans led to regurgitation indices of less than 5% in all cases studied.

Advances in the video-technique in the last few years allowed us to use video-densitometry, with big contoured windows covering the silhouette of the whole left ventricle or of other chambers. With these contoured windows, one can measure the absolute or relative amount of indicator present at a given moment in the total cavity of the heart, and study its changes in correct temporal sequence.[3,10,11]

If an adequate copper filter is used to restrict the X-radiation to short wavelengths, the transmission is related exponentially to the amount of contrast medium, expressed as the product of concentration (c) and depth (d), as given by Lambert-Beer's law:

$$T = e^{-k \cdot c \cdot d}$$

In order to obtain video-densitometric signals that are proportional to the total amount of the contrast medium within an area of the X-ray image, e.g., a cardiac chamber, the video signal has therefore to be converted logarithmically before summing up by the densitometer. The problem of photo scattering in the image transfer system can be considered by taking brightness measurements during zero transmis-

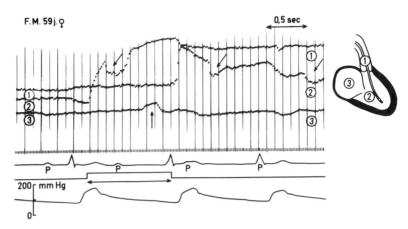

Figure 1. Atriogenic diastolic reflux in a 59 year old woman with total atrioventricular block. During the interval indicated by the double-ended arrow, 15 ml Rompacon 440 were injected into the left ventricle.

380

sion of X-rays produced by means of a piece of lead inserted over the area of interest, and by subtracting this black level.

Taking into consideration these conditions we have approached the problem of quantitative measurements of regurgitant flow. Detection of the total quantity of indicator in the atrium by adjusting the sampling window to the left atrial silhouette allowed us to measure the total amount of radio-opaque medium present at each instant in the chamber during angiocardiography. Thus the degree of mitral incompetence can be calculated from the increase of contrast medium in the left atrium during systole.

Another principle proposed initially by Bürsch and associates[3] seemed even more promising for quantitation of mitral and aortic regurgitation. One window is adjusted over the left ventricle, the other equisensitive window over both the left ventricle and the left atrium. In the case of competent valves, after injection of contrast medium into the left ventricle both curves are identical; there is no change during diastole, since the amount of contrast in the left ventricle stays the same during diastole. The decrease of contrast medium during systole is proportional to the forward stroke volume.

Figure 2 shows schematically the contrast dilution curves that are found in cases of mitral incompetence. The decrease of the amount of contrast medium during systole in the left ventricle is due to mitral regurgitation and forward stroke volume. The systolic decrease in the window encompassing the left ventricle and the left atrium is due only to forward stroke volume. Mitral regurgitation is the difference between total and net forward stroke volume. There-

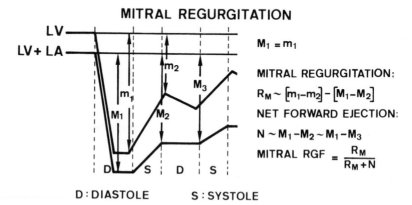

MITRAL REGURGITATION

$M_1 = m_1$

MITRAL REGURGITATION:

$$R_M \sim [m_1 - m_2] - [M_1 - M_2]$$

NET FORWARD EJECTION:

$$N \sim M_1 - M_2 \sim M_1 - M_3$$

$$MITRAL\ RGF = \frac{R_M}{R_M + N}$$

D : DIASTOLE   S : SYSTOLE

Figure 2. Schematic equisensitive density curves obtained over the left ventricle (LV) and over left ventricle and left atrium together (LV + LA) after diastolic injection of contrast medium into the left ventricle. RGF = regurgitation fraction.

fore, mitral regurgitation can be calculated as the difference between the systolic emptying of the left ventricular window and the combined window. $R_M = (m_1 - m_2) - (M_1 - M_2)$. Net forward ejection N equals $M_1 - M_2 = M_1 - M_3$. Regurgitation fraction is defined as the relation of regurgitant flow to total flow of the left ventricle, and therefore:

$$RGF = \frac{R_M}{R_M + N} = 1 - \frac{M_1 - M_2}{m_1 - m_2}$$

The measurement of regurgitation if both mitral and aortic incompetence are present is also possible by using a modified formula. In actual densitograms a systolic-diastolic phasic variation in the density signals occurs even before the injection of contrast medium. Assuming steady state conditions, i.e., a repetitive heart cycle, these density changes are corrected for by subtraction of the oscillatory base line at every moment during which a density measurement is to be made.

To check the accuracy of this roentgendensitometric regurgitation measurement, a valid reference method was necessary. An electromagnetic flow probe for production and measurement of acute mitral regurgitation flow in dogs had to be constructed in our laboratory.[4] The flow probe is equipped with tipmanometer, a thermistor, and a balloon inside the probe. The probe is introduced in the mitral valve through the left atrial appendage so that it does not necessitate open heart surgery. The amount of regurgitant flow through the mitral valve from slight to high degrees of valvular incompetence could be changed very quickly by deflating or inflating the balloon inside the electromagnetic flow probe.

The question of whether the mitral leaflets would fit closely around the mitral flow probe during ventricular systole was checked by injection of cold saline into the left ventricle. Since no temperature change was detected in the atrium when the balloon was occluded, it was concluded that no significant regurgitation occurred around the probe.

By using this electromagnetic reference and simultaneously measuring the amount of contrast medium in the left ventricle and together in the left ventricle and left atrium, we obtained roentgendensitograms during 90 injections in 8 dogs with a wide variation of backflow. The correlation coefficient between both regurgitant fractions amounted to 0.89. If the regurgitant fraction as obtained by roentgendensitometry is termed y and the regurgitant fraction as obtained by electromagnetic flowmetry is termed x, the best straight line was $y = 0.02 + 0.88 x$.

At present the roentgendensitometric method described above is applied to humans in our catheterization laboratory. Figure 3 shows the contoured windows in position in a 48 year old patient with slight mitral incompetence. Regurgitant fraction by thermodilution was 0.20; roentgendensitometry gave a value of 0.16. In other patients the agreement was not always as close. In the 17 patients in which until now mitral insufficiency was estimated by thermodilution and roentgendensitometry, the correlation does not seem to be strong (r = 0.7). The main reason is probably that thermodilution has a considerable error due to the measurement at one point in the left atrium. Furthermore, these measurements have not been simultaneous, but rather at the middle and the end of a catheterization procedure with different heart rates. An error in the video-densitometric procedure may also arise from over-projection of the descending aorta with enlarged left atria in several cases, as well as from the backflow of the contrast medium in the pulmonary veins in cases of marked mitral incompetence. At the moment we do not know exactly the degree of inaccuracy related to thermal and roentgendensitometric regurgitation measurement in humans. This comparison shows clearly that a new method can only be validated if it is compared to the most accurate available method.

SUMMARY

The usefulness and limitation of roentgendensitometric quantitation of mitral regurgitation has been demonstrated in experimental studies in both dogs and humans. The method does not require left

LEFT VENTRICLE

LEFT VENTRICLE
AND LEFT ATRIUM

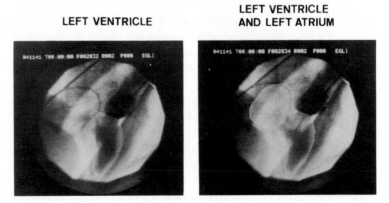

Figure 3. Shape and position of sampling windows in a 48 year old patient with slight mitral regurgitation (12%).

atrial catheterization, as do the classic upstream sampling techniques. The changes in total amount of contrast material in the left ventricle, and in the left atrium together with the left ventricle, were measured continuously. The regurgitant fraction can be calculated from the difference between the systolic decrease of left ventricular contrast medium and the systolic decrease in both left atrium and left ventricle. This method, which can be applied during angiocardiography and needs insertion of only one instead of three catheters, showed a good correlation with an absolute and accurate mitral flow measurement. However, the comparison of the method in humans using thermodilution as a reference presently underway in our laboratories shows less consistent results.

REFERENCES

1. von Bernuth, G., Tsakiris, A.G., and Wood, E.H. Quantitation of experimental aortic regurgitation by roentgen videodensitometry. *Am. J. Cardiol.* 31: 265 (1973).

2. Bloomfield, D.A., Battersby, E.J., and Sinclair-Smith, B.C. Use of indicator dilution techniques in measuring combined aortic and mitral insufficiency. *Circ. Res.* 18: 97 (1966).

3. Bürsch, J.H., Heintzen, P.H., and Simon, R. Videodensitometric studies by a new method of quantitating the amount of contrast medium. *Europ. J. Cardiol.* 14: 437 (1974).

4. Kléber, A.G., Simon, R., and Rutishauser, W. Probe for production and measurement of acute mitral regurgitant flow in dog. *J. Appl. Physiology* (in print).

5. Lacy, W.W., Goodson, W.H., Wheeler, W.G., and Newman, E.V. Theoretical and practical requirements for the valid measurement by indicator-dilution of regurgitant flow across incompetent valves. *Circ. Res.* 7: 454 (1959).

6. Newcombe, C.P., Sinclair, J.D., Donald, D.E., and Wood, E.H. Detection and assessment of mitral regurgitation by left atrial indicator-dilution curves. *Circ. Res.* 9: 1196 (1961).

7. Rutishauser, W. *Kreislaufanalyse mit Roentgendensitometrie.* Bern, Switzerland: Huber, 1969.

8. Rutishauser, W., Wirz, P., Gander, M., and Lüthy, E. Atriogenic diastolic reflux in patients with atrioventricular block. *Circulation* 34: 807 (1966).

9. de Sépibus, G., Vecht, R. and Rutishauser, W. Requirements for accurate measurement of valvular regurgitation by indicator dilution. *Basic. Res. Cardiol.* 68: 545 (1973).

10. Simon, R., Callensen, C. und Heintzen, P.H. Bestimmung der Regurgitationsfraktion von Pulmonalinsuffizienzen durch videodensitometrische Indikator-Mengenmessung. *Basic. Res. Cardiol.* 68:509 (1973).

11. Simon, R., Steiger, U., Wirtz, P., Krayenbühl, H.P., Schönbeck, M. und Rutishauser, W. Quantifizierung von Aortenklappeninsuffizienzen durch videodensitometrische Kontrastmittelmessung. *Schw. Med. Wschr.* 104:1562 (1974).

12. Tsakiris, A.G., Sturm, R.E. und Wood, E.H. Experimental studies on the mechanisms of closure of cardiac valves with use of roentgen videodensitometry. *Amer. J. Cardiol.* 32:136 (1973).

13. Williams, J.C.P., Russel, A., Vandenberg, T., O'Donovan, P.B., Sturm, R.E. and Wood, E.H. Roentgen video densitometer study of mitral valve closure during atrial fibrillation. *J. Appl. Physiol.* 24(2), 217 (1968).

14. Williams, J.C.P. and Wood, E.H. Application of Roentgen videodensitometry to the study of mitral valve function. Ed. P.H. Heintzen. In *Roentgen-, Cine- and Videodensitometry.* Stuttgart: Georg Thieme Verlag, 89-98 (1971).

33 The Pre- and Post-Operative Evaluation of the Hemodynamic State in Patients with Mitral Insufficiency

P.G. Hugenholtz, M.D.
R.W. Brower, Ph.D.
G.T. Meester, M.D.
M. van den Brand, M.D.
Mrs. I. Tiggelaar-de Widt
R.E. Ellison, M.D.

INTRODUCTION AND DESCRIPTION OF AIMS

"The impression is that the life history of patients with mitral valve incompetence is long, but that left ventricular performance deteriorates gradually and tends to be advanced by the time symptoms are prominent."[6] Few interested in the function of the mitral valve will dispute the fact that much remains to be understood before we can predict the outcome of a valve replacement operation in a given individual patient. The main problem today is no longer the technical replacement of the valve, although surgical techniques will undoubtedly improve further. Nor is it the design of an artificial valve that is physiologically better, which also will happen. The present problem resides in the determination of the optimal moment for surgery. For the patient whose ventricular function has already progressed to a point where fibrosis and other degenerative changes

385

have replaced an optimally performing muscle mass can only partially, and at times not at all, be helped by even the most able of surgeons.

Briefly reviewing the literature between 1972 and 1975, one can state that early mortality still ranges from as low as 5% to as high as 24% with an additional late mortality of 10%.[1-5] Kirklin[6,7] states that the figures in his hospital still are considerably higher for mitral valve replacement than for aortic valve replacement, where mortality even in the presence of cardiomegaly now tends to run as low as 5%. In our institution in Rotterdam too, the death rate for mitral valve replacement over the past five years has been 8.7%.[8]

Why Is the Incidence of Early Post-Operative Death Still Too High?

The hypothesis is that a sudden return of competence of the mitral valve at the time of surgery and the resulting sudden increase in afterload (or the stress in the cardiac wall per unit of cross-sectional area) has a deleterious effect on cardiac performance.[3-5] This is particularly detrimental in those patients in whom decreased cardiac compliance is already present preoperatively. The results are increased wall-stress, reflected in increased end-diastolic and systolic pressure, which, in turn, in those not dying postoperatively from cardiac decompensation, can lead to augmented cardiac muscle mass and possibly fibrosis. It is this hypothesis, as yet unproved but also suggested by Kirklin, that I would like to explore further; if it is true, it should lead to a postoperative management aimed at a continued low afterload by means of actively decreasing peripheral vascular resistance and/or cardiac mechanical assistance by balloon-pumping. A second aim would be to improve the selection of the optimal moment of surgery through timely and detailed analysis of cardiac performance, particularly of its hydraulic function.

To achieve this goal we have culled our patient material at the Thoraxcenter in Rotterdam, which consists of 195 patients who were operated upon for valvular replacement in the past five years. Of these, 80 had mitral valve replacement only, and of these 80 a subset of 7 patients was selected in whom pre- and post-operative studies were carried out in great detail under virtually identical circumstances.

We may best explore the hypothesis by emphasizing the findings in a few well studied patients who did not show the expected improvement clinically. In addition, we have reviewed the extensive experience at the Children's Hospital in Boston in the period between 1962 and 1968, where similar, although less sophisticated studies

were carried out in patients mainly with congenital mitral insufficiency.

METHODS, MATERIALS, AND RESULTS

A concise graphical description of the volume overload to the left
ventricle secondary to increasing degrees of regurgitation through the
mitral valve is given in Figure 1, taken from the study by Lewis and
Gotsman.[9] Details of the methodology employed in these and related
measurements are given in references 10 and 11. The initial approach
was to evaluate the clinical course in 65 young patients with left
ventricular volume overload by comparing the ejection fraction (EJF)
and the resting end-diastolic volume (EDV) in two groups: one that
required surgery (16 patients) and one that did not (49 patients). While
EDV was higher, with a mean of 250 ml/m² in the 9 patients who died,
and with a mean of 210 ml/m² in the 8 patients that had difficulties in
the post-operative period, than in the 8 who did well after surgery
(mean 130 ml/m²) or who required no surgery (120 ml/m²), individual
values shared a high degree of overlap. The same applies to the EJF,
which was lower—58% in the 8 deaths, 60% in the 8 with postoperative difficulties—than the 68% in the 41 patients who did not
require surgery. Thus neither EDV nor EJF could be employed to
predict outcome in the individual case.

As shown in Figure 1, the regurgitant fraction, a regurgitant
volume as percentage of EDV, is a quantitative expression of the
degree of regurgitation. This measurement in 19 patients with mitral
valve regurgitation also failed to separate those who ultimately had a
poor postoperative result or death from those who did not. Also V_{pm},
(dp/dt/p)max in sec⁻¹, an indicator of the contractile state of the
myocardium, while lower on average (35 sec⁻¹ and 34 sec⁻¹) in those
who had either severe symptoms or evidence of congestive heart
failure when compared to the control groups who had neither (48 sec⁻¹
and 49 sec⁻¹ respectively), did not permit the identification of individual cases with a poor prognosis because of the degree of overlap
mentioned earlier.

Detailed analysis of cardiac mechanical performance, including
peak wall stress, cardiac wall mass, and circumferential fiber shortening, shows, however, that in one patient whose clinical state improved from class III (NYHA) to class II in the 6 month postoperative period these measurements reflect the clinical correlations.
Analysis of Table 1 (patient KMH) shows the expected decrease in
EJF and EDV, as the heart does not regurgitate significant amounts of

388

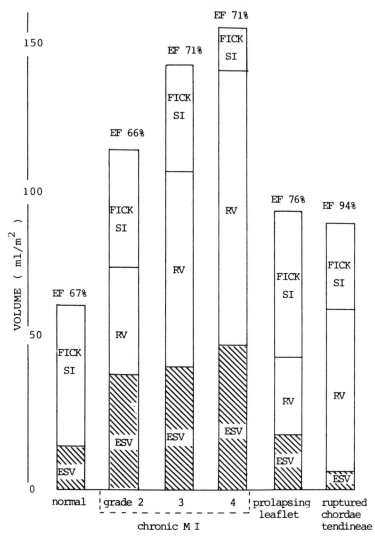

Figure 1. Left ventricular volumes (normalized for body surface area) in normal subjects and in patients with mitral incompetence. The patients with chronic mitral incompetence are classified into three subsets (grades 2, 3, and 4) based on their functional disability (New York Heart Association classification); patients with a prolapsing leaflet and ruptured chordae tendineae are shown separately. Each column shows the total end-diastolic volume, which is subdivided into end-systolic volume (EVS, black zone) and angiographic stroke index (SI, white zone). The angiographic stroke index is further subdivided into two fractions: forward stroke index (Fick SI) and regurgitant stroke index (RV). The ejection fraction (EF) is shown at the top of each column. A normal ejection fraction is maintained in each group, and the ventricle handles the large volume load by an increase in end-diastolic volume and angiographic stroke index. Patients with a larger regurgitant volume (RV) had greater disability. The patient with acute chordal rupture had an increase in ejection fraction.

Table 1
Diagnosis: Mitral Insufficiency, gr. III, coarc. Patient KMH

	Pre-Operative	Post-Operative
H.R., b/min	63	61
Pk LVP, mm Hg	136	148
LVEDP, mm Hg	20	16
Pk stress, gm/cm²	319	244
wall mass, gm/m²	199	230
EDV, ml/m²	156	135
Ej.Fr., %	67	62
CFSR, 1/s	1.17	0.93

blood after valve replacement. A lower total stroke volume requires less EDV as well as a lower velocity of circumferential fiber shortening (CFSR), and leads to a return of the preoperatively elevated EJF towards normal. Also, wall stress has decreased, which is reflected in a lower end-diastolic pressure. In this case wall mass did not (yet) return to normal, since peak left ventricular pressure actually increased. Such salutary effects were, however, not observed in all patients.

Of the 7 studied in detail whose clinical status pre- and postoperatively is given in Figure 2, many actually showed one or more

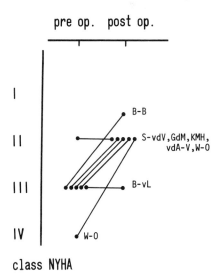

Figure 2. Change in clinical validity from preoperative to postoperative state. Details of the hemodynamic state in patients KMH and BB are given in Tables 1 and 2.

signs of deterioration in terms of hemodynamics. In all 7 there was a gratifying decrease in EJF (mean 68 to 56%) and CFSR (mean 1.01 to 0.72%) (Fig. 3), and also in wall stress (mean 317 to 281 gm/cm²) (Fig. 4). All these changes were significant to at least the 1% level (p < 0.1). On the other hand in all 7 patients left ventricular peak pressure rose from 151 to 169 mm Hg (Fig. 4), while left ventricular end-diastolic

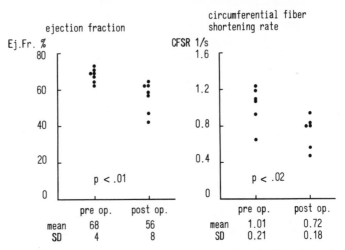

Figure 3. Distribution of ejection fraction and circumferential fiber shortening rate pre- and postoperatively. The decreases in mean values are statistically significant.

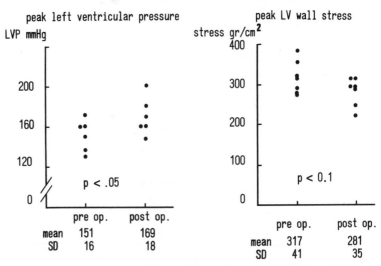

Figure 4. Distribution of peak left ventricular pressure and peak left ventricular wall stress pre- and postoperatively. The changes in the mean values are statistically significant.

pressure and volume, stress-time index, and wall mass showed variable results, in some actually increasing (Table 2, patient B-B).

DISCUSSION

While this series is very small and actually represents data on a subgroup of patients with mitral valve disease who did not improve to class I in the 6 months after the operation, the data obtained show that the expected decrease in peak wall stress associated with the anticipated improvement in EJF and CFSR is associated with a number of unsatisfactory observations, such as the increase in ventricular peak systolic pressure and the variable responses in end-diastolic pressure, volume, and cardiac mass.

These data and other experimental and clinical evidence support the idea that sudden ablation of mitral incompetence in a subject with chronic heart failure immediately depresses left ventricular function by increasing afterload. In patients with decreased compliance this may be fatal, although the present data obviously do not establish this latter hypothesis. It therefore might be advisable to keep the surviving troubled patients at low systolic pressures by means of drugs which lower systemic vascular resistance. The "low-output" syndrome so familiar in some patients with mitral valve syndrome might be effectively prevented if such therapy were timely instituted.

Along with the data now available concerning the efficacy of present operative techniques and prosthetic devices, our data also indicate that serious consideration must be given to advising much earlier operation for many patients with mitral incompetence than is presently done, so as to minimize the secondary cardiomyopathy that develops in long-standing disease. One indicator may simply be increasing cardiomegaly while significant symptoms remain absent. Additional research into more accurate ways of assessing ventricular

Table 2

Diagnosis: Mitral Stenosis-Mitral Insufficiency, gr. III. Patient BB

	Pre-Operative	Post-Operative
H.R. b/min	90	63
Pk LVP mm Hg	150	180
LVEDP mm Hg	10	16
Pk stress gm/cm²	289	292
wall mass gm/m²	116	128
EDV ml/m²	56	50
Ej.Fr. %	71	42
CFSR 1/s	1.07	0.46

compliance is necessary in order to determine whether a given patient has lost his left ventricular reserve mechanisms. If a patient with advanced mitral incompetence can be identified as having lost his reserve mechanisms and has decreased compliance, special intra- and postoperative techniques (such as cardiac assistance with balloon pumping) will probably be required if he or she is to be operated upon at the low risk that mitral valve replacement should carry today.

REFERENCES

1. Bonchek, Lawrence I., Anderson, Richard P., and Starr, Albert. Mitral valve replacement with cloth-covered composite-seat prostheses. *Journal of Thoracic and Cardiovascular Surgery*, 67: 1, 1974.

2. Kochoukos, N.T. Problems in mitral valve replacement. Edited by J.W. Kirklin. In *Advances in Cardiovascular Surgery*. New York: Grune Stratton Publisher, 1973.

3. Braunwald, E., Welch, G.H., and Sarnoff, S.J. Hemodynamic effects of quantitatively varied experimental mitral regurgitation. *Circulation Research* 5: 539, 1957.

4. Urschel, C.W., Covell, J.W., and Sonnenblick, E.H. Myocardial mechanics in aortic and mitral valvular regurgitation: the concept of instantaneous impedance as a determinant of the performance of the intact heart. *J. Clin. Invest.* 47: 867, 1968.

5. Miller, G.A.H., Kirklin, J.W., Swan, H.J.C. Myocardial function and left ventricular volumes in acquired valvular insufficiency. *Circulation* 31: 374, 1965.

6. Kirklin, John W., and Pacifico, Albert D. Surgery for acquired valvular heart disease. *New Engl. J. Med.* 288: 194, 1973.

7. Kirklin, John W. Replacement of the mitral valve for mitral incompetence. *Surgery* 72: 827, 1972.

8. Meester, G.T., Brower, R.W., vd Brand, M., Tiggelaar- de Widt, I., and Hugenholtz, P.G. The Effect of Cardiac Valve Replacement in the Heart. In preparation.

9. Lewis, Basil S., Gotsman, Mervyn S. Left ventricular function during systole and diastole in mitral incompetence. *Am. J. Cardiol.*, 34: 635, 1974.

10. Brower, R.W., Meester, G.T., and Hugenholtz, P.G. Quantification of ventricular performance: a computer based system for the analysis of angiographic data. *Catheterization and Cardiovascular Diagnosis*. 1: 33, 1975.

11. Meester, G.T., Bernard, N., Zeelenberg, C., Hoare, M.R., and Hugenholtz, P.G. A computer system for real time analysis of cardiac catheterization data. *Catheterization and Cardiovascular Diagnosis*. 1: 113, 1975.

12. Bristow, J.D. and Kremkau, L. Hemodynamic changes after valve replacement with Starr-Edwards prosthesis *Am. J. Cardiol.*, 35: 716, 1975.

34 Left Ventricular and Left Atrial Function Assessment in Mitral Valve Disease*

Harold T. Dodge, M. D.

Mitral valve stenosis (MS) impedes the flow of blood into the left ventricle, resulting in a pressure overload on the left atrium. Mitral valve regurgitation (MR) imposes a volume overload on the left ventricle, which is associated with reduced impedance and a volume and pressure overload on the left atrium. Quantitative angiocardiographic methods have been applied to assess left ventricular and atrial volumes, volume changes, and left ventricular mass in humans with mitral valve disease. In addition, these volume measurements have been related to chamber pressure to determine pressure-volume characteristics of the left ventricle and atrium.

In 85% of subjects with MS, left ventricular (LV) end-diastolic volume (EDV) is within the normal range, and in 15% it is less than normal.[1,2] Accordingly, an enlarged EDV in a patient with MS suggests the presence of a complicating lesion, such as mitral or aortic valvular regurgitation, or myocardial disease of the LV.

The systolic ejection fraction (EF) is reduced below 50% in approximately one-third of subjects with mitral stenosis and is below

* Supported in part by NHLI grant number HL 13517-04.

40% in 15% of subjects.[1,2] The reduced EF is a consequence of a reduced stroke volume in the presence of a normal EDV. In most conditions in which a reduced EF indicates myocardial disease, EDV is increased. The reason for the depressed EF in MS is not clear. Myocardial fibrosis from rheumatic myocardites, or extension of fibrosis into the LV myocardium from the diseased mitral valve annulus, have been postulated as possible causes. However, it may be a consequence of a long-standing reduced preload. In this regard it is of interest that in postoperative studies performed an average of approximately one year following surgery for mitral stenosis, the ejection fraction was usually increased over preoperative values, although not necessarily to the normal range.[3]

Left ventricular mass is usually normal in subjects with mitral stenosis, but is occasionally reduced when mitral stenosis is severe and of long duration.[1,2] In mitral valve regurgitation (MR) the LVEDV is usually increased proportionate to regurgitant flow, and in chronic mitral insufficiency the LV dilatation is associated with a proportionate increase of LV mass, so that the ratio LVM/EDV remains normal.[2] In a comparison of hemodynamic data from 24 subjects with relatively acute MR from ruptured chordae tendineae and 25 subjects with chronic rheumatic MR, values for LVEDV, SV, regurgitant flow, and LV mass were less (Table 1), although forward stroke volumes were similar and left atrial pressures higher in the group with ruptured chordae tendineae (4). The lower mass values observed with acute MR are associated with a low EDV/LVM ratio, suggesting that the mechanism of hypertrophy has incompletely compensated for the large LVEDV and SV.[2] In chronic mitral insufficiency the extent of regurgitant flow, as well as the magnitude of

Table 1
Mitral Insufficiency

	Ruptured Chordae (n = 24)		Chronic Rheumatic (n = 25)	
	mean ± 1 SD	Range	mean ± 1 SD	Range
Regurgitant Flow/stroke (ml/m²)	59 ± 29	(19-132)	81 ± 49	(29-238)
Regurgitant Flow/Min (l/m²/Min)	5.19 ± 2.9	(1.9-12.9)	6.37 ± 3.9	(2.1-16.5)
LVSV (ml/m²)	86 ± 29	(32-157)	109 ± 50	(48-269)
LVEDV (ml/m²)	142 ± 43	(54-256)	188 ± 75	(96-399)
LV Mass (gm/m²)	133 ± 27	(96-183)	166 ± 50	(95-244)

LVSV and EDV enlargement, are great and occasionally massive (Table 1).

The LV ejection fraction in subjects with mitral regurgitation (MR) is usually normal. When low, the ejection fraction indicates depressed myocardial performance. However, because of the reduced afterload with mitral insufficiency, the ejection fraction in this condition may not provide a very accurate index of depressed myocardial function.[2] In this regard it is of interest that studies performed at approximately one year following surgical correction of MR showed a fall of EF and the circumferential fiber shortening rate, although end-diastolic pressure, LVEDV, and SV were reduced.[3] This suggests that the reduced impedance to ejection was a factor in elevating the EF.

The maximum volume of the normal left atrium (LA) is 36 ± 8.7 ml/M^2, or approximately half the normal LVEDV, and occurs just prior to mitral valve opening at a time which corresponds to the peak of the "v" wave of LA pressure. The cylic changes of volume of the normal left atrium have been shown to be 18 ± 7.4 ml/M^2, or approximately half of the maximum volume and 38% of the LV stroke volume.[5] The remaining 62% of volume inflow is not reflected by LA volume change.[6] Left atrial contraction contributes approximately 21% to mitral valve inflow. These relationships between atrial volume changes and LV inflow volume are influenced by changes of heart rate, P-R interval, and mitral valve disease.

In one reported series of patients with mitral stenosis, the mean maximum left atrial volume was 117 ± 57 ml, which is approximately three times normal.[2] The left atrial stroke volume is usually normal, whereas the portion of LV volume inflow that occurs during atrial systole is reported to be increased to an average of 33% from the usual 21% in normal subjects.[1,2]

The left atrial maximum volume in subjects with chronic mitral regurgitation (MR) is usually larger than with mital stenosis or with acute MR as occurs with ruptured chordae tendineae. This is shown in Table 2. This table also shows that the LA stroke volume is also larger with chronic MR than with acute MR. Because the left atrium is stiffer and less compliant in acute MR, left atrial peak pressure and pulse pressure are usually higher than in subjects with chronic rheumatic MR, although the volume changes are less.[4]

It is of interest that in subjects with significant MR, the volume of mitral valve regurgitant flow often exceeds the left atrial volume changes. In one study, regurgitant flow exceeded LA volume change by an average of 20 ml/m^2 and 21 ml/m^2 in groups of subjects with

Table 2
Left Atrial Volumes

	Normal Values (± S.D.)	MS (n = 25)	MS + MR (n = 27)	MR Ruptured Chordae (n = 25)	MR RHD (n = 25)
L.A. Max Vol. (ml/m²)					
Mean	35 ± 9	117 ± 57	180 ± 106	119 ± 47	267 ± 131
Range		44-288	84-596	62-277	110-605
L.A. Vol. Change (ml/m²)					
Mean	18 ± 7	14 ± 9	23 ± 11	39 ± 15	60 ± 36
Range		1-45	4-50	11-70	25-176

L.A. = left atrium; MS = mitral stenosis; MR = mitral regurgitation; RHD = rheumatic heart disease

ruptured chordae and chronic rheumatic MR respectively.[4] Accordingly, the pulmonary venous bed must accept a portion of the regurgitant flow in many subjects with MR.

Abnormalities of atrial rhythm, and particularly atrial fibrillation, frequently occur with mitral valve disease and alter atrial contraction, but the atrium continues to function as a passive volume reservoir with appreciable cyclic volume changes in both mitral stenosis and MR.[6,7] It is likely that the volume changes with atrial fibrillation are reduced from what would occur with normal rhythm. With MR, very large cyclic volume changes may occur, even in the presence of atrial fibrillation.[7]

Another method for analyzing left atrial performance is in terms of its pressure-volume characteristics. In Figure 1 are shown left atrial pressure and volume curves which have been related with respect to time to construct a left atrial pressure-volume curve. This curve has a figure-eight type of configuration in contrast to the relatively simple "loop" which characterizes the left ventricular pressure-volume curve. The right hand portion of this curve occurs during atrial diastole, with the maximum pressure and volume occurring at the peak of the "v" wave. With opening of the mitral valve, atrial pressure and volume decrease until the onset of atrial systole. At this point atrial pressure rises with a further decrease of volume as illustrated by the loop on the left hand portion of Figure 1. With closure of the mitral valve, atrial pressure and volume increase to the peak of the "v" wave.

The above atrial pressure and volume changes can be analyzed in terms of pressure-volume work as has been previously described.[6] During atrial filling while the mitral valve is closed, pressure-volume

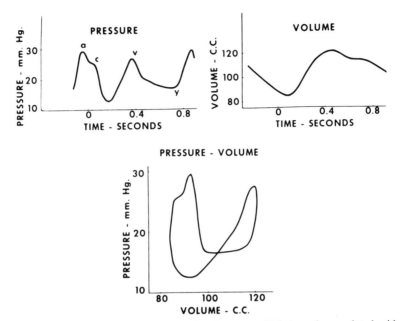

Figure 1. Left atrial pressure and volume curves which have been related with respect to time to construct the pressure-volume curve.

work is expended on the left atrium in distending it. In the absence of mitral valve insufficiency, this work which is performed in distending the left atrium is generated by the right ventricle. In the presence of MR, a portion of this work comes from the left ventricle.

With opening of the mitral valve, energy stored in the distended left atrium is released as pressure-volume work during the passive phase of atrial emptying.[6] Additional work is performed with atrial contraction. Pressure-volume work performed by the left atrium can be computed as:

$$\int_{\text{min. atrial V}}^{\text{max. atrial V}} P dV$$

where P is left atrial pressure during the period of ventricular diastole which is related to the atrial volume changes during this same time interval. Work performed by the left atrium during passive atrial emptying can be computed as:

$$\int_{\text{V at onset "a"}}^{\text{max. atrial V}} P dV$$

Where P and dV are atrial pressure and volume changes during passive atrial emptying prior to atrial contraction. Similarly work performed by the atrium during atrial systole can be computed from atrial pressure and volume changes.

In mitral stenosis, pressure-volume stroke work performed by the left atrium for ventricular filling is elevated to the range of 600 to 1500 gm cm. Approximately one-half of this work is generated during atrial systole, except when there is atrial fibrillation. It is of interest that nearly as much work is expended in distending the left atrium as is released by the left atrium, and accordingly atrial contraction per se does not contribute much work.[6]

The total work expended in ventricular filling can be computed by relating the left ventricular volume change during diastole (dV) to the left atrial pressure during the period of ventricular filling (Pd) as:

$$\int_{LV\ min.\ V}^{LV\ max.\ V} Pd\ dV$$

In mitral stenosis this is elevated to the range of 1500 to 2500 gm cm. per beat, or nearly to the range of systolic work of the right ventricle in normal persons. Approximately half of this work is generated by pressure-volume changes in the left atrium, while the remainder comes directly from the right ventricle through the pulmonary vasculature without being reflected by atrial pressure-volume changes. In mitral stenosis the major portion of the work of filling is expended in overcoming mitral valve resistance and a lesser amount on actually distending the diastolic left ventricle.

In mitral valve insufficiency there are large atrial pressure and volume changes which absorb energy through distension of the elastic atrium during ventricular systole and contribute work to ventricular filling during ventricular diastole. An example of left atrial and ventricular pressure and volume curves, as well as work computations for the left atrium and ventricle, is shown in Figure 2. The left ventricular stroke volume is 180 ml, and left atrial volume change in excess of 100 ml is associated with a left atrial pressure which rises to over 60 mm Hg at the peak of the "v" wave. The total energy absorbed by the left atrium during ventricular systole and with atrial distension is not computed, but will be in excess of the total atrial work value of 2713 gm cm. The latter is the atrial contribution to the work expended in distending the diastolic left ventricle during ventricular diastole (44.3 gm m or 4430 gm cm). Accordingly, approximately half the work expended in distending the diastolic left ventri-

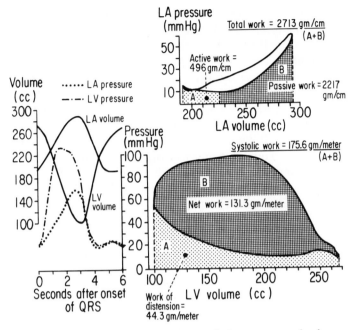

Figure 2. On the left are the left atrial and ventricular pressure and volume curves. These atrial and ventricular pressure and volume curves respectively have been related to construct the atrial and ventricular pressure-volume curves as illustrated on the right. Work components are computed from areas beneath these curves as illustrated.

cle comes from the left atrium and the remainder from the pulmonary vasculature and right ventricle. Less than one quarter of the left atrial work occurs during atrial systole. This illustrates the striking atrial pressure and volume changes that occur with severe mitral insufficiency, and illustrates a method for quantifying certain features of atrial performance under these conditions.

In summary, this has been a brief review of some of the effects of mitral valve disease on left atrial and ventricular performance. The pressure-volume characteristics of the left atrium are greatly altered in mitral stenosis, and as are the characteristics of both the left atrium and ventricle in mitral regurgitation. Methods are described for analyzing these pressure-volume changes in man with mitral valve disease.

REFERENCES

1. Kennedy, J.W., Yarnall, S.R., Murray, J.A., and Figley, M.M. Quantitative angiocardiography IV. Relationships of left

atrial and ventricular pressure and volume in mitral valve disease. *Circulation* 41: 817, 1970.

2. Dodge, H.T., Kennedy, J.W., and Peterson, J.L. Quantitative angiocardiographic methods in the evaluation of valvular heart disease. *Progress in Cardiovascular Diseases* 16: 1, 1973.

3. Doces, J., and Kennedy, J.W. Quantitative assessment of left ventricular function following successful mitral valve surgery. (Abst.) *Amer. J. Cardiology* 35: 132, 1975.

4. Baxley, W.A., Kennedy, J.W., Feild, B., and Dodge, H.T. Hemodynamics in ruptured chordae tendineae and chronic rheumatic mitral regurgitation. *Circulation* 48: 1288, 1973.

5. Murray, J.A., Kennedy, J.W., and Figley, M.M. Quantitative angiocardiography II. The normal left atrial volume in man. *Circulation* 37: 800, 1968.

6. Grant, C., Bunnell, I.L., and Greene, D.G. The reservoir function of the left atrium during ventricular systole. *Am. J. Med.* 37: 36, 1964.

7. Hawley, R.R., Dodge, H.T., and Graham, T.P. Left atrial volume and its changes in heart disease. *Circulation* 37: 989, 1966.

DISCUSSION: PART VII

Dr. Yellin: I have one slide of a dog in acute mitral regurgitation (approximately 25%) (Fig. 1). Upon removal of incompetence the systolic LVP and stroke volume increase; mitral inflow and diastolic filling period both decrease. Within several beats (Panel B), systolic LVP and stroke volume return to the values during regurgitation. The animal was obviously in a state of compensated volume load, and removal of incompetence removed a parallel path and increased the total impedance seen by the ventricle. After this condition was met, reflex mechanisms intervened to provide only the needs of the animal. The chronically ill patients studied by Dr. Hugenholtz may not have this capacity to return to normal conditions after the repair of a regurgitant valve.

Dr. Dodge: I am sure you also mean that if the ventricle is normal it can adapt to the increased impedance and presumably in a matter of days it will set its control mechanisms back to normal in the surviving patients. But the poorly functioning left ventricle may not be able to adapt to the increased impedance, and adaptation may be impossible.

Dr. Lyngborg: I think Dr. Hugenholtz' remarks regarding mitral regurgitation and the effect of operation were very interesting. One

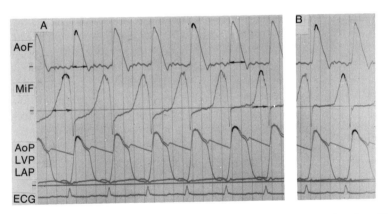

Figure 1. An oscillographic record of the hemodynamic measurements in a dog with acute reversible mitral regurgitation. Panel A: Following a stable sequence of incompetent beats, the regurgitation is reversed and there is an immediate increase in LVP and stroke volume. Panel B: Within several seconds of no regurgitation the animal returns to its initial conditions. The peaks of selected curves have been delineated to accentuate the significant changes. AoF = aortic flow; MiF = mitral flow, AoP, LVP, LAP = Aortic, left ventricular, and left atrial pressures; ECG = electrocardiogram. The peaks of the pressure and flow curves have been accentuated.

thing I wonder about is the effect of work in a patient with mitral regurgitation, as the total left ventricular output in patient with severe mitral regurgitation at rest is similar to that of a normal patient during exercise: Does the regurgitation increase or decrease during exercise? I also would like to ask Dr. Hugenholtz whether any exercise test had been made in his patients before and after operation.

Dr. Hugenholtz: The answer is simple: no, we did not do this kind of measurement at the time of exercise. Are you proposing to use physical exercise to see what the reserve mechanisms of the heart in a given situation are?

Dr. Sonnenblick: The question of ventricular reserve in pathological situations is an intriguing one. While it is often possible to define the performance of the ventricle under resting condition, there is commonly a large reserve of contractility which may not be manifest. For example, the depressed heart may respond with an increase in contractility following an extrasystole. This increment may be very substantial. Moreover, such extrasystoles help to distinguish akinetic from depressed but still viable heart muscle in the presence of ischemic heart disease. We have been studying the phenomenon of extrasystoles in chronic heart failure and feel that this may be a useful tool for ascertaining which hearts may improve with further therapeutic interventions.

Another point which Dr. Hugenholtz has alluded to is the question of reversibility of the depressed heart, especially following chronic overloads imposed by valvular heart disease. The work of Dr. Gault and others would suggest that contractility is not improved in some patients with severe aortic insufficiency, although ventricular performance may be bettered by removing the hemodynamic load which an insufficient valve creates. However, these studies involved only a small group of patients, and the entire question of reversibility and its relationship to the abnormal loading conditions and the duration of the lesion needs to be explored and answered.

Now, I have a question for Dr. Hugenholtz. I am interested to know how you calculated the increase in ventricular mass. I am also interested to know, since this seems to me a rather unusual circumstance, whether these seven cases were possibly treated differently at the operating table from the other patients that you followed. Were they for instance treated with ischemic arrest or potassium arrest?

Dr. Hugenholtz: No, there are no obvious factors in surgical techniques that would explain these observations. I cannot deny that taking 7 patients who do not improve out of a group of 80 is not a statistically acceptable way of handling it. I simply wanted to illustrate the mechanisms which I think are operative in patients who do not do well after surgery. I would rather believe that we should continue to look in the direction of altered compliance preoperatively.

Dr. Dodge: It was mentioned that with exercise the elevated cardiac output may be similar to what is observed in mitral valve insufficiency. This really is not the case. The large cardiac output in mitral insufficiency is a consequence of the large stroke volume of the left ventricle, whereas in exercise by and large the cardiac output goes up because of an increase in the heart rate, and these are remarkably different phenomena. We have made observations on the effects of surgery for mitral insufficiency on left ventricular work, volumes, and mass. Although left ventricular volumes and work are reduced, left ventricular mass does not change. This is different from what occurs with aortic valve surgery. Following aortic valve surgery, there is frequently a regression of hypertrophy.

Dr. Reid: I enjoyed Dr. Hugenholtz's paper very much. Various authors have looked and tried to identify risk factors in cardiac surgery, and they all indicate that the most consistently reliable risk factor prognostically is ejection fraction. The heart either pumps well or it doesn't. The conclusion quantitatively of most workers has been that if you have an ejection fraction of only 20 or 30% you are going to do badly after cardiac surgery. I wonder whether the 7 patients who did badly in fact have ejection fractions in that range? I am also disconcerted to find that ejection fractions fell following mitral valve surgery in some of the cases you presented.

Dr. Hugenholtz: I do not think you should be disturbed by a fall in ejection fraction, because I think it is a proper thing to do for a ventricle which had a leaky valve. When you consider the low afterload acts as a "sink" in which the LV empties itself, this will, by definition, increase the ejection fraction beyond control values. Each of the seven cases acted like the classical examples that Gotsman or Urschel had in acute preparations, with ejection fractions above 70%. In fact, I believe that you can have already depressed muscle function in the presence of elevated ejection fractions. Then, when you suddenly increase afterload by placing the artificial competent valve, ejection fractions may become abnormally low.

Dr. Reid: May I also ask whether your calculations of ventricular wall muscle mass were made acutely or some months after surgery?

Dr. Hugenholtz: These studies all are done approximately 8 to 10 months after the surgical correction had taken place, so as to try to give the patients time to adapt to the new load.

Dr. Barlow: I am just interested also in the technical point here, which perhaps Dr. Sonnenblick or Dr. Dodge might answer: the business of measuring ejection fraction as a cardiac assessment after the injection of radio-opaque dyes. It would seem to me that this had the exact opposite effect on ventricles as your experiments in dogs with ruptured chordae. In fact, this could result in an increase of the ventricular area and obviously decrease the ventricular function.

Dr. Dodge: This is a bit of a problem actually, because the injected contrast medium is a volume load. The other aspect is that the depressive effects take place after several beats, and the measurements are made in the first few beats.

It would be rather intriguing to know if by use of echocardiography, a non-invasive way of determining ejection fraction, these observations can be made over the immediate postoperative period.

Dr. Hugenholtz: Doctor Barlow, I am a member of the group of people who have always believed in angiocardiography as a quantitative measurement. This matter of injection of contrast is an old issue. I think that you will find ample evidence now with very careful studies in the recent literature that the detrimental effect in terms of chemical influence through the coronary circulation comes well after the volume measurements have been made. The added volume load is not a really very large one for various reasons such as regurgitation itself and the fact that the injection is over a few cycles and so forth. So I do not think, apart from it being a systematic error, that it brings a very large additional error.

Dr. Carpentier: I would like to congratulate Dr. Hugenholtz for his brilliant and lucid exposé, especially for having stressed the importance of myocardial function. When results following surgery are not up to expectations, one tends to incriminate either the valve or the surgeon, all too often forgetting poor myocardial performance.

I have a question concerning the calculation of myocardial wall stress. According to the Laplace's law, stress is directly proportional to the radius. As the left ventricle presents different curvatures, stress must necessarily vary from one area to the next. My question then is: to arrive at your calculations, did you select a particular area on the myocardial wall or did you take an average of several measurements from different areas of the left ventricle?

Dr. Hugenholtz: You are quite right: for wall thickness, we took one predetermined point on the free lateral wall. We have to assume that the ventricle is symmetrical. In the model we calculate volume and stress, the radius is derived from the measured area and the longest axis. Generally speaking, with an error of about 10%, these data should give you pretty good results.

Dr. Krayenbuehl: I think after all these pros and cons, could you perhaps define for all of us, for the surgeon especially, who is now a patient with mitral insufficiency on whom we should operate? What are the important parameters of the hydraulic and isovolumic studies, and what patients would you recommend for surgery?

Dr. Hugenholtz: This is a dangerous kind of discussion to get into for two reasons: firstly, it smacks of what I call "side-walk" consultation; and secondly I throw out the challenge: I do not think I know! I only have pointed out that if a ventricle handles its volume load adequately by the parameters I have shown, such as a high ejection fraction and a high end-diastolic volume, and utilizes its Starlings' law optimally, with adequate compliance, and this patient has beginning symptoms, and *most important* beginning cardiomegaly, then I would start thinking of a valve. It depends of course who the surgeon is, which valve we have, where we are, what the patient wants (do not forget!). Most important is our attitude, which I think you allude to. We cannot wait for him or her to complain of severe symptoms, because then decompensation has taken place, pulmonary vascular resistance is up, left atrial pressure is very high, etc., and it is too late. The optimal moment is *before* that time and can be determined from the calculations which I have shown.

Dr. Krayenbuehl: How about peripheral systemic resistance? Because when you have increased peripheral resistance it may be very harmful in the post-operative period. In fact you showed patients who had a systolic pressure after surgery above 180 mm Hg.

Dr. Hugenholtz: That is correct. We also should employ all the drugs in the post-operative period which can reduce vascular resistance and thus this aspect of elevated afterload.

Dr. Denolin: I think that the question put by Mr. Krayenbuehl is very basic a question. We don't accuse surgeons too much, we do accuse valves and the heart muscle quite a lot, but on a relatively simple basis we can choose what appears to be the optimal time for surgery.

SUMMARY: PART VII

H. P. Krayenbuehl, M.D.

In essence this session dealt with the alterations of left ventricular size, shape, and performance that occur with abnormal mitral valve function. When mitral regurgitation was acutely induced in the dog, the size of the left ventricle and especially the end-diastolic basilar diameter were found to be the major determinants of the extent of regurgitation, regardless of the actual systolic pressure gradient between the left ventricle and atrium. Thus, these experimental studies of Dr. Sonnenblick and his coworkers confirm the older clinical impression that by the progressive increase of the size of the left ventricular cavity, "mitral insufficiency begets mitral insufficiency."

In humans, mitral regurgitation can be quantitated either from the volumetric analysis of left ventricular cineangiograms combined with Fick or dye cardiac output measurements, or by indicator dilution methods. Dr. Rutishauser and his colleagues reported on their experience with one specific form of dilution technique, namely roentgenvideodensitometry. In normal dogs the extent of regurgitation evaluated by this technique compared favorably with the electromagnetically metered regurgitant flow. However, in humans with the occasional great enlargement of the left atrium that complicates integral indicator sampling, the accuracy of roentgenvideodensitometry for evaluating regurgitant flow remains to be determined.

Left ventricular performance in patients with mitral regurgitation was analyzed pre- and postoperatively by Dr. Hugenholtz and his colleagues. Despite successful correction of abnormal mitral valve function, ventricular ejection fraction decreased postoperatively. This decrease does not, however, necessarily imply an impairment of intrinsic left ventricular contractile function, since the postoperative increase in mean aortic pressure and the decrease in left ventricular end-diastolic dimensions tend in themselves to decrease ejection fraction. Although no hemodynamic parameter appears to be predictive of the postoperative outcome in patients with mitral regurgitation, Dr. Hugenholtz feels that surgery should be undertaken before left ventricular diastolic compliance is increased. This conclusion remains, however, speculative since left ventricular compliance was not assessed in terms of diastolic changes in volume per changes in pressure.

Finally, Dr. Dodge pointed out that in long standing mitral stenosis, left ventricular size and mass as determined by angiography

408

may be lower than normal. Then he outlined some important differences in left atrial dynamics of patients with acute and chronic mitral insufficiency. In acute mitral regurgitation from ruptured chordae tendineae, the left atrial size was found to be moderately increased and the left atrial cyclic volume changes were significantly smaller than in chronic mitral insufficiency. Hence the pulmonary veins must accept an appreciable amount of the regurgitant flow in these patients.

PART EIGHT

PROSTHETIC
VALVE
REPLACEMENT

35 Mitral Valve Replacement with Ball Valve Prosthesis: A Current Appraisal of Late Results

Albert Starr, M.D.

The surgical management of valvular heart disease has progressed considerably since the first successful clinical implantation of a ball valve prosthesis in 1960.[1,2] Operative mortality and the incidence of prosthesis-related complications have both decreased substantially.[3,4] Nonetheless, the proper timing of operations is not definitely established, and discussion continues among proponents of various prosthetic and biologic valves in regard to the best device for valve replacement. It is likely that no single valve substitute will be ideal in all circumstances. The assessment and selection of prostheses must therefore depend upon precise evaluations of their early and late results, with proper consideration of the clinical settings in which they are applied.

Experience in our own clinic has been almost entirely with the ball valve prosthesis. During the past 14 years, careful analyses of clinical data and of the results of animal and in vitro tests have resulted in a sequence of orderly changes in valve design. The Stellite poppet, introduced in 1967, eliminated concern for ball variance. The extended cloth covering of the orifice, introduced in 1965 and now

413

414

available in the model 6120 prostheses, substantially decreased the incidence of emboli. The complete cloth covering, first used in 1967, further reduced the incidence of emboli. However, in the earliest fully cloth-covered valves (model 6300), hydraulic performance was inferior to that of the valves not covered with cloth, and the first composite seat prostheses were therefore introduced in 1968.

This report reviews the results of valve replacement with cloth-covered, composite seat prostheses; compares these results with those of the current-model noncloth-covered valves (model 6120); and discusses their clinical implications. In order to facilitate comparisons of different prostheses, attention is confined to isolated valve replacement. The validity of such comparisons is enhanced by the application of advanced actuarial techniques to a discrete group of patients followed up closely and contacted at regular intervals.[5,6]

PROSTHESES

The noncloth-covered mitral prosthesis (model 6120) has been virtually unchanged during the past 10 years (Fig. 1). It consists of a highly polished cage of Stellite 21 and a ball of silicone rubber. The

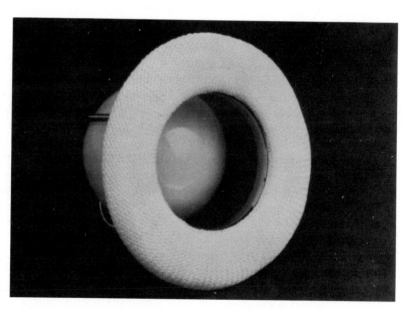

Figure 1. Noncloth-covered mitral valve prosthesis (model 6120).

cloth-covered prosthesis (models 6310-6320), in use since 1968, contains a Stellite poppet and a composite orifice of alternating Teflon fibers and metallic studs. The 6310 has a double layer of Teflon cloth covering the struts. The 6320 has an inner layer of Teflon and an outer layer of polypropylene as a cloth covering. The polypropylene cloth does not "cold flow" as does Teflon, and because of its "memory" it has the superior ability to stay in place around the strut (Fig. 2).

The sewing ring in all currently available prostheses, both cloth-covered and noncloth-covered, is designed to provide flexibility and compressibility to enhance coaptation at the valve-tissue interface. This is achieved with a molded foam insert incorporated between layers of folded Teflon and polypropylene cloth to provide an "upholstered" effect.

While complete strut cloth tear has not been seen with the cloth-covered mitral prosthesis (model 6310-6320), there has been evidence of flattening of the cloth fibers or some fraying of the fibers on the inner surface of the struts. In some rare instances there has been circumferential tear of the orifice cloth. Modifications of design were therefore made with the development of the composite strut prosthesis to diminish the possibility of these problems.

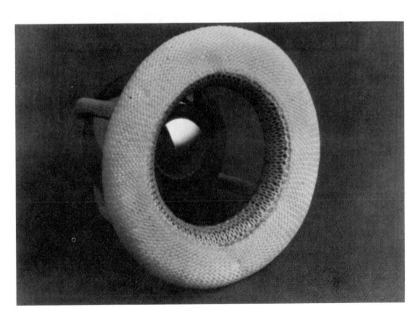

Figure 2. Cloth-covered, composite seat mitral valve prosthesis (model 6310-6320).

Composite Strut Prosthesis

This prosthesis, commonly referred to as the "track valve" and designated model 6400-mitral, has been under clinical evaluation in our center since November 1972. It has a single layer of loosely knit, relatively thin Dacron cloth stretched over highly polished struts (Fig. 3). The strut cloth is completely protected from injury by a Stellite track on the inside of each strut. The construction of the orifice and hydraulic function of the valve resemble those of the other composite seat prostheses.[7,8] However, stud height is increased and the orifice cloth has been changed from Teflon to run-resistant (lock-stitch) Dacron to lessen the chance of circumferential orifice cloth tears.

Experience with this prosthesis is still in its early phase. However, the results obtained at this time (September 1975) on statistical analysis are similar to the earlier composite seat prosthesis (models 6310 and 6320) in terms of thromboembolic complications.

Clinical Experience

Mitral Valve Replacement The extended cloth orifice prosthesis with bare metal struts (model 6120) has been used for mitral

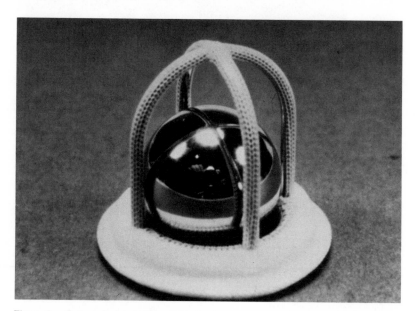

Figure 3. Composite strut ("track") mitral valve prosthesis (model 6400).

valve replacement in 86 patients since March 1965; of the survivors, 64 received continuous warfarin therapy postoperatively, 8 did not, 3 were enrolled in a double-blind study of the effectiveness of anticoagulation that is now being terminated, and 2 have been lost to follow-up study.

The cloth-covered, composite seat prosthesis (models 6310 and 6320) has been used in 220 patients since December 1968; of the survivors, 171 received continuous warfarin therapy postoperatively, 4 received antiplatelet drugs, 24 received no anticoagulant agents or antiplatelet drugs continuously, and 14 patients were enrolled in the double-blind study referred to earlier. Ninety patients received a track valve prosthesis (model 6400). Of the 84 survivors, 77 have been followed beyond 6 months and are available for late analysis. In this group there were various anticoagulant programs with 48 patients on continuous warfarin therapy postoperatively.

The clinical characteristics of these patients are listed in Table 1. Eighty-three (27 percent) with pure or predominant mitral stenosis received a ball valve prosthesis without incident. We have not experienced the difficulties with "small left ventricle" that others have reported.[9,10] A total of 44 patients (11%) required size 1M prostheses, whereas 158 (40%) received 2M, 150 (40%) received 3M, and 36 (9%) received 4M prostheses.

Indications for operation generally were disabling symptoms of exercise intolerance or fatigue associated with hemodynamic evidence of significant mitral valve disease. A recent detailed analysis of

Table 1
Mitral Valve Replacement: Preoperative Clinical Findings in 363 Patients[*]

	No.	%
Sex:		
Male	139	35
Female	257	65
Hemodynamic lesion:		
Mitral stenosis	107	27
Mitral insufficiency	103	26
Mixed lesion	186	47
Cause:		
Rheumatic	364	92
Congenital	12	3
Ruptured chordae tendineae	20	5
Functional class:		
II	44	11
III	293	74
IV	59	15

[*] Age range 15 to 74 years (mean 50).

late functional results in our patients indicated a significant correlation between postoperative functional class (New York Heart Association criteria) and preoperative duration of symptoms and response to medical management.[4] As a result, patients in "early" class III whose condition has recently deteriorated are seriously considered for operation, as will be further discussed subsequently. Of the 44 patients (11%) in class II preoperatively (Table 1), 12 were patients with mitral stenosis whose primary indication for operation was preoperative emboli; 8 of these had been receiving warfarin. Prosthetic valve replacement was required because the valves were not amenable to repair—usually as a result of calcification. The remaining patients were in late class II; their functional impairment had previously been more severe but had lessened with stringent medical management. They accepted operation because they were not content with their exercise capacity. The vast majority of patients had preoperative left and right heart catheterization, and patients over age 40 now also have coronary arteriography by the Judkins technique.

Operative technique includes a brief period of aortic cross-clamping and electrical fibrillation at mild hypothermia (30° to 32° C), during which the left atrium is opened, the valve excised, and simple interrupted sutures are placed (2-0 Tevdek; Deknatel, Inc.). We continue to believe that when the annulus is calcified, peribasilar leaks are best prevented by thorough debridement to provide a pliable bed for valve seating, rather than by elaborate suture techniques. If operative exposure permits, the aortic cross-clamp is then removed and the sutures are passed through the sewing ring of the prosthesis. The sutures are then tied, with the aortic clamp reapplied if necessary for exposure.

The operative mortality rate was 10% (9 of 86) with the 6120 prosthesis, 3% (7 of 220) with the 6310-6320 prostheses, and 7% (6 of 90) with the 6400 prosthesis (Table 2). These figures include deaths within the first month after operation, and hospital deaths from complications that started in the first month even if death occurred later (for example, from postoperative respiratory insufficiency). The track valve series includes 11 patients with aortocoronary bypass grafts and 5 patients with previous mitral valve replacement. The increase in survival between 1965 and 1968 resulted from advances and refinements in our established techniques of operative and postoperative management rather than from restricted case selection that excluded patients with advanced ventricular dysfunction. Although operation has recently been offered to class III patients earlier in their course than previously and to a few patients in late class II, the limits of operability have been extended in both directions; that is, the low operative mortality rate has encouraged us to accept patients whose condition might previously have been considered inoperable. It should be noted parenthetically that changes in prosthetic design cannot account for the changes in operative mortality rate.

Analyses of late results include only data on patients who survived operation. Excluded are data on patients who for various reasons did not receive continuous warfarin therapy, since the group is too small to contribute statistically meaningful information.

An actuarial analysis of late deaths and various complications in 64 patients with the model 6120 prosthesis is depicted in Figure 4. There were 14 late deaths (Table 3): 7 were definitely unrelated to the prosthesis, and 4 were prosthesis-related (3 from cerebral emboli and 1 from endocarditis); in 3 other cases autopsy was not performed.

An identical actuarial analysis of late deaths and complications in 171 patients with model 6310-6320 prostheses who received warfarin is displayed in Figure 5. There were 24 late deaths (14%); none were due to emboli (Table 4). The late actuarial results of the 6400 compared to the 6310-6320 series are virtually identical (Fig. 6). There were 6 late deaths. Two are prosthesis-related, one from cerebral embolus, and one from cerebral hemorrhage (Table 5).

Table 2
Mitral Valve Replacement: Causes of Operative Death

Cause	Deaths (no.)
6120 (86 implants):	
Low cardiac output	2
Pneumonia	2
Myocardial infarction	1
Cerebrovascular accident	1
Technical	3
Total	9 (10%)
6310-6320 (220 implants):	
Arrhythmia	4
Myocardial infarction	2
Respirator malfunction	1
Total	7 (3%)
6400 (90 implants):	
Low cardiac output	3
Injury to left ventricle	1
Arrhythmia	1
Cerebrovascular accident	1
Total	6 (7%)

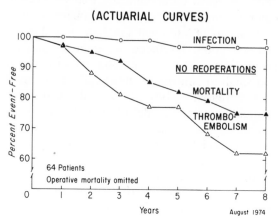

Figure 4. Mitral valve replacement with model 6120 prosthesis (noncloth-covered), March 1965 to August 1975. Actuarial analysis of individual event-free curves in patients who survived operation and received warfarin. Vertical bars denote standard errors.

The actuarial analyses in Figures 4 and 5 indicate a reduced incidence of thromboemboli with the cloth-covered prostheses, and this difference becomes statistically significant 3 years after operation ($P < 0.01$). With the cloth-covered prostheses most emboli occurred in the first year, and all within the first 3 years, but with the noncloth-covered prostheses the threat of emboli persisted up to 7 years.

Table 3

Mitral Valve Replacement with Noncloth-Covered Prosthesis (Model 6120): Causes of Late Death in 64 Survivors of Operation[*]

Cause	Deaths (no.)

Nonprosthesis-related
  Congestive heart failure: 4
  Probable arrhythmia: 2
  Suicide: 1
	7

Prosthesis-related
  Cerebrovascular accident: 3
  Subacute bacterial endocarditis: 1
	4

No autopsy:	3
Total	14

[*] All patients receiving warfarin.

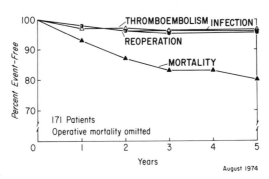

MITRAL VALVE REPLACEMENT:
CLOTH-COVERED, COMPOSITE SEAT PROSTHESES
UNIVERSITY OF OREGON MEDICAL SCHOOL

December 1968 - August 1974   Model 6310-20

(ACTUARIAL CURVES)

Figure 5.   Mitral valve replacement with model 6310-6320 prostheses (cloth-covered, composite seat). Actuarial analysis as in Figure 4.

Further analysis of embolic events with the noncloth-covered prostheses (model 6120) in terms of the severity of embolism is shown in Figure 7. The chance for a fatal embolus is only 2% and the chance for an embolus with residual neurologic damage is 8% at the end of 9 years following implantation. The remainder of the embolic episodes, including all occurring after 5 years, were transient ischemic attacks without residual abnormality.

Table 4
Mitral Valve Replacement with Cloth-Covered, Composite Seat Prostheses (Model 6310-6320): Causes of Late Death in 171 Survivors of Operation*

Cause	Deaths (no.)
Nonprosthesis-related	15
Probable arrhythmia: 4	
Congestive heart failure: 4	
Pulmonary: 2	
Hemorrhage: 1	
Miscellaneous: 4†	
Prosthesis-related:	2
Subacute bacterial endocarditis: 2	
No autopsy:	7
Total	24

* All patients receiving warfarin.
† Asthma, drug reaction, renal failure, emphysema.

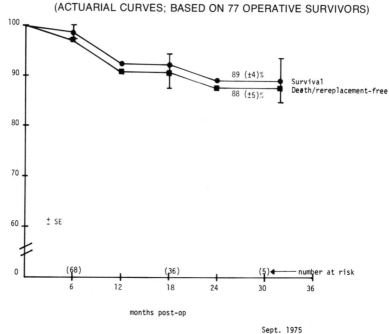

ISOLATED MITRAL VALVE REPLACEMENT:

Model 6400

(ACTUARIAL CURVES; BASED ON 77 OPERATIVE SURVIVORS)

Figure 6. Mitral replacement with model 6400 prostheses (composite strut). Actuarial analysis as in Figure 4.

Table 6 analyzes the incidence of thromboembolism in terms of embolic episodes per 100 patient years of follow-up. With the noncloth-covered prosthesis, there were 6 emboli per 100 patient years while with the 6310-6320 series, the incidence was 1.9 episodes per 100 patient years. Such calculations for the track valve (Model

Table 5

Mitral Valve Replacement with Composite Strut ("Track") Prosthesis (Model 6400): Causes of Late Death in 84 Survivors at Operation

Cause	Deaths (No.)
Nonprosthesis-related	3
Probable arrhythmia: 3	
Prosthesis-related	2
Cerebral Hemorrhage: 1	
Cerebral Embolus: 1	
No Autopsy	1
Total	6

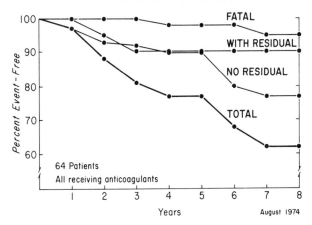

INCIDENCE OF THROMBOEMBOLIC COMPLICATIONS
(ACTUARIAL CURVES)

Figure 7. Mitral valve replacement with model 6120 prosthesis. Actuarial analyses of thromboembolic complications according to severity in patients receiving anticoagulant therapy.

6400) are not comparable, since the mean follow-up is much shorter for the current standard prosthesis. (There are no currently acceptable statistical methods for assessing the significance of differences reported in this manner.)

In patients with the model 6120 prosthesis there were no reoperations. Five patients (3 percent) with model 6310-6320 prostheses receiving warfarin required reoperation; operative findings are listed in Table 7. This table also displays the findings in four patients with model 6310-6320 prostheses who were not receiving warfarin. Problems such as periprosthetic leaks and prosthetic valve endocarditis occur with any prosthesis in a small percentage of cases. Orifice stenosis due to thrombus has primarily been seen in patients not receiving warfarin. However, two patients receiving warfarin had

Table 6
Mitral Valve Replacement: Incidence of Emboli

	Noncloth-Covered (model 6120)	Cloth-Covered (model 6310-6320)
Patients (no.)	64	171
Total patient years of follow-up	384	428
Average years of follow-up per patient	6.0	2.5
Emboli/100 patient years	6.0	1.9

thrombus that interfered with proper seating of the poppet and caused regurgitation.

Of note is that catastrophic malfunction due to thrombus on the valve requiring emergency operation was not seen. In such instances, the diagnosis can be made by clinical and hemodynamic studies with elective reoperation and small operative risk.

There were no cases of poppet variance, wear, or disruption with either prosthesis. Orifice cloth wear in one patient with an early model 6310 prosthesis that had flow stud height prompted replacement of the prosthesis (Table 7). In one other patient a mild degree of orifice cloth wear was observed when the valve was inspected 15 months postoperatively during reoperation for tricuspid insufficiency; replacement was not required. Stud height has been increased in more recent prostheses, and with the lock stitch in the orifice cloth, this complication is less likely. Strut cloth tear with model 6310-6320 prostheses was not observed at reoperation. However, some valves recovered at autopsy had flattening and some fraying of the cloth at the base of the struts. The track valve configuration obviates the possibility of strut cloth wear.

Hemolytic anemia has not occurred with either prosthesis in the absence of peribasilar leaks. No patient required transfusion or reoperation for hemolysis. Several patients with normal hematocrits receive oral iron therapy at the suggestion of their family physicians; their continued need for iron is uncertain.

The incidence of prosthetic valve endocarditis is displayed actuarially in Figures 4 and 5 and is quite similar for both models 6120 and 6310-6320 prostheses. We have recently reviewed this general prob-

Table 7
Mitral Valve Replacement with Model 6310-6320 Prostheses: Findings at Reoperation

	With Anti-coagulant Therapy (5 patients)	Without Anti-coagulant Therapy (4 patients)	Total (9 patients)
Thrombotic obstruction	1	4	5
Thrombotic regurgitation	2	0	2
Perivalvular leak	1	1	2
Suture impingement	1	0	1
Orifice cloth tear	1	0	1
Strut cloth tear	0	0	0
Total	6*	5*	11*

* The number of findings exceeds the number of patients because some patients had more than one finding.

lem, and have noted several cases of apparent "cure" when there was no peribasilar leak to complicate the situation and the causative organism was sensitive to antibiotic agents.[11]

DISCUSSION

The early mitral prosthesis in use from 1960 to 1965 (model 6000) demonstrated the feasibility of mitral replacement with the ball valve prosthesis, but carried with it an unacceptable incidence of serious thromboembolic complications. In addition, fatty infiltration of the silicone rubber ball with swelling of the poppet, while rare, was seen in 2 patients in our series and other instances were reported to the manufacturer. The change in configuration of the noncloth-covered prosthesis in 1965 resulting in the current prosthesis (model 6120) greatly reduced the embolic complication rate, and ball variance has not been seen with this prosthesis with follow-up to 10 years. The effectiveness of this design change, while obvious now in retrospect, could not have been known in 1967, and it seemed reasonable at that time to take an alternative path, namely the development of cloth-covered prostheses. In the mitral series this has decreased the incidence of thromboembolic complications enormously but has, at the same time, introduced new problems with regard to thrombosis and cloth injury.

A selection of one prosthesis over the other must depend on both the relative incidence of various complications and a value judgment on the significance of one complication vs. another, since no prosthesis is completely free of complications. A comparison of the noncloth-covered prosthesis (model 6120) to the cloth-covered prosthesis (model 6310-6320) is shown in Figure 8. The percentage of patients alive and complication-free at 5 years is similar with both prostheses as is the late mortality rate. The incidence of embolism is significantly greater with the noncloth-covered valve, while the need for reoperation is greater with the cloth-covered valve. It is noteworthy that at least half of the embolic complications with the noncloth-covered prosthesis leave no residual damage. It is likely that the reoperation rate for the track valve (model 6400) due to cloth injury will be reduced, but the thromboembolic potential of this valve is not so well established because of the relatively short followup. An actuarial comparison of the incidence of this complication between the 6310-6320 prostheses and the 6400 prosthesis is shown in Figure 9. At 30 months there is no statistical difference.

On balance, there is no statistical difference then in the results that one can achieve at least at the end of 5 years with cloth-covered

426

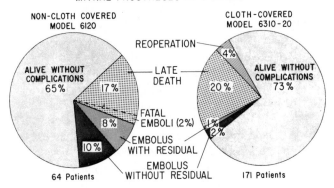

MITRAL VALVE REPLACEMENT
UNIVERSITY OF OREGON MEDICAL SCHOOL

ACTUARIAL COMPARISON OF CLOTH-COVERED VS. NON CLOTH-COVERED
MITRAL PROSTHESES AT 5 YEARS*

NON-CLOTH COVERED
MODEL 6120

CLOTH-COVERED
MODEL 6310-20

REOPERATION
LATE DEATH
ALIVE WITHOUT COMPLICATIONS 65%
17%
ALIVE WITHOUT COMPLICATIONS 73%
4%
20%
FATAL EMBOLI (2%)
8%
1%
2%
10%
EMBOLUS WITH RESIDUAL
EMBOLUS WITHOUT RESIDUAL
64 Patients
171 Patients

*ALL PATIENTS RECEIVING ANTICOAGULANTS
OPERATIVE MORTALITY OMITTED

Figure 8. Actuarial analysis of comparative complications of mitral valve prostheses (models 6120 vs. 6310-6320).

vs. noncloth-covered prostheses. These results must, of course, be interpreted cautiously, since noncloth-covered prostheses may pose a continuing threat of embolic complications beyond the 5 year period, while this is unlikely with cloth-covered prostheses. In our clinic, the reduction in embolism with cloth-covered valves has been considered an overriding long-term advantage; we have accepted the

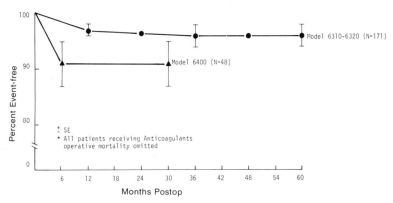

ISOLATED MITRAL VALVE REPLACEMENT

Comparative Thromboembolism*

Model 6310-6320 (N=171)

Model 6400 (N=48)

‡ SE
* All patients receiving Anticoagulants
operative mortality omitted

Percent Event-free

100

90

80

0

6   12   18   24   30   36   42   48   54   60

Months Postop

Figure 9. Actuarial analysis of comparative thromboembolism with mitral valve prostheses (models 6310-6320 vs. 6400).

increased incidence of reoperation and the need for more careful followup of the patient in this regard as a reasonable price to pay for this advantage.

Hemodynamically, the cloth-covered and noncloth-covered prostheses are similar.[12,14] However, the possibility of narrowing of the orifice of a cloth-covered prosthesis by thrombis material must be taken into consideration in selecting the suitable prosthesis for a particular patient. At present we continue to use both series of valves, with the cloth-covered preferred in the larger sizes (size 3 and 4M) and the noncloth-covered in the smaller sizes (size 1 and 2M). We recommend anticoagulant treatment for all of our patients as standard medical care with either series of valves in the absence of specific contraindications to such a program.

Statistical Analysis of Late Results

The foregoing discussion, in which the late results with two ball valve prostheses are compared, relies upon an appraisal of closely followed patients by means of current actuarial techniques that provide a true perspective of time-related risks.[5,6] Whereas randomized studies are ideal for comparing prostheses, they are rarely feasible. It is therefore crucial that clinical reports of results with various prostheses carefully define the patient population under analysis, and present late results in a statistically meaningful manner that facilitates comparison with other reports. In recent years, it has been recognized that actuarial (life-table) methods best satisfy these criteria, and should be employed routinely. However, the actuarial method is not standardized[15,16] and a report of survival rates should also be accompanied by a clear description of the method of calculation employed, or by a reference to such a description, with clarification of any modifications introduced by the investigators.

Unfortunately, reports frequently appear in which short-term follow-up is presented and incidence rates of late death and specific complications are described only as simple percentages. Such practices tend to obscure rather than to illuminate experience because they ignore the distribution of patients in time. Since accurate analyses of late results are vital to an assessment of valve substitutes, the choice of a prosthesis must inevitably be influenced by the quality of available information.

Timing of Operation

The timing of operation in patients with significant valvular heart disease depends upon a comparison of the risks of operation and prostheses with the risks of uncorrected disease. In patients with heart disease of the type that requires valve replacement, operation has traditionally been deferred until symptoms were far advanced and refractory to medical management. Because of the heart's compensatory mechanisms, severe hemodynamic abnormalities and significant ventricular dysfunction can exist without striking clinical disability, particularly in the case of aortic or mitral regurgitation. Indeed, experimental evidence suggests that acute mitral regurgitation, by increasing ventricular preload and decreasing ventricular afterload, acutely enhances certain isolated parameters of left ventricular performance while increasing myocardial oxygen consumption a modest, but definite, amount.[17]

In the early 1960's, the mortality rate for valve replacement was relatively high. In addition, long-term functional results were influenced significantly by valve-related complications. However, with improvement in cardiac surgical techniques and prosthetic devices, more patients with advanced valvular disease have survived. Long-term follow-up of those survivors with poor cardiac reserve has demonstrated the consequences of delaying operation. In a previous study[4] of late functional results after mitral valve replacement with model 6310-6320 prostheses in our clinic, preoperative hemodynamic variables and functional class had little or no correlation with postoperative functional class. For example, approximately half the patients in preoperative class III and half in class IV were in class I postoperatively, so that preoperative functional class could not be used for prognosis. Instead, a "prognostic classification" derived from the preoperative duration of symptoms and their response to medical management had a highly significant correlation with postoperative functional class. It was concluded that in view of long-term results with current prostheses, mitral valve replacement can reasonably be offered to moderately disabled patients with recent clinical deterioration who respond to medical treatment, rather than being restricted only to those with severe disability who can no longer respond to medical therapy.

REFERENCES

1. Harken, D.E., Soroff, H.S., Taylor, W.J., et al. Partial and complete prostheses in aortic insufficiency. *J. Thorac. Cardiovasc. Surg.* 40:744, 1960.

2. Starr, A., Edwards, M.L.: Mitral replacement: clinical experience with a ball valve prosthesis. *Ann. Surg.* 154:726, 1961.

3. Herr, R.H., Starr A., Pierie, W.R., et al. Aortic valve

replacement: a review of six years' experience with the ball valve prosthesis. *Ann. Thorac. Surg.* 6:199, 1968.

4. Bonchek, L.I., Anderson, R.P., Starr, A. Mitral valve replacement with cloth-covered composite-seat prostheses: the case for early operation. *J. Thorac. Cardiovasc. Surg.* 67:93, 1974.

5. Anderson, R.P., Bonchek, L.I., Grunkemeir, G.L., et al. The analysis and presentation of surgical results by actuarial methods. *J. Surg. Res.* 16:224, 1974.

6. Grunkemeier, G.L., Lambert, L.E., Bonchek, L.I., Starr, A. An improved statistical method for assessing the results of operation. *Ann. Thorac. Surg.* 20:289, 1975.

7. Research and Development Group, Technical Data Analyses, Edwards Laboratories, Santa Ana, Calif.

8. Hodam, R., Anderson, R.P., Starr, A., et al. Further evaluation of the composite seat cloth-covered aortic prosthesis. *Ann. Thorac. Surg.* 12:621, 1971.

9. Roberts, W.C., Morrow, A.G. Mechanisms of acute left atrial thrombosis after mitral valve replacement: pathologic findings indicating obstruction to left atrial emptying. *Am. J. Cardiol.* 18:497, 1966.

10. Kay, E.B., Suzuki, A., Demaney, M., et al. Comparison of ball and disc valves for mitral valve replacement. *Am. J. Cardiol.* 18:504, 1966.

11. Slaughter, L., Morris, J.E., Starr, A. Prosthetic valvular endocarditis: a 12 year review. *Circulation* 47:1319, 1973.

12. Bristow, J.D., Kloster, F.E., Herr, R., Starr, A., Colin, W.M., and Griswold, H.E. Cardiac catheterization studies after combined tricuspid, mitral and aortic valve replacement. *Circulation* 34:437, 1966.

13. Kloster, F.E., Farrehi, C., Mourdjinis, A., Hodam, R.P., Starr, A., Griswold, H.E. Hemodynamic studies in patients with cloth-covered composite-seat Starr-Edwards valve prostheses. *J. Thorac. Cardiovasc. Surg.* 60:879, 1970.

14. Russell, T., Kremkau, E.L., Kloster, F.E. and Starr, A. Late hemodynamic function of cloth-covered Starr-Edwards valve prostheses. Suppl *Circulation* 45 & 46:I-8-U-13, 1972.

15. Armitage P.: The comparison of survival curves. *J. R. Stat. Assoc.* 122:12, 1959.

16. Kuzma, J.W. A comparison of two life table methods. *Biometrics* 25:51, 1967.

17. Urschel, C.W., Covell, J.W., Graham, T.P., et al. Effects of acute valvular regurgitation on the oxygen consumption of the canine heart. *Circ. Res.* 23:33, 1968.

36 Long-Term Results After Mitral Valvular Prosthetic Replacement: Causes and Results of Reoperations

C. Cabrol, M.D.
A. Cabrol, M.D.
I. Gandjbakhch, M.D.
G. Guiraudon, M.D.
C. Christides, M.D.
M.F. Mattei, M.D.
M.H. Cappe, M.D.

INTRODUCTION

When properly selected prior to operation, correctly operated upon, and given a suitable prosthesis, patients having mitral valve replacement should experience a dramatic improvement. If not, the patient must have a complete reassessment of his or her cardiac condition, including history of the disease, physical examination, hemodynamic studies, radiological explorations (angiography, coronary arteriography) to detect the reasons for the heart failure.

MATERIAL

Since 1964, we have operated upon 2100 patients for heart valve replacement. Among them 720 patients had a mitral prosthesis, 461 for an isolated mitral replacement, 180 with an associated aortic prosthesis, 50 with an associated tricuspid replacement, and 29 with an associated aortic and tricuspid replacement. We implanted 618

431

Starr-Edwards valves, 90 Björk-Shiley valves, 10 Lillehei-Kaster valves, and 2 Beall valves.

During the same time, we did 27 reoperations (3.7%) on patients with a mitral valve prosthesis. Reasons for severe cardiac failure and subsequent reoperation were prosthetic complications (17 cases), as well as neglected associated valvular disease (5 cases), other cardiac defects created or not detected at the first operation (2 cases), associated coronary disease (2 cases), and myocardial dysfunction (1 case).

Prosthetic Complications

These include 8 thromboses, 8 paravalvular leaks, 6 infections, 3 deteriorations, and 2 hemolyses. These complications were frequently combined. Thrombosis and infection were encountered in 3 cases, and infection caused paravalvular leaks in 2 cases; hemolysis was the consequence of a prosthetic deterioration in one case, and of a paravalvular leak in 2 cases.

Prosthetic complications were well described elsewhere, and we will here concern ourselves with only the most severe of them: thrombosis. We observed 8 cases of prosthetic and atrial thrombosis after mitral valve replacement: 5 on Björk valves, 3 on Starr-Edwards valves. Two were of the "toilet seat" type. They appear on the atrial wall near the mitral orifice, and move suddenly and occasionally to close the orifice of the mitral prosthesis, giving a sudden systemic hypotension and syncop; this often can be cured by changing the position of the patient. Quite different is the clinical aspect of a thrombosis developed on the prosthesis itself. The diagnosis is often difficult and is suspected because of the occurrence of multiple emboli, the modifications of the cardiac sounds on the phonocardiogram, and the abnormal motion of the poppet on a movie X-ray of the valve. These thromboses have definite predisposing factors, and were often seen in our experience on disc-valve (Björk) patients, and on patients having a chronic low cardiac output before operation. The treatment consists in the replacement of the previous prosthesis by a new one (preferably a ball valve or a xenograft). The prognosis for this reoperation is poor, and we lost 5 of our 8 patients in this group. The reason for this peculiar high risk is the poor preoperative condition of these patients, who are often admitted at the hospital in emergency, sometimes after a cardiac arrest and in cardiovascular shock.

Other Reasons for Reoperation

More interesting because less familiar are the other causes of reoperation on patients with mitral prostheses. One of the most frequently seen is an associated valvular disease not detected or neglected at the first operation. For such lesion we had to reoperate on six patients: one aortic insufficiency, one aortic stenosis, two tricuspid insufficiencies alone, and two tricuspid insufficiencies associated with a mitral prosthetic complication (paravalvular leak). It is now our policy to treat any tricuspid insufficiency, even if it is reversible, when it is observed in the preoperative course. For the cure we use our semicircular annuloplasty, which is a simple, fast, safe, and reliable technique (Fig. 1). For the same reason the aortic valve is

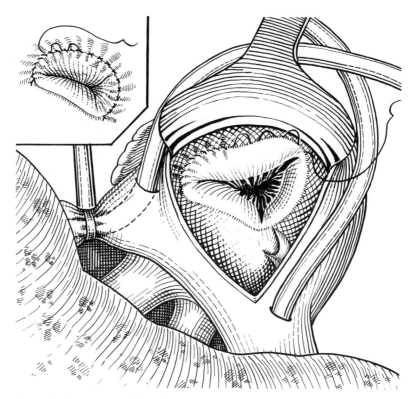

Figure 1. Semicircular Tricuspid Annuloplasty. The right atrium, between the two encircled venae cavae, is opened transversely. A running suture is threaded in the distensible part of the tricuspid annulus (along the attachment of the anterior and the inferior leaflets), respecting the fixed part on the septum and so avoiding injury to the Bundle of His.

carefully examined at the time of operation during each mitral replacement, and is replaced if the releasing of the aortic clamp after the onset of the cardiac bypass is followed by a drop of the aortic pressure over 20 mm Hg, or by an aortic regurgitation, appreciated by the intracardiac suction, over 800 cc/min, and if the aortic valve palpated by an intraventricular finger appeared severely damaged.

Other cardiac lesions were missed prior to and during the first intervention, and this explained the poor results observed. In one case a persisting left coronary artery-coronary sinus fistula was misinterpreted as a tricuspid insufficiency, and only recognized after the completion of an efficient tricuspid annuloplasty, which was, nevertheless, unable to correct the clinical signs of a right cardiac diastolic overloading.

In another case the lesion was created at the first operation performed for mitral insufficiency due to a left atrial myxoma. The myxoma was resected with a portion of the atrial septum, and a badly damaged mitral valve was replaced by a prosthesis. The closure of the septum was not perfect, and it caused the persistence of an interatrial septal defect which had to be closed six months later.

Sometimes a poor post-operative result after mitral valve replacement is explained by an associated coronary disease not diagnosed or neglected at the first operation (one case in this series). The coronary disease can appear after the initial operation. We experienced one case of post-cannulation coronary stenosis after a double mitral and aortic replacement, and one case of coronary thromboembolism after mitral valve replacement alone. The two first cases were given a saphenous-vein aortocoronary bypass upon reoperation, with one good result and one death.

It is only when, after a careful and complete cardiac evaluation, one cannot detect any prosthetic complications, associated valvular disease, other cardiac defects, chronic pericardial tamponade, or coronary artery disease, that one may suspect an "isolated" myocardial failure. This is sometimes easily explained by a poor myocardial protection during the first operation leaving a large myocardial infarct.

The reason for complications is also often the existence of an advanced and chronic myocardial failure before intervention. Some patients of that group regain a good left-ventricular contractility after mitral replacement, but most of them remain in congestive failure. This emphasizes the necessity of earlier operation in this long-term, slow-degrading disease.

In that group must also be mentioned some patients in an advanced stage of cardiomyopathy with functional mitral insufficiency who are presented to the surgeon for the correction of that "symptomatic" regurgitation. The functional improvement after the mitral valvular replacement is usually of short duration, and death rapidly follows. In such a case we performed a cardiac transplantation (which is the only logical treatment), with a lasting success a year and a half later.

RESULTS

Of this total number of 27 reoperations, we have lost 7 patients. This operative mortality of 25% is high, and is mostly due to the left atrial thrombosis, which accounted for 5 of the 7 deaths.

CONCLUSIONS

For the reasons mentioned above, we advocate a careful followup after mitral valve replacement, but in addition we strongly recommend a *complete* cardiac reassessment of patients with poor results in order to detect the prosthetic, valvular, pericardial, coronary, or muscular lesion which explains the observed failure instead of the expected improvement. Once diagnosed, the causal lesion must be treated by reoperation as soon as possible in order to lower the spontaneous or "post-reoperation" mortality, which is still too important in the long-term results of mitral valve replacement.

SUMMARY

Out of a total number of 720 mitral replacements, we did 27 reoperations (3.7%). Reasons were the familiar prosthetic complications in 17 cases, but in 10 cases other cardiac lesions were found: associated valvular disease (5), other cardiac defects (2), associated coronary disease (2), and myocardial dysfunction (1). These lesions explain the percentage of poor results and the relatively high mortality observed in the long-term results of mitral replacement. They suggest the complete reassessment of patients who do not experience a dramatic improvement after such operations.

REFERENCES

1. Acar, J., Duron, F., Luxereau, P., Grunberg, F., Lainee, R., Auperin, A., and Farah, E. Indications et résultats des réinterventions chez les opérés de prothèses mitrales et aortiques. *Coeur*, n° spécial, Journées de Deauville, 487, 1975.

2. Christides, D., Cabrol, C. and A., Guiraudon, G., Gandjbakhch, I., Mattei, M.F., Luciani, J. and Akrout, J. Réinterventions sur prothèses valvulaires mitrales. *Coeur*, n° spécial, 515, 1975.

3. Widne, B., and Levy, M. Thromboembolism following heart valve replacement by prosthesis: survey of 365 consecutive patients. *Chest* 63:713, 1973.

4. Engelman, R.M., Chase, R.M., Boyd, A.D., and Reed, G.E. Lethal post-operative infections following cardiac surgery. Review of four years experience. *Circulation* 48, supplem. III, 111, 1973.

5. Kirklin, J.W., and Pacifico, A.D. Surgery for acquired valvular heart disease (second of two parts). *New Eng. J. Med.*, 288:194, 1973.

37 Hemodynamic Data and Left Ventricular Function of Diseased Mitral Valves Replaced by Prostheses

Postoperative Change and
Prognostic Value

P. Luxereau, M.D.
F. Herreman, M.D.
J. Carlet, M.D.
G. Lutfalla, M.D.
J. Acar, M.D.

The change in hemodynamic parameters after mitral valvular replacement has been the subject of a certain number of papers, in part devoted to evaluation of individual prostheses.[1-12] Certain points concerning the quality and rate of improvement and changes in the cases with a steep increase in pulmonary-vascular resistance and pressure are still little known, as well as the prognostic value of preoperative hemodynamics, whose analysis has given varying results. The purpose of this study is to contribute to the knowledge of the aforementioned points.

MATERIAL AND METHODS

Out of 450 observations of valvular replacements made between 1968 and 1975, we have selected 96 patients operated on for mitral monovalvular replacement, and explored by catheterization. The average age of these patients when operated was 50 years (distribution, 24 to 66). There were 47 men and 49 women. There were 27 cases of mitral stenosis (MS), 24 cases of mitral regurgitation (MR), and 45 cases with associated stenosis and regurgitation (MS + MR).

In 23 cases, a functional tricuspid insufficiency was corrected by conservative annuloplasty during the same operation.

A Starr prosthesis with a silastic poppet model 6120 was used 75 times (78%) and with a stellite poppet 10 times (eight model 6320, two model 6300) a Björk valve seven times, a Smeloff-Cutter valve two times, and a Beall valve two times.

All patients had right or right and left heart catheterization with measurement of cardiac output before the operation. Fifty-four underwent a second postoperative catheterization within an average of 19 months (distribution, 1 month to 98 months). In most cases, the right heart was catheterized with a floating Swan-Ganz catheter. The following prostheses were used in these 54 cases: Starr 6120, 45, Starr 6320, 3, Starr 6300, 1, Björk, 3, Smeloff-Cutter, 1, Beall 1.

Twenty-seven iterative postoperative investigations were made of 12 patients over a period of 24 months.

A comparative preoperative and postoperative study of the left ventricular function was made on eight patients 26 to 55 years of age (MR: 4; MS: 1; MS + MR: 3). This study, using the data from catheterization and biplane cineangiography at 100 frames per second, is based on the estimate of the left ventricular end-diastolic volume (EDV), ejection fraction (EF), amplitude (Δ lf), and average velocity of fiber shortening ($\overline{Vf}$). The results were compared with those for a group of eight subjects with no malfunction of the left heart.*

Thirty-five patients had preoperative mean pulmonary artery pressure greater than or equal to 40 mm Hg. They were the subject of a separate clinical study. Nineteen were recatheterized after the operation. There were 19 men and 16 women in the group, with an average age of 49 (distribution, 26 to 66). They suffered from the following valvular diseases: MS, 12; MR, 10 (8 with ruptured chordae tendineae); MS + MR, 13. The following prostheses were used: Starr 6120, 27; Starr 6320, 4; Starr 6300, 1; Björk, 3.

The pressures are expressed in mm of Hg and pulmonary arteriolar resistance in international units per m²:

$$\frac{\text{mean AP} - \text{mean wedge mm Hg}}{\text{CI l/min/m}^2}$$

Cardiac output is measured by the method of dye dilution curves.

The statistical methods used included a comparison of averages by tests of matched series and t test (Student and Fischer).

---

* Average normal values EDV: 73 ± 16 cm3/m2, EF: 60 ± 5%, Δ lf: 22 ± 2% Vf: 0.70 ± 0.14 muscle length/sec (ML/S).

RESULTS

Changes in hemodynamic parameters for entire series

The preoperative and postoperative hemodynamic data appear in Figure 1. A marked decrease in lesser circulation pressures and an increase in the cardiac index can be seen. All of these variations are statistically very significant.

The change over time is seen in Figure 2. It was evaluated on the basis of 27 iterative postoperative catheterizations in 12 patients (two mitral regurgitations due to ruptured chordae tendineae, four mitral stenoses, and six stenoses with regurgitation). With but a few exceptions, the evolution is favorable. What is remarkable, however, is that the improvement in pulmonary wedge and arterial pressures and, to a lesser degree, in the cardiac index is more noticeable from one examination to the next, and continues gradually until at least the second postoperative year.

Changes in ventricular function

Before the operation (Table 1) the left ventricular end-diastolic pressure is normal except in one case of acute infectious MR (II);

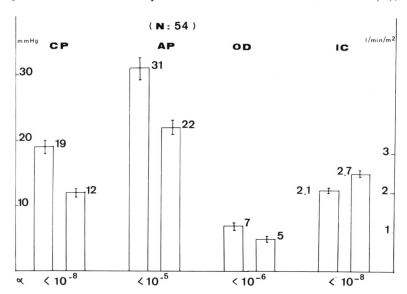

Figure 1. Preoperative (left columns) and postoperative (right) hemodynamic results, average values. CP: pulmonary wedge pressure (mean). AP: pulmonary artery pressure (mean). OD: right atrial pressure. IC: cardiac index, α: statistical significance.

440

cardiac output falls in all cases. Left ventricular dilatation is more marked in pure MR than in MS + MR. On the other hand, EDV is normal in the MS (VIII). The left ventricular function indexes are normal or moderately lowered in five cases (EF $\geqslant$ 50%, Δ1f $\geqslant$ 15%, and $\overline{Vf}$ > 50 ML/S). In three cases (III, IV, VI), left ventricular performance seems to be considerably altered.

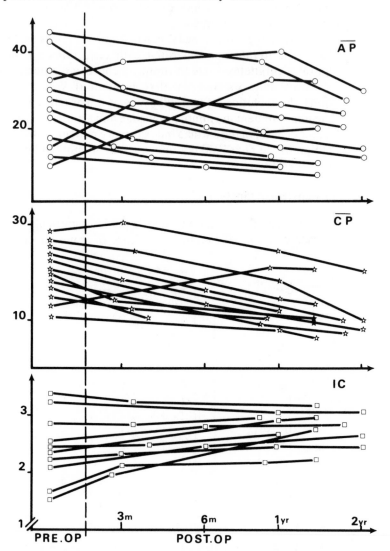

Figure 2. Results of iterative catheterizations up to the second postoperative year (12 patients). CP: pulmonary wedge pressure (mean). AP: pulmonary artery (mean). IC: cardiac index.

Table 1
Pre and Post Operative Left Ventricular Function Indexes (See Text)*

No.	Age	Valvular Lesion	Pre Op							Post Op					
			PAP	LVEDP	CI	LVEDV	EF	Δ Lf	V̄f	PAP	CI	LVEDV	EF	Δ 1F	V̄f
I	33	MR	22/10	10	2.0	185	54	23	.65	25/6	3.7	115	62	22	.80
II	26	MR	80/40	20	2.0	155	68	28	.95	30/12	3.3	70	75	33	1.20
III	34	MR	30/15	8	2.1	180	40	8	.20	22/9	2.2	90	54	15	.55
IV	53	MR	40/10	12		270	38	13	.45	25/10	2.9	80	54	19	.75
V	33	MS + MR	32/12	12	2.2	145	62	20	.60	33/10		115	64	26	1.10
VI	42	MS + MR	32/17	9		120	29	10	.35	30/7	3.1	110	45	12	.40
VII	55	MS + MR	45/25	12	2.1	100	50	19	.60	35/12	3.3	190	38	12	.50
VIII	47	MS	75/30	10	2.3	80	50	15	.50	35/15	2.8	70	61	22	.85

* LVEDP: left ventricular end-diastolic pressure. PAP: pulmonary artery pressure. CI: cardiac index. EF: ejection fraction. Δ Lf: amplitude of fiber shortening. V̄f: average velocity of fiber shortening. LVEDV: left ventricular end-diastolic volume.

After the operation, cardiac output returns to normal, and the EDV decreases significantly in the presence of dilatation. In one patient (VII), however, the EDV, which was subnormal before the operation, increased greatly afterwards. The left ventricular function indexes improved in all cases except one (VII), resulting in values which were normal or only slightly below normal in six cases. In one case, finally, the performance indexes improved but still were considerably lower than normal after the operation (VI).

Cases with high pulmonary hypertension

In preoperative terms, the functional disability was important. Only one patient was in functional class II (New York Heart Association), 18 in class III, and 16 in class IV. Thirty showed clear signs of right-sided heart failure. The average cardiothoracic ratio was 0.60 (distribution 0.50 to 0.70). The ECG showed signs of right ventricular hypertrophy 27 times and atrial fibrillation 23 times.

Preoperative hemodynamics were severely altered:
Mean pulmonary artery pressure (mm Hg) 40 to 62 (average 51)
Mean pulmonary wedge pressure (mm Hg) 18 to 38 (average 27)
Mean right atrial pressure (mm Hg)   4 to 21 (average 9)
Arteriolar resistance (IU/m^2 4.5 to 27 (average 11)
Cardiac index (1/min/m^2)   1.1 to 3.3 (average, 2.1)

Operative death totaled four cases (11.4%). The survivors were seen 1 month to 10 years later (average, 24 months). Four remain in functional class III, 17 in class II, and 10 in class I.

The clinical signs of congestive heart failure disappeared or decreased in 24 patients and remained unchanged in three. The average cardiothoracic ratio changed from 0.60 to 0.56.

The change in hemodynamics in 19 recatheterized patients is shown in Figure 3. In most cases there is a notable, significant reduction (< 0.001) in pressure and resistance.

In four cases, however, the results are incomplete or insignificant. In each of these cases, an additional cause may explain the failure. One 63-year-old patient was operated on for mitral regurgitation due to fibrocalcific transformation of a papillary muscle due to an anomalous left coronary artery arising from the pulmonary artery. The total absence of improvement may be attributed to the old, long-standing left-to-right shunt. In three other cases of incomplete improvement, postembolic pulmonary arterial obliterations were responsible in one case, and the model or small size of the prosthesis (6300, No. 2, 6120, No. 1) in two cases.

Prognostic value

The comparison of the percentages of operative deaths, depending on whether the mean pulmonary artery pressure is lower (61 cases) or higher (35 cases) than 40 mm of Hg, or whether the arteriolar resistance is lower (44 cases) or higher (28 cases) than 7 international units per m², showed no significant differences. Similarly, we found no significant differences between the group of early deaths and that of good results for average values of pulmonary wedge pressure (respectively, 19 and 21), mean pulmonary arterial pressure (34 and 34), right atrial pressure (5 and 7), pulmonary resistance (6.1 and 6.5), and the cardiac index (2.3 and 2.1).

DISCUSSION

On the whole, this study confirms the very significant improvement in hemodynamic parameters following the replacement of mitral valves. It should be pointed out that these results were obtained in most of our patients with Starr prostheses using a Silastic poppet (model 6120).

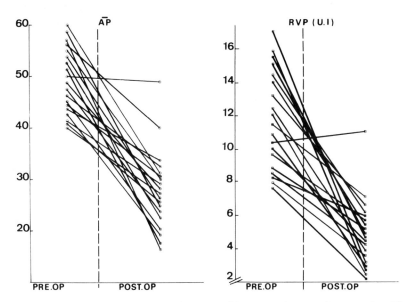

Figure 3. Hemodynamic changes in cases with steep pulmonary hypertension (19 patients). AP: pulmonary artery (mean pressure). RVP: arteriolar resistances (international units/m²).

Independent of the type of valvular disease, the trend appears to be similar. In particular, a comparison between mitral stenosis and mitral regurgitations due to ruptured chordae tendineae showed no statistically significant differences over time.

On the other hand, a comparison with a similar group of aortic replacements showed improvements which were not as complete in the group of mitral valves whose pressures decrease less and whose output remains significantly lower. These results are probably due to several factors: 1) the frequent coexistence of irregular rhythm and, in particular, atrial fibrillation (found in 78% of the patients operated on in the present series), and 2) the different influence on hemodynamics of a prosthesis depending on whether it is placed on an atrioventricular orifice where it acts during diastole as an obstacle to blood flow,[9] or on the aortic orifice, where it only acts indirectly by means of the left ventricular function.

Long-term changes in hemodynamics after mitral replacement had not been studied. Some authors[10] have suggested that postoperative improvements could take place gradually in certain cases. The present series uses iterative catheterization to show that this improvement can continue up to the second postoperative year, not only for the pulmonary arterial pressure, which is easily understandable given the reduction in resistance, but also for the wedge pressure and cardiac index. This suggests a slowly regressive preoperative modification of the left ventricular function, even in the cases of pure mitral stenosis. This gradual change appears specific to cases of mitral cardiopathy and different for cases of aortic cardiopathy whose return to normal values takes place very quickly, as was seen in the parallel study of a group of aortic cardiopathy cases.

This study confirms the reversible nature of severe pulmonary hypertension and increase in resistance.[11-13] As for the other patients in the series, the improvement in pressures and cardiac index takes place gradually. The improvement in hemodynamics is accompanied by a clinical improvement.

The incomplete improvements are all explained in this series by the associated pathology or the prosthesis used.

LEFT VENTRICULAR FUNCTION

Complete surgical repair of the valve defect leads to a clear improvement in hemodynamics in all cases, with a decrease in the left ventricular volume when there is a volume overload.

Little is known about changes in the contractile value of the myocardium after valve surgery. In five cases of aortic regurgitation,

Gault[14] observed no postoperative changes. Hildner,[15] on the other hand, saw improvements in certain cases, in particular in cases of considerable preoperative dilatation. Herreman[16] observed the same phenomenon.

Our series of eight mitral valvular diseases proves that the ventricular function can improve after radical repair of valvular lesions. However, if the myocardial insufficiency is severe, myocardial alterations appear to be irreversible (case VI), especially when the heart is only slightly dilated before the operation.

Finally, on the other hand, a myocardial insufficiency can appear after the operation, raising the issue of the role of the surgical traumatism.

PROGNOSTIC VALUE

The prognostic value of preoperative hemodynamics has been disputed. Litwak,[17] on the basis of a series of 110 mitral replacements between 1962 and 1968, attributes a predictive value of operative death to certain parameters. Other authors[2,4,11] see no influence of the same variables on short- and long-term results. Zener,[13] studying 19 mitral replacements with extreme pulmonary hypertension (greater than 100 mm of Hg for systolic pressure), found that the increased operative risk is more a function of pulmonary vascular resistance than pressure. Simonsen[18] arrived at the same conclusions. Despite the presence of a large proportion of severe pulmonary hypertension in our series, none of the parameters considered, including pulmonary resistance, could be credited with a statistically significant prognostic value. Lowering of operative death during the last 10 years may explain certain points of disagreement between works performed in the past and more recently because of progress in surgery that has eliminated some or all of the aggravating character of certain factors.

CONCLUSION

The study of 96 cases of mitral monovalvular replacement, 54 of which were recatheterized post-operatively, confirms the usual improvement of hemodynamic parameters.

Iterative catheterization shows that improvement takes place gradually and continues up to the second post-operative year.

Unless there is an additional problem, patients with high

pulmonary pressure and resistance show a favorable post-operative hemodynamic course.

Studies of left ventricular function performed post-operatively in 8 patients demonstrate the possibility of great improvement of ejection fraction, amplitude, and velocity of fiber shortening.

REFERENCES

1. Beck, W., Fergusson, D.J.G., Barnard, C.N., and Schrire, V. Hemodynamic findings following replacement of the mitral valve with the University of Cape Town Prosthesis. *Circul.* 32: 721, 731, 1965.

2. Bonchek, L.I., Anderson, R.P., Starr, A. Mitral valve replacement with cloth-covered composite seat prostheses. The case for early operation. *J. Thorac. Cardiovasc. Surg.* 67: 93, 106, 1974.

3. Hultgren, H., Hubis, H., Shumway, N. Cardiac function following mitral valve replacement. *Am. Heart J.* 75: 302, 1968.

4. Levine, F.H., Copeland, J.G., Morrow, A.G. Prosthetic replacement of the mitral valve: continuing assessments of the 100 patients operated upon during 1961-1965. *Circul.* 47: 518, 1973.

5. Matloff, J.M., Dalen, J.E., Dexter, L., Harken, D.E. Hemodynamic response to discoid mitral valve replacement. *Circul.* 37, 38, supp. II: 94, 1968.

6. Morgan, J.J. Hemodynamics one year following mitral valve replacement. *Am. J. Cardiol.* 19: 189, 1967.

7. Reid, J.A., Stevens, T.W., Sigwart U., Fulweber, R.C., Alexander, J.H. Hemodynamic evaluation of the Beall mitral valve prosthesis. *Circul.* 45, 46, supp. I, 1, 1972.

8. Hawe, A., Frye, R.L., Ellis, F.H. Late hemodynamic studies after mitral valve surgery. *J. Thor. Cardiovasc. Surg.* 65: 273: 509, 1965.

9. Glancy, D.L., O'Brien, K.P., Reis, R.L., Epstein, S.E., Morrow, A.G. Hemodynamic studies in patients with 2 M and 3 M Starr Edwards prostheses: evidence of obstruction to left atrial emptying. *Circul.* 39, 40, suppl. I: 113, 1969.

10. Braunwald, E., Braunwald, N.S., Ross, J. Jr., Morrow, A.G. Effects of mitral valve replacement on the pulmonary vascular dynamics of patients with pulmonary hypertension. *N. Eng. J. Med.* 273: 509, 1965.

11. Dalen, J.E., Matloff, J.M., Evans, G.L., Hoppin, F.G., Bhardwaj, P., Harken, D.E. Early reduction of pulmonary vascular

resistance after mitral valve replacement. *N. Eng. J. Med.* 277: 387, 1967.

12. Hollinrake, K., Baidya, M., Yacoub, M.H. Hemodynamic changes in patients with high pulmonary vascular resistance after mitral valve replacement. *Brit. Heart J.*. 35: 1047, 1973.

13. Zener, J.C., Hancock, E.W., Shumway, N.E., Harrison, D.C. Regression of extreme pulmonary hypertension after mitral valve surgery. *Am. J. Cardiol.* 30: 820, 1972.

14. Gault, J.H., Covell, J.W., Braunwald, E., Ross, J. Left ventricular performance following correction of free aortic regurgitation. *Circul.* 42: 773, 1970.

15. Hildner, F.J., Javier, R.P., Cohen, L.S., Samet, P., Nathan, M.J., Yahr, W.Z., Greenberg, J.J. Myocardial dysfunction associated with valvular heart disease. *Am. J. Cardiol.* 30: 319, 1972.

16. Herreman, F., Brun, P., Cannet, G., Savin, E., Nitenberg, A., Luxereau, P. Etude de la fonction ventriculaire gauche dans les cardiopathies valvulaires avant et après cure chirurgicale. *Coeur* No. spécial: 775, 1975.

17. Litwak, R.S., Silvay, J., Gadboys, H.L., Lukban, S.B., Sakurai, H., Castro Blanco, J. Factors associated with operative risk in mitral valve replacement. *Am. J. Cardiol.* 23, 335, 1969.

18. Simonsen, S., Forfang, K., Andersen, A., Efskind, L. Hospital mortality after mitral valve replacement. Prognostic significance of preoperative clinical and hemodynamic factors. *Acta Med. Scand.* 195: 243, 1974.

38 Results of Mitral Valve Replacements with the Björk-Shiley Tilting Disc Valves

Viking Olov Björk, M.D.

INTRODUCTION

Artificial heart valves in the mitral area have now been used for 13 years. Because of technical improvements, the size of the valve has been diminished to a low-profile version. The gradient and the blood damage have been brought to a minimum in the Björk-Shiley valves, which were introduced in 1969.

MATERIAL

The Björk-Shiley tilting disc valve has now been used 1023 times at the Karolinska Sjukhuset in Stockholm: 615 times in the aortic, 353 in the mitral, and 55 in the tricuspid area. The disc tilts open 60°; the occluder fits within the ring and gives a central, nearly laminar flow (Fig. 1). The gradient does not diminish if it is opened more at flows as high as 26 liters per minute.

449

DURABILITY

Wear testing of the disc of Pyrolite as well as the struts of Stellite has shown a durability of many hundred years. I have not had one single valve failure in 1023 cases over a 6½-year period. I have heard of three instances of breakage of the larger leg or strut of the Björk-Shiley mitral valve after 8 weeks, 11 weeks, and 21 months respectively. Two were in No. 29 and one in No. 31.

If on X-ray a fracture is shown on a strut, the valve has to be exchanged, as otherwise the disc will shortly embolize. A detailed analysis of the three valves has indicated a rare combination of factors relating to the weld area as the probable cause of fracture. Corrective actions have been implemented to provide an ever greater safety margin and to reduce the probability of future fractures. The struts on the 29 and 31 mm valves are being made stronger (reinforced). In one case during operation, early in the series, the valve was somewhat forcefully rotated with forceps with the consequence that the struts were slightly disturbed. The disc came loose and the valve had to be exchanged. Such a case was described by Messmer and Senning. I therefore recommend that, before insertion, the valve be rotated with the valve holder. It is then loose, and after being sutured in place, it is easy to rotate, if necessary. It is most important that the surgeon should gently loosen up the rotation for the disc with a valve holder, and never use forceps or clamps for adjusting the

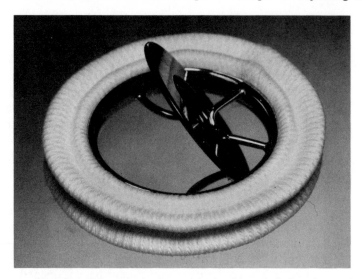

Figure 1. The Björk-Shiley mitral valve prosthesis with a pyrolytic carbon occluder and a double flange Teflon sewing ring.

position of the disc. This does not exclude the possibility of a fault in material or welding technique in the fractures reported.

I saw the autopsy of my first case with three Björk-Shiley valves in a giant heart of a 60-year-old man who was operated on 4 years and 9 months ago. He was then in failure with edema up to his groin. Even the delrin discs and the struts appeared in an excellent condition in all three valves.

INSUFFICIENCY

The valve insufficiency due to the small space between the disc and the ring is dependent on the systolic pressure; it amounts to only 2% of the forward stroke volume for valves Nos. 21 and 23, and to about 5% for the largest valves.

SURGICAL TECHNIQUE

I prefer to suture the valve in a subannular position with 20 isolated mattress sutures (Fig. 2 A). The mitral valve prosthesis has a Teflon sewing ring with two flanges which may be placed intra-annularly, so that the sutures can be buffered on both sides by these suture ring flanges to prevent the sutures from cutting through if the valve base is thin, edematous, or calcified (Fig. 2 B). I recommend orienting the big hole posteriorly, as it gives the smallest gradient during higher flow (Figs. 3 A and B). In Figure 4 the dotted (inter-rupted) lines show this posterior orientation of the big opening, as

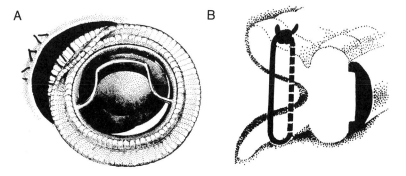

Figure 2 A. The mattress sutures were passed first through the sewing ring and then through the rim of the mitral valve from the ventricular side, starting in the anterolateral commissure, going first anteriorly. The big hole is oriented against the posterior wall of the left ventricle.

Figure 2 B. The two flanges used to buffer the sutures on both sides of the valve base.

452

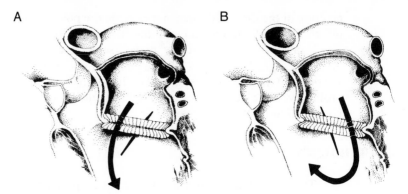

Figure 3 A. Prosthesis oriented with the large opening against the ventricular septum (group I).
Figure 3 B. Prosthesis with the preferred orientation with the large opening against the posterior wall of the left ventricle (group II).

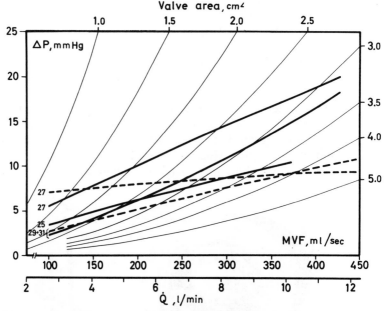

Figure 4. Driving pressure ΔP (mm Hg) across mitral prosthesis in vivo in relation to mitral valve flow, MVF (ml/sec), and cardiac output, $\dot{Q}$ (l/min), after mitral valve replacement at rest and during exercise. The relationship between MVF and $\dot{Q}$ was obtained with least-squares linear regression. Thin curved lines indicate valve area (cm²) using the Gorlin formula, which assumes a squared relationship between ΔP and MVF. Thick straight lines indicate least-squares regression for the observations in group I with orientation of the large hole anterior against the ventricular septum (26 patients) for the different prosthesis sizes; dashed lines indicate least squares regression for the observations in group II with orientation of the large hole posterior against the posterior wall of the left ventricle (24 patients). The 29 mm and the 31 mm prostheses have the same orifice area.

compared to an orientation of the big hole against the septum. The difference is not obvious at low flows, but becomes significant at higher flows during an exercise test. My explanation for this is the inward movement of the upper portion of the ventricular septum during diastole. This narrowing of the inflow to the left ventricle can be avoided by orienting the big hole posteriorly (Fig. 5). Flow visualization of this valve in Dr. Wright's test machine in Liverpool has shown laminar flow, with vortex formation that helps to close the valve at the end of diastole.

The Björk-Shiley valve in the tricuspid area should be oriented with the large opening to the diaphragmatic surface of the right ventricle. If the base of the septal tricuspid leaflet is thin, the sutures are usually buffered on both sides by the two flanges (Fig. 6).

LONG-TERM RESULTS

Eighty-three cases of isolated mitral valve replacement followed for 12 to 48 months have had an early mortality of 2% and a late mortality of 16% . The main cause of the deaths was myocardial insufficiency in 10% of the patients and thromboembolism in 6%. The total for thromboembolism was 4 cases during 1000 patient-months at risk. Of those, 6% were fatal and 4% nonfatal; 1% occurred during operation, 1% had recurrent embolism with 4 episodes, and 5% had thrombotic encapsulation of the disc. One of the four patients was successfully operated on with simple thrombectomy from the valve with a nerve hook and strong suction during stepwise rotation of the valve, utilizing the valve holder. Although a simple thrombectomy of

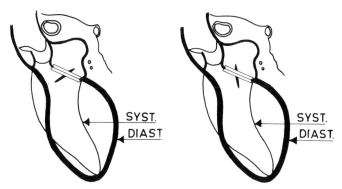

Figure 5. Diagram of the movements of the ventricular septum during the cardiac cycle. With the anterior orientation of the big hole (to the left), the inflow of blood into the left ventricle is somewhat narrowed. With the posterior orientation of the big hole (to the right), the bulging ventricular septum will not narrow the inflow to the left ventricle.

a clotted valve is a good operation in the aortic position, it is not recommended for the mitral area, where a new valve replacement is preferable.

The actuarial curve shows an 89% 4-year-survival with most deaths occurring within the first year, and an actuarial freedom of thromboembolism of 94% after 4 years. All patients are anticoagulated. Of the surviving patients, 96% showed a subjective improvement, which could only be proved by function tests in 80%. The functional capacity improved one or two classes (NYHA) after the operation.

DISCUSSION

The Björk-Shiley tilting disc valve with its low profile and its large orifice-to-tissue-diameter ratio can be used in small hearts and in children where other valves, including tissue valves, cannot be used. Mechanical valves in the mitral area should always be used with anticoagulation. Approximately half of the emboli after mitral valve replacement come from the large fibrillating left atrium. We have also found it easy to carry through an adequate anticoagulation therapy for small children. One child with corrected transposition and mitral insufficiency, operated on at age 4 with a Björk-Shiley valve, has now had anticoagulant treatment with a blood control once a month for 5½ years without problems.

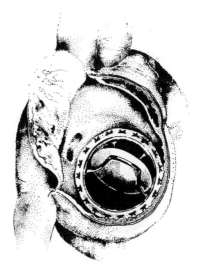

Figure 6. In the tricuspid area the large opening should be oriented against the diaphragmatic surface of the right ventricle.

CONCLUSION

As long-term degenerative changes, such as calcification, rupture, and shrinkage of the tissue valves, are virtually unknown, the low-profile Björk-Shiley tilting disc valves are preferred, since they result in the lowest possible blood damage and transvalvular gradient. An adequate anticoagulation therapy is an important part of the treatment—and accepted for a better long-term result than with tissue valves.

REFERENCES

Björk, V.O.   A new tilting disc valve prosthesis. *Scand. J. Thor. Cardiovasc. Surg.* 3: 1, 1969.

Björk, V.O.   The central flow tilting disc valve prosthesis (Björk-Shiley) for mitral valve replacement. *Scand. J. Thor. Cardiovasc. Surg.* 4: 15, 1970.

Björk, V.O.   The pyrolytic carbon occluder for the Björk-Shiley tilting disc valve prosthesis. *Scand. J. Thor. Cardiovasc. Surg.* 6: 109, 1972.

Björk, V.O., Böök, K., Cernigliaro, C., and Holmgren, A.   The Björk-Shiley tilting disc valve in isolated mitral lesions. *Scand. J. Thor. Cardiovasc. Surg.* 7: 131, 1973.

Björk, V.O., Böök, K., and Holmgren, A.   Significance of position and opening angle of the Björk-Shiley tilting disc in mitral surgery. *Scand. J. Thor. Cardiovasc. Surg.* 7: 187, 1973.

Böök, K., Holmgren, A., and Szamosi, A.   The left atrial v-wave after mitral valve replacement. *Scand. J. Thor. Cardiovasc. Surg.* 9: 9, 1973.

Böök, K.   Mitral valve replacement with the Björk-Shiley tilting disc valve. *Scand. J. Thor. Cardiovasc. Surg.,* Suppl. 12., 1974.

Messmer, B.J., Okies, J.E., Hallman, G.L., and Cooley, D.A.   Mitral valve replacement with the Björk-Shiley tilting-disc prosthesis. *J. Thor. Cardiovasc. Surg.* 62: 938, 1971.

Messmer, B.J., Okies, J.E., Hallman, G.L., and Cooley, D.A.   Early and late thrombo-embolic complication after mitral valve replacement. *J. Cardiovasc. Surg.* 13: 281, 1972

Messmer, B.J., Rothlin, M., and Senning, Å.   Early disc dislodgment. An unusual complication after insertion of a Björk-Shiley mitral valve prosthesis. *J. Thor. Cardiovasc. Surg.* 65: 3, 1973.

Wright, J.T.M.   Personal communication. 1975.

39 Clinical and Hemodynamic Results of the Beall Valve

Arthur C. Beall, Jr., M.D.

Clinical introduction of the pump oxygenator in 1953 provided the means for direct surgery on the mitral valve.[1] The far advanced disease state of most mitral valves requiring operation, however, prevented satisfactory restoration of function. Introduction of the caged-ball mitral valve prosthesis in 1960[2] allowed for total replacement of these diseased valves, and clinical experience with use of these prostheses demonstrated significant hemodynamic improvement in most instances.[3]

Long-term experience with these caged-ball mitral prostheses demonstrated a significant incidence of thromboembolic complications, even with the use of anticoagulants. In a five and one-half year follow-up of one large group of patients undergoing prosthetic replacement of the mitral valve, deaths due to thromboembolism were not exceeded by any other cause of late death.[4] For this reason, attempts were made to design a mitral valve prosthesis that would not be associated with such a high incidence of thromboembolic complications.[5]

Since it is believed that most thrombus formation associated with

457

mitral valve prostheses originates at the junction between the cloth sewing ring and the metal of the prosthetic base,[6] this cloth-metal interface was eliminated by covering the entire base and sewing ring of a mitral valve prosthesis with Dacron velour, a loop-pile which encourages the ingrowth of fibrous tissue.[7] Thus, once the prosthetic base is incorporated by host tissue, only the Teflon disc and Teflon-covered cage legs remain in the bloodstream. Long-term clinical experience with this prosthesis, the Beall-Surgitool Mitral Valve Prosthesis Models 102-104, demonstrated a thromboembolic incidence of only 4.5% even without use of anticoagulants.[8]

This low incidence of thromboembolic complications was verified in a number of centers,[9-14] and is comparable to the incidence of thromboembolism associated with mitral annuloplasty[15] and open mitral commissurotomy.[16] Improvement in this first generation of prostheses consisted in changing from a thin, extruded Teflon disc (Model 102) to a thicker, compression-molded Teflon disc (Model 103) because of reports of wear problems,[17] and in increasing the primary and secondary orifice areas in the smaller sizes (104), due to reports of undesirably high gradients across these sizes.[18] Throughout the world more than 18,000 of these first-generation prostheses have been used to date.

In an effort to further diminish the possibility of wear associated with these prostheses, development of a second generation was begun with use of Pyrolite carbon as a coating for both the cage legs and disc.[19] The Dacron velour-covered base and sewing ring was unchanged, and after host tissue encapsulation, only the electronegative Pyrolite carbon-covered cage legs and disc remain in the bloodstream. Wear studies in calves with scanning electron microscope analysis demonstrated less than 0.8% penetrating of the Pyrolite carbon in one year, leading to a prediction of more than 140 years wear.[19] Clinical experience with this prosthesis (Model 105) also demonstrated an exceedingly low incidence of thromboembolism (1 fatal and 3 non-fatal episodes in 175 patients).[20]

Increases in primary and secondary orifice areas included in the smaller sizes of the Model 104 were incorporated into all sizes of the Model 105, and 17 patients underwent repeat cardiac catheterization 6 months or more following isolated mitral valve replacement with one of these prostheses.[20] With one exception there had been a significant increase in cardiac index after operation, and mean diastolic gradients across the prostheses varied from 2 to 7 mm Hg, usually without end-diastolic gradient. Such findings appear to indicate no clinically significant obstruction caused by these prostheses, even with use of a central occluder, which is necessary if the entire base and sewing ring are to be cloth-covered.

However, a problem developed which was not anticipated and has yet to be seen in the three centers in which original clinical trials were conducted. As a material is made harder in order to reduce wear, ductility is decreased and the material becomes more brittle. If Pyrolite carbon is mishandled, for example by dropping or bending the cage legs, it can be cracked, which then concentrates stresses on the wire of the cage leg in the area underlying the crack. This phenomenon resulted in six instances of fatigue fracture of a cage leg with escape of the disc.[21, 22] In order to prevent such mishaps, the diameter of wire of the cage legs underlying the Pyrolite carbon was increased, resulting in three times more force being required to crack the Pyrolite carbon (Model 106 – Fig. 1). Additionally, a package for the Model 106 prosthesis was developed in which the prosthesis may be sterilized by either steam or ethylene oxide, and which protects the prosthesis until the time of implantation (Fig. 2). As long as the prosthesis remains in the package, it cannot be damaged, and the package cannot be opened without breaking the seal. Thus, if the seal on the package has been broken previously, the prosthesis should not be used but returned to the manufacturer for reinspection.

The Model 106 prosthesis now has been in use since February of 1974 and not a single broken cage leg has been noted. Thus, it would appear that the changes in the Model 106 and its packaging have been effective in preventing mishandling, but the prosthesis still should not be grasped by the cage legs. As with any delicate instrument, proper handling remains important.

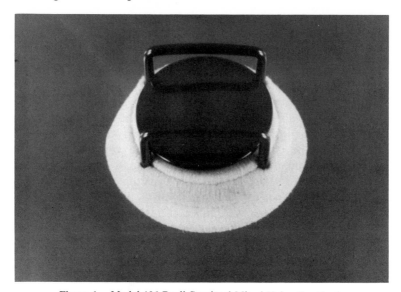

Figure 1.   Model 106 Beall-Surgitool Mitral Valve Prosthesis.

460

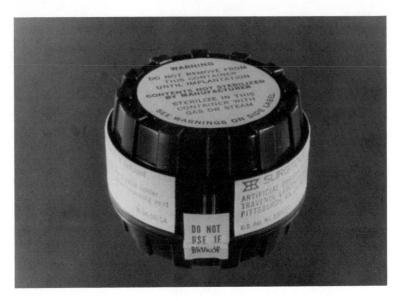

Figure 2. Protective container within which Model 106 is sterilized and stored prior to use.

SUMMARY

Development of the pump oxygenator for cardiopulmonary bypass provided direct access to diseased mitral valves, but effective surgical therapy for these patients was not possible until the development of caged-ball prostheses for valve replacement. However, early mitral valve prostheses were associated with a high incidence of thromboembolic complications. To prevent such complications a mitral valve prosthesis was developed in which the entire base and sewing ring were covered with Dacron velour, in order to eliminate the cloth-metal interface from which most thromboembolic phenomena are believed to originate. Clinical experience in numerous centers then demonstrated that this design achieved an extremely low incidence of thromboembolism. Subsequent modifications in this prosthesis have been aimed at improving hemodynamic characteristics and preventing wear. The current Model 106 has excellent wear characteristics and a low incidence of thromboembolism, even without anticoagulants, comparable with that seen after mitral annuloplasty or commissurotomy.

REFERENCES

1. Gibbon, J.H., Jr.   Application of mechanical heart and lung apparatus to cardiac surgery. *Minnesota Med.* 37:171, 1954.

2. Starr, A., and Edwards, M.L.   Mitral replacement: Clinical experience with a ball-valve prosthesis. *Ann. Surg.* 154:726, 1961.

3. Beall, A.C., Jr., Bricker, D.L., Cooley, D.A., and DeBakey, M.E.   Ball-valve prostheses in surgical management of acquired valvular heart disease. *Arch. Surg.* 90:720, 1965.

4. Beall, A.C., Jr., Bloodwell, R.D., Bricker, D.L., Okies, J.D., Cooley, D.A., and DeBakey, M.E.   Prosthetic replacement of cardiac valves: Five and one-half years' experience. *Am. J. Cardiol.* 23:250, 1969.

5. Beall, A.C., Jr., Bloodwell, R.D., Liotta, D., Cooley, D.A., and DeBakey, M.E.   Elimination of sewing ring-metal seat interface in mitral valve prostheses. *Circ.* 37 (Suppl. II):184, 1968.

6. DeBakey, M.E., Jordan, G.L., Jr., Beall, A.C., Jr., O'Neal, R.M., Abbott, J.P., Halpert, B.   Basic biological reactions to vascular grafts and prostheses. *Surg. Clin. N. Amer.* 45:477, 1965.

7. Beall, A.C., Jr., Bloodwell, R.D., Arbegast, N.R., Liotta, D., Cooley, D.A., DeBakey, M.E.   Mitral valve replacement with Dacron-covered disc prosthesis to prevent thromboembolism: Clinical experience in 202 cases. Edited by Brewer, L.A., III. *Prosthetic Heart Valves.* Springfield, Ill.: Charles C. Thomas, 1969.

8. Beall, A.C., Jr., Bricker, D.L., Messmer, B.J.   Results of mitral valve replacement with Dacron velour-covered Teflon-disc prosthesis. *Ann. Thoracic Surg.* 9:195, 1970.

9. Javier, R.P., Hildner, F.J., Berry, W., Greenberg, J.J., and Samet, P.   Systemic embolism and the Beall mitral valve prosthesis. *Ann. Thoracic Surg.* 10:20, 1970.

10. Messmer, B.J., Okies, J.E., Hallman, G.L., and Cooley, D.A.   Early and late thromboembolic complications after mitral valve replacement. *J. Cardiovasc. Surg.* 13:281, 1972.

11. Nichols, H.T., Fernandez, J., Morse, D., and Gooch, A.S.   Improved results in 336 patients with the isolated mitral Beall valve replacement. *Chest* 62:266, 1972.

12. Ramsey, H.W., Williams, J.C., Jr., Vernon, C.R., Wheat, M.W., Daicoff, G.R., and Bartley, T.D.   Hemodynamic findings following replacement of the mitral valve with the Beall valve prosthesis. *J. Thorac. Cardiovasc. Surg.* 62:624, 1971.

13. Stanford, W., Lindberg, E.F., and Armstrong, R.G.   Implantation of heart valve prostheses without anticoagulants. *J. Thorac. Cardiovasc. Surg.* 63:648, 1972.

462

14. Vogel, J.H.K., Paton, B.C., Overy, H.R., Pappas, G., Davies, H., and Blount, S.G., Jr. Advantages of the Beall valve prosthesis. *Chest* 59:249, 1971.

15. Messmer, B.J., Gattiker, K., Rothlin, M., and Senning, A. Reconstruction of the mitral valve. *Ann. Thoracic Surg.* 16:30, 1973.

16. Mullin, M.J., Engelman, R.M., Isom, O.W., Boyd, A.D., Glassman, E., and Spencer, F.G. Experience with open mitral commissurotomy in 100 consecutive patients. *Surgery* 76:974, 1974.

17. Robinson, M.J., Hildner, F.J., and Greenberg, J.J. Disc variance of Beall mitral valve. *Ann. Thorac. Surg.* 11:11, 1971.

18. Reid, J.A., Stevens, T.W., Sigwart, V., Fulweber, R.C., and Alexander, J.K. Hemodynamic evaluation of Beall mitral valve prosthesis. *Circ.* 45 (Suppl II):394, 1972.

19. Beall, A.C., Jr., Morris, G.C., Jr., Noon, G.P., Guinn, G.A., Reul, G.J., Jr., Lefrak, E.A., and Greenberg, S.D. An improved mitral valve prosthesis. *Ann. Thorac. Surg.* 15:25, 1973.

20. Beall, A.C., Jr., Morris, G.C., Jr., Howell, J.F., Jr., Guinn, G.A., Noon, G.P., Reul, G.J., Jr., Greenberg, J.J., and Ankeney, J.L. Clinical experience with an improved mitral valve prosthesis. *Ann. Thorac. Surg.* 15:601, 1973.

21. Nathan, M.J. Strut fracture: A late complication of Beall mitral valve replacement. *Ann. Thorac. Surg.* 16:610, 1973.

22. Gold, H., and Hertz, L. Death caused by fracture of Beall mitral prosthesis. *Am. J. Cardiol.* 34:371, 1974.

40 The Medium-Term Follow-Up of Beall Prosthetic Valves in the Mitral or Mitro-Tricuspid Position

C. Rioux, M.D.
J.Y. Neveux, M.D.
E. Hazan, M.D.
A. Dequirot, M.D.
J. Mathey, M.D.

In 1969, Professor Mathey and the members of his surgical team decided to use Beall's prosthetic valve in the mitral or tricuspid positions. This choice was based on three considerations: 1) good quality hemodynamic performances; 2) small intra-ventricular bulk; and 3) the reputation for a low rate of thrombo-embolic accidents. Our study involved 100 consecutive patients operated on between November 1969 and February 1972 who received a Beall valve in the mitral or mitro-tricuspid position, excluding a combination with any other type of prosthesis.

This population of 100 patients differed little from the usual groups of mitral or mitro-tricuspid patients. The female sex was predominant; there were 58 women and 42 men. The average age was 46.5 years; 29 patients were over 60. One-half of the patients had mitral valve disease.

In 40 cases an associated tricuspid failure was present, and in two cases a tricuspid disease. It should be emphasized that in two cases the mitral lesion was congenital; in one patient it was combined with an aorto-pulmonary fistula and in the other with complete agenesis of the arch of the aorta. According to the criteria of the New York Heart Association, 12 patients were in class II, 51 in class III, and 37 in class IV. Twenty-seven of these patients had undergone a commissurotomy, on the average 7 years previously; 26 of these were blind procedures, and one an open-heart procedure.

The prosthetic valve implant was carried out with extracorporeal circulation, under hemodilution and normothermia, and with a beating heart. Aortic clamping, when it was used, did not exceed 15 minutes. After an average stay of 2.5 days in our intensive care unit, the operated patients remained in the surgical department for an average of 12 days. Anticoagulant treatment by subcutaneous calcium heparinate was applied from the 72nd post-operative hour and continued for three weeks. The K antivitamin back-up was then taken up under the supervision of the doctors of the original cardiology department.

HOSPITAL MORTALITY (First 30 days)

This mortality was considerable: 14 deaths. However, certain specific facts must be taken into account when analyzing these results (Table 1): Two deaths in fact involved the two congenital mitral malformations which required the correction of an associated major anomaly in young children. Infection, too, took a heavy toll. Three deaths involved an extra-cardial cause (a hepatic necrosis, a renal failure, and a massive cerebral hemorrhage). In the 6 deaths apparently due to myocardial causes, it is impossible to incriminate the prosthetic valve in any way.

DISTRIBUTION OF SURVIVORS

We lost track of 17 of our 86 survivors. Of those remaining, 18 died; these deaths occurred after a mean period of 8.5 months (range 2

Table 1
Causes of Immediate Deaths

14 Deaths (< 30 Days) 8 Grade III, 6 Grade IV	
"Cardiac" Causes	8
Renal Failure	1
Hepatic Necrosis	1
Cerebral Hemorrhage	1
Septicemia	3

to 25 months). The Beall prosthetic valve could be suspected only once, though no anatomical check was carried out. The death occurred at home 10 months after surgery in a patient who had to that point been recovering from his operation; he was in a state of acute pulmonary edema, leaving a doubt as to the possibility of sudden thrombosis of the valve (Table 2).

The last 51 patients were all reexamined, either by their own cardiologist or in the cardiology department that passed them on to us. Seven were examined between 6 and 12 months, 27 between 13 and 24 months, 13 between 25 and 36 months, and 4 between 37 and 42 months.

EVOLUTION OF THE 51 REEXAMINED PATIENTS

Clinical improvement

Of these 51 patients, 84% were considered by themselves and by their cardiologist to have improved. Almost all of them had a functional improvement (Fig. 1). However, the cardiothoracic index remained high, around 0.60 in about 4 out of 5 patients.

Frequency of thromboembolic accidents

Selecting only those observations in which proof of thrombosis was provided by anatomical examination, or those in which the clinical and evolutionary context appeared sufficiently conclusive, we note that: Among the 18 patients who died through secondary effects, 2 suffered characteristic embolic accidents (obliteration of the aortic bifurcation, multiple cerebral embolism, and embolism of the members); however, these embolic accidents were not the cause of death, which occurred much later (three months and eleven

Table 2
Cause of Late Deaths

18 Late Deaths 2 Months to 25 Months	
Cardiac Failure	5
Respiratory Failure	1
Cerebral Stroke	2
Septicemia	3
Hepatitis	2
Cancer	2
Unknown	3

months). Six of the 51 survivors were victims of an embolic accident. All these accidents, however, were resolved.

Hemolysis

In addition to the clinical evaluation, we have taken into account the figure for the red blood cells, the hematocrit reading, and the level of reticulocytes. Out of 51 patients studied, 15 had manifest hemolysis and 5 slight hemolysis. Among the 15 cases of manifest hemolysis, 3 required repeated blood transfusions and 6 others tolerated their hemolysis rather badly. Contrary to the usual information given in literature, the hemolysis did not seem to us to diminish with time, since the incidence of this hemolysis was the same for the patients followed for over 2 years as for those followed for less than 2 years.

Wear

Two of those operated on showed a clinical picture combining major hemolysis and patent mitral leakage. Upon re-intervention, we found abnormal wear on the edges of the disc, which made it stick intermittently to the bars of the cage.

CONCLUSION

The Beall valve we used, i.e., one comprising a Teflon disc, is unquestionably appealing for use in small ventricular cavities and

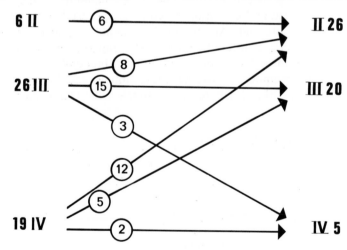

Figure 1. Functional evolution in 51 patients

especially in children. The functional improvement of the patients is the proof of a hemodynamic quality comparable to that of ball replacement valves. Though all our patients underwent anticoagulant treatment, the incidence of thromboembolic accidents did not seem to us distinctly lower than those observed with other types of prosthetic valve.

There were, however, two drawbacks which appear to us to be major ones. One is the high frequency of hemolysis, which constitutes a definite handicap for the patients who are affected by it. The other is the unpredictable wear of the disc; sometimes it wears out within a very short time. This seems to us to condemn this type of prosthesis.

SELECTED READINGS

Beall, A.C., Bloodwell, R.D., Liotta, D., Cooley, D.A., DeBakey, M.E.   Clinical experience with a Dacron velour covered Teflon disc mitral valve prosthesis. *Ann. Thorac. Surg.* 5:402, 1968.

Beall, A.C., Morris, L., Moon, F., Swinn, E., Reul, E., Lefrak, E., Greenberg, S.D.   An improved mitral valve prosthesis. *Ann. Thorac. Surg.* 15:25, 1973.

Carcone, P.   Complications thrombo-emboliques après mise en place de prothèses mitrales. *Thèse* Paris 1971.

Goudard, A., Monties, J., Baille, Y., Jausseran, J.M., Sicard, M.P., Avierino, C., Henry, E.   La prothèse de Beall. Son emploi dans le traitement chirurgical des valvulopathies mitrales. *N. Presse Mèd.* 1:1069, 1972.

Indeglia, R., Shea, M., Varco, R., Bernstein, E.   Erythrocyte destruction by prosthetic heart valves. *Circulation* 37:86, 1968.

Kay, E., Suzaki, A., Demany, M., Zimmerman, H.   Comparison of Beall and disc valves for mitral valve replacement. *Amer. J. Cardiol.*, 18: no. 4, 1966.

Messmer, B.J., et Coll.   Early and late thromboembolic complications after mitral valve replacement. 10th Cong. Inter. Card. Vasc., Moscow, August 26-28, 1971.

Nichols, H., Fernandez, J.   Improved results in 336 patients with the isolated mitral Beall valve replacement. *Chest* 62:3, 1972.

Penther, P., Bensaid, J., Maurice, P., LeNegre, J.   Les complications thrombo-emboliques après remplacement valvulaire par la prothèse de Starr-Edwards. *Arch. Mal. Coeur* 61:1278-1289, 1968.

Weily, H., Steele, P., Genton, E.   Platelet survival in patients with a Beall valve. *Amer. J. Cardiol.* 30:229, 1972.

Williams, J.C.   Hemolysis following mitral valve replacement with the Beall valve prosthesis. *J. Thor. Surg.* 61:392, 1971.

Vogel, J., Patton, B., Overy, H., Pappar, G., Davies, A., Blount, G.   Advantages of the Beall valve prosthesis. *Chest* 59:249-253, 1971.

DISCUSSION: PART VIII

Dr. Acar: I'd like to commend Dr. Starr for the remarkable quality of his paper which was quite novel, given the number of years of his follow-up. I have several questions to address him. First of all, as regards valve 6120: in my series, the percentage of thrombotic incidents is a bit higher than yours (6.45/1000 months of treatment). So, my first question is the following: Did you associate the platelet function inhibitors — such as pyrimidamol or sulfine-pyrazone — to Coumadin? and if you did, what are your own results? My second question has to do with the model 6320 valve: with this more recent valve, the follow-up is shorter, but we wonder if the patients are not exposed to two risks: 1) The risk of progressive stenosis because of deposit of fibrine; and I would like to know if, by iterative catheterization, you have noticed such a complication. 2) The risk of cloth tear: Can you tell us the percentage of cloth tear you found during re-operation or at autopsy amongst the model 6320 valves? Are the wear and tear unusual? or fairly frequent? Have you dropped the 6320 model and is it the reason why you started using the 6400 model?

Dr. Starr: I think that those are very important questions. With regard to the non-cloth-covered mitral valve, the 6120, mentioned in my presentation, we had to reoperate on two such patients out of approximately 100 for late thrombotic stenosis occurring about 9 years after operation. One of these patients died at reoperation; he was in very poor condition. The other survived the operation. So although up until a few months ago I thought that thrombotic stenosis of the non-cloth-covered valves simply did not occur, it apparently does. It must involve a very small percentage of patients, however, because it is not a common complication.

With regard to the use of anticoagulant drugs, all of our non-cloth-covered valve patients, except for a few children, have been on Coumadin. It is our practice that if while receiving Coumadin the patient has an embolic episode, we would consider the use of an antiplatelet drug in addition to Coumadin, and would use aspirin, Persantine, or sulfinpyrazone. This is a somewhat dangerous step to take, because it exposes the patient to significant bleeding problems. So if the patient had multiple embolic episodes, I think that would be an indication for re-operation. But if he has a single episode it may be worthwhile to use an antiplatelet drug in addition to Coumadin. Certainly Dr. Harken and his group have demonstrated that to be of value with the use of his particular disc valve.

469

Now with regard to the cloth-covered valves, the question was: does progressive restenosis occur in a cloth-covered mitral valve? I think we have to distinguish that from thrombosis. We have never seen a patient who had progressive fibrotic stenosis of the cloth-covered orifice, but we have had reoperations for thrombotic stenosis, and we had five patients who were reoperated on for thrombotic stenosis of the valve. This is a significant complication of a cloth-covered valve. That is one of its imperfections. Now if that occurred often and could not be easily prevented by anticoagulant treatment, it would be a very serious drawback to the use of cloth-covered valves. Fortunately, of our five cases, only one occurred in a patient who was receiving anticoagulants; therefore, this seems to indicate that anticoagulants are very protective against the occurrence of thrombotic stenosis. I might add that when regarding the problem of thrombotic stenosis, one has to consider whether it imposes a catastrophic event on a patient or simply a slowly progressive mitral restenosis that is easily amenable to evaluation and re-operation. This is a very important point, then. The patients that we have re-operated on for thrombotic stenosis have had a gradual return of symptoms; these patients were not rushed to the operating room in the middle of the night.

Another important question was why we found so few cloth tears at re-operation or at autopsy. I think here the difference between aortic and mitral valve replacement is very great, because in aortic autopsies with cloth-covered valves, strut-cloth tear is found in at least 3 out of 4 cases, whereas in the mitral position it is very unusual to find any. We have seen at the most some flattening of the fibers near the base of the cage. However, in the mitral there is more of a risk of orifice-cloth tear, and while this is not common, it has been a cause for reoperation in one of our patients and in another series at other clinics. This has been a more common cause of reoperation. For this reason we felt that it was important to make some minor modification of the orifice cloth. In the model 6400 valve (track valve) the orifice cloth has a lock-stitch which prevents it from unravelling if one fiber is cut. In addition the height of the stud has been raised so that the cloth will not ride up on the top of the stud and then be cut by the ball, and that, coupled with the track which prevents any possibility for injury of the cloth on the remainder of the valve, has produced a very attractive prosthesis, as I mentioned. The results that we have had with 150 such implantations done during the last three years have been the same as with the previous cloth-covered valve except for an absence of complications due to the cloth. I did not show the actual curves for that particular valve because the mean follow-up time is about a year, although the series began three years ago, and the results are not yet significant enough to warrant being pinned down exactly as to what to expect. But it seems to preserve the low incidence of embolism which is characteristic of cloth-covered valves.

Dr. Oury: Dr. Starr, I wonder whether the complications associated with anticoagulation shouldn't rightfully be considered complications of the valve itself, and my question is: What complications have you seen from the use of Coumadin? Are bleeding problems secondary to Coumadin usage in the series of patients that you reported?

Dr. Starr: That is a very good point. We have seen significant complications from anticoagulants; we had at least one death in the series of mitral patients from what we considered to be cerebral hemorrhage rather than embolism. Also, we have done three or four operations for retroperitoneal hematoma in patients who have had Coumadin therapy. That is why I mentioned in my opening remarks that we still have problems related to artificial valves, even though the incidence of complications of embolism has been markedly reduced. As long as we use anticoagulants we will have a dangerous situation from just that kind of complication. The incidence is small, however, and when we reviewed this the complication rate due to anticoagulants was considerably less than 1% per year.

Dr. Popp: Dr. Starr, in regard to the correlation between prognosis and the persistence of symptoms in response to medical therapy, was the degree of left ventricular enlargement, particularly in patients with mitral regurgitation, correlated as well? Would this not possibly correlate well with both of those factors and also prognosis?

Dr. Starr: Yes, certainly we have the clinical impression that massive cardiomegaly is related to a poor prognosis. I certainly have that with aortic valve disease, but in the mitral series we ran more than a hundred variables through a program with our computer and we were not able to come up with a correlation with the heart size. The only other feature that correlated well was the presence or absence of functional tricuspid regurgitation, which was a very important determinant, and also the presence of previous valvular surgery. I think the Mayo Clinic group performed a similar study and also showed that those two features are an important prognostic sign.

Dr. Popp: Dr. Starr, on the same problem: the Mayo Clinic people have looked at the left atrial size; they think it is a very important prognostic sign and that one should follow it. When there is an increase in the size of the left atrium, that is the time to operate. What do you think about it?

Dr. Starr: Well, I have seen that report and we have not been able to make that correlation ourselves. However, I would not argue about it; I am sure that it must be a valid correlation. I think that using that as a means of determining the time of operation is another question. It is very difficult in the present state of the art of valve replacement to recommend mitral valve replacement in patients who do not have significant disability. The prognosis in such patients is good without surgery. In aortic valve disease it is different. I mean, we do lots of aortic insufficiency cases simply on the basis of alarming and rapidly progressive cardiomegaly. I think it is hard to do that at this time with the present state of the art with mitral valve cases.

Dr. Acar: Well, what are the conclusions that can be drawn from this session? I have 3 conclusions.

1) In the final analysis it was seen that Dr. Starr's prostheses are good ones. Yesterday it was said that these patients led a dangerous life, but still one should point out that three quarters of the patients who survived operation are still alive after 8 years; we know what the Silastic ball prostheses are worth, but there is a greater degree of uncertainty regarding the 6320 valve and especially greater uncertainty with regard to the 6400 valve. I think Dr. Starr will agree.

2) Some complications can be cured through reoperation, for instance thrombosis and loosening; this means that these patients really have to be followed up, and Dr. Popp told us how interesting echocardiography is in detecting such complications.

3) Most of the late complications that come up don't stem from prosthetic complications per se but simply from some sort of other valvular disease that was overlooked, for instance tricuspid disease. Or the complication may come from myocardial failure; and many patients, true enough, are operated on much too late indeed. They should be operated on at an earlier stage. But still it must be stressed that at present we haven't got a precise, accurate, hemodynamic criterion which would really enable us to say in specific cases that it is too late to operate, because the postoperative evolution is sometimes unpredictable.

Dr. Frater: I want to ask a question of Dr. Beall. Presumably a large number of patients with mitral valve disease needing much of a replacement must have atrial fibrillation. I don't believe it is possible to follow a group of people with normal mitral valves and atrial fibrillation without anticoagulation without getting a certain incidence of thromboembolism. So I would find it very difficult to avoid putting any patient with atrial fibrillation on anticoagulation, whether he had a prosthesis or not. I wonder whether Dr. Beall could comment on this?

Dr. Beall: We were not able to correlate any difference in our group between anticoagulants and no anticoagulants. It is more our theory that certain of these patients are going to have thromboemboli whether or not they are given anticoagulants, and I raise the issue: Perhaps we are treating ourselves with anticoagulants. If the patient is receiving anticoagulants and has an embolus, then there is nothing we could have done about that. We did the best we could, whereas, if the same patient were not on anticoagulants and had the same embolus, we would feel that maybe if we had given him anticoagulants he wouldn't have had it. There are certain patients who are going to have thromboembolism that anticoagulants will not prevent. Of more importance, as I mentioned, is the high rate of death, 1% per year, from anticoagulants, plus many patients, as Dr. Starr mentioned, with retroperitoneal hematoma, patients that lose a kidney, patients who get Volkmann's contracture of the arm where they bleed into a muscle; all of these are in addition to the mortality rate.

Dr. Somerville: I wonder would the speakers mind explaining in very simple terms to someone who is not a surgeon how it comes about that the results obtained by people who did not invent an operation are never quite as good as the results obtained by the inventor of the operation? Is this to be explained entirely on the grounds that the person who did the operation in the first instance has greater experience? Or is there some secret factor that perhaps you'd be good enough to reveal to us?

Dr. Björk: Well, I would say that first of all I am very proud that wherever I come now other speakers always have better results with my valve than I have. When a doctor is introducing a new valve, he will, perhaps, being a senior fellow, do the procedure himself on the first hundred cases, before he lets his younger doctors come along. Then, there will necessarily be a few more complications regarding the operative mortality. But as far as late mortality goes, it will not have any influence. I think it is important to have 100% follow-up. I am working in a system where every patient comes back to me. You lose a lot of information if you get your follow-up secondhand or even thirdhand, instead of talking directly to the patients as I did in these series.

Dr. Silver: Mr. Chairman, I'd like to draw attention to a particular complication I have seen associated with the rotation of a mitral Björk prosthesis when it is in situ. If this is done with too much enthusiasm one can, apparently, generate tremendous shear forces that tear the myocardium at the junction between the left ventricle and atrium. Then, a hemorrhage occurs instantaneously or develops two or three days later following dissection through the area. Fortunately, this complication is rare, but the risk exists.

Dr. Björk: The first time I ever put in a prosthesis like this, the disc did not move due to calcific episodes. I had to take it out and put it in another way. Therefore, the disc is made in such a way so that you cannot take it back directly after being autoclaved. That is why it is so important to do these ten rotations yourself to get it loose, and not to rely on others. So you should have the valve loose in its sewing ring before you put it in. Then you do not need to use force to rotate it. But I'd like to say that we have encountered rupture of the left ventricle even if we have not rotated the prosthesis.

Dr. Burger: Dr. Beall, I am intrigued by your finding that there is no difference in the incidence of thromboembolism with and without anticoagulation. Can you tell us whether this is a prospective randomized study and whether you think that the finding of no statistically significant difference is due to the insufficient number of cases? Or do you really believe that the presence or absence of anticoagulation does not affect this?

Dr. Beall: In actuality the way it worked out was this: one third of the cases were my own; I did not use anticoagulants. One third of the cases were Dr. Cooley's; he used anticoagulants for six months and then stopped. One third were Dr. DeBakey's, and he kept them anticoagulated permanently. Dr. Somerville has brought up the question about results of developers. I might throw the question to Dr. Bruno Messmer from Zurich who was with us for two years at the time, and he, rather than I, actually worked up the data. So I have an impartial observer! Bruno, could you speak to that?

Dr. Messmer: Thank you for calling me "an impartial observer." We did our best at that time to find out which of all those prostheses worked really the best, and I must agree still today: In a patient whom I cannot put on anticoagulants for some reason, and mostly geographical reasons, I would put a Beall valve.

Dr. Barlow: The question of hemolysis from the Beall valve has been written about in the literature, and we have heard of a unit which has abandoned the use of the valve because of hemolysis. Could Dr. Beall please comment?

Dr. Beall: In my experience, there has been the requirement of an average of one additional bottle of blood during the period of hospitalization, until the cloth becomes incorporated by tissue. There has been relatively little hemolysis after that unless a mechanical defect has occurred. One such defect is notching of the Teflon disc, and our reason for going to the Pyrolite was to prevent that complication. The other cause of this has been a perivalvular leak, and it is my contention that you cannot tell a perivalvular leak unless you re-catheterize the patient, since he or she may not have a mitral systolic murmur. So you must recatheterize to make sure that it is not a perivalvular leak. In our experience this has been the troublesome hemolysis. Another thing that can occur, and I keep stressing this, is that if too large a prosthesis is put in, you have obstruction in the tertiary orifice. This will also cause hemolysis. The article in the literature referring to hemolysis was by the group in Gainesville, Florida, and if you look at their definition of severe hemolysis, included in the definition were patients with a red-cell half life of less than 20 days. The majority of the patients they referred to as having hemolysis were on this basis, even though the hematocrits were in the range of 42, 43, 44, 45. This is hemolysis that the body can compensate for, and I am willing to accept it to achieve low thromboembolism without anticoagulants.

Dr. Ranganathan: I'd like to ask Dr. Beall to comment on a distressing complication that we have encountered in a small series of patients with disc prostheses. This has not been commented upon earlier here. In addition to the notching that has been described, we have had three actual cases of dislodgement of the disc; one was successfully reoperated and two died in intractable pulmonary edema. We have had to substitute other prostheses because of this early bad experience. Now I wonder whether this sort of thing can ever happen with the new Pyrolite coating. I'd like to ask Dr. Beall his comment on this.

Dr. Beall: Are you referring to dislodgement of a Teflon disc? This has occurred in 4 cases that I know of. In one of these, too large a valve was put in a patient with mitral stenosis, and the septum impinged upon the cage leg. You could see a ridge in the septum at autopsy, where the cage leg had been pressed on every beat and it eventually caused fatigue failure. The other three cases occurred because of cloth cutting in the orifice. This was prior to putting a Dacron felt pad in that area of the orifice, and those discs then were against metal. Teflon against metal will cause this problem. We have not seen disc wear since we began using the Pyrolite carbon. I can give you overall statistics of more than 18,000 of the Teflon prostheses distributed. We know of cases of disc wear in 16.

Dr. Kinsley: We believe that mild aortic incompetence might be important in the proper functioning of the Björk valve. Recently we have had two patients with mild aortic incompetence who had Björk-Shiley mitral valve replacements, and in both these patients, immediately after operation, there were significant gradients across the mitral valve. In one of the patients we merely rotated the disc of the Björk valve such that the major orifice was posterior. In the other patient we replaced the aortic valve. In both these patients, with different forms of treatment, the gradient across the mitral valve disappeared.

Dr. Yacoub: I have a question for both Dr. Björk and Dr. Beall. Dr. Björk mentioned gradients across the prosthesis. Can I ask him where these were taken? Were the patients at rest? Were they end-diastolic gradients or mean gradients, and were the patients in atrial fibrillation? Was this measurement taken over a number of beats, superimposing the wedge pressure and the left ventricular pressure?

Dr. Björk: All these were done both at rest and during exercise. The same tests were done before operation and after operation, using transseptal catheterization for the measurements of pressures simultaneously in the left atrium and the left ventricle. The mean gradients were determined by planimetry.

Dr. Yacoub: Over several beats?

Dr. Björk: Oh, yes.

Dr. Yacoub: And actually the gradients varied between?

Dr. Björk: Well, I showed that the gradient is different for different sizes of prostheses and will increase with the cardiac output, from average of 5 mm Hg for a cardiac output of 5 l/m, rising to up above 10 mm Hg for a cardiac output of 10 l/m. That was the rough estimation.

Dr. Beall: These were done predominantly at rest; we have some exercise studies but not enough to draw accurate conclusions. They were, as I mentioned, both mean diastolic gradients and occasional end-diastolic gradients. Basically, the technique was superimposing wedge pressure over left ventricular pressure.

Dr. Yacoub: And what was the average gradient?

Dr. Beall: Mean gradients at rest of 2, 3, occasionally 4 mm Hg. End-diastolic gradients were rarely seen.

Dr. Kaster: I would like to comment briefly on the subject of valve complications. During the early years of prosthetic valve surgery, the ball valve was found to be a very durable prosthesis. Later, as new and improved valve designs were introduced, there was a certain incidence of valve complications due to mechanical failure of the prosthesis. Some of the problems that were experienced clinically, I believe, were introduced by mishandling of the prosthesis between the time the valve left the manufacturer and the time it was implanted. Today mishandling of the prosthesis is a prominent cause of valve-related complications—regardless of design or construction materials.

For the most part, valve complications due to mishandling can be eliminated if the surgeon, and especially those that handle the prosthesis prior to implantation, understand and exercise the proper techniques and precautions when handling the valve.

Mr. Taylor: With regard to the attempts to compare different prosthetic valves by measuring either the mean pressure drop or the end-diastolic pressure difference derived from pressure data alone in a catheter laboratory, I would like to remind speakers of some points raised earlier. Firstly, the cross-over points on pressure curves do not correspond to the start and end of flow. We are dealing with a phasic flow system, and therefore flow lags behind pressure difference; with prosthetic valves this lag can be relatively greater than in the healthy valve. Secondly, whereas in the normal valve closure occurs without flow reversal, the prosthetic valves behave like the diseased mitral valve and all close after flow reversal with a regurgitant fraction. Lastly, at equivalent heart rate and cardiac output the proportion of the cardiac cycle for which diastolic filling occurs varies depending on the types of prosthesis. If we are to make a valid comparison between the fluid mechanics across different prostheses, flow and time should be taken into account, and we must try to develop measures of energy loss or power loss capable of being carried out in patients.

SUMMARY: PART VIII

C. Dubost, M.D.

The ideal mitral prosthesis remains to be discovered. Various models of artificial valve prostheses in use today have their respective disadvantages, and all are plagued by the risk of thromboembolic complications.

Two main types of valves are used in the mitral position: The ball valve of the Starr type, and the disc valve of the Björk type.

Ball valves have undergone a series of modifications since their invention. The initial metal prosthesis with a Silastic ball has been supplanted by fabric-covered cages with a metal ball. A radical decrease in thromboembolic complications has been reported with the latter valves by their developer.

The disc valves have an improved hydraulic performance, but are more prone to valve thrombosis and thromboembolic complications due to the eccentric displacement of the disc. Nevertheless, the latter are our current choice for mitral valve replacement.

One unmistakable conclusion remains: Mitral valve replacement by an artificial prosthesis is less than ideal. It must not be undertaken until all other possibilities have been ruled out. This underlines the importance of reconstructive surgery of the mitral valve.

Research undertaken in the laboratory with bioprostheses should in the not too distant future bring forth a more satisfactory solution to the serious problem of mitral valve replacement.

PART NINE

TISSUE VALVES

41 Long-Term Results of Tissue Valve Grafts for Mitral Replacement*

William W. Angell, M.D.

Techniques originally described for aortic homografts have been applied to mitral valve replacement since 1967.[1] The inverted transplanted semilunar valve has been shown to be an acceptable replacement for irreparably damaged mitral valves. The basic method is one which we first described in 1967 using stent-mounted aortic homografts where mitral valve leaflets and mechanisms were so destroyed that neither commissurotomy nor annuloplasty was feasible. This fresh, viable homograft tissue has functioned for eight years (Fig. 1), showing little tendency for thrombosis, small measured gradients, a low incidence of postoperative infection, and impressive tissue durability. However, the late and persistent regurgitation rate has resulted in only 40% of the original valves still functioning, thus making this valve no longer acceptable for clinical use. The variability of these results is primarily due to nonviability in portions of the donor valve. The pre- or post-implantation loss of functional donor fibro-blasts prevents the formation of new collagenous tissue in the functional

* Supported in part by the National Institutes of Health Grant HL 14845 and the American Heart Association Grant 72 901.

481

valve leaflet, and results in thinning, stretching, and sometimes disruption of these untreated, nonviable tissues. Contrarily, exuberant viable homograft donor cell activity has also been a problem, with some cases of shortening, thickening, and scarring similar to that seen with autogenous fascial valves.[2] It is important to note that none of these processes resulting in valve failure has been sudden or devastating in onset, and in virtually every instance accurate, timely diagnosis and repeat surgical intervention have been possible.

These plus the logistical problems associated with the use of fresh tissue valves prompted us to examine the use of tanning agents. While the results with the formalin-tanned valves were well known,[3] and contributed to an initial skepticism, we began in 1970, following Carpentier's work,[4] a clinical series utilizing the tanning and bactericidal properties of glutaraldehyde. The encouraging long-term follow-up of an initial series of six patients receiving these grafts in both the aortic and mitral positions led to our efforts to further refine this technique.

Glutaraldehyde serves to tan, sterilize, and stabilize the tissue in concentrations from 0.1% to 5%. Figure 2 illustrates the basic

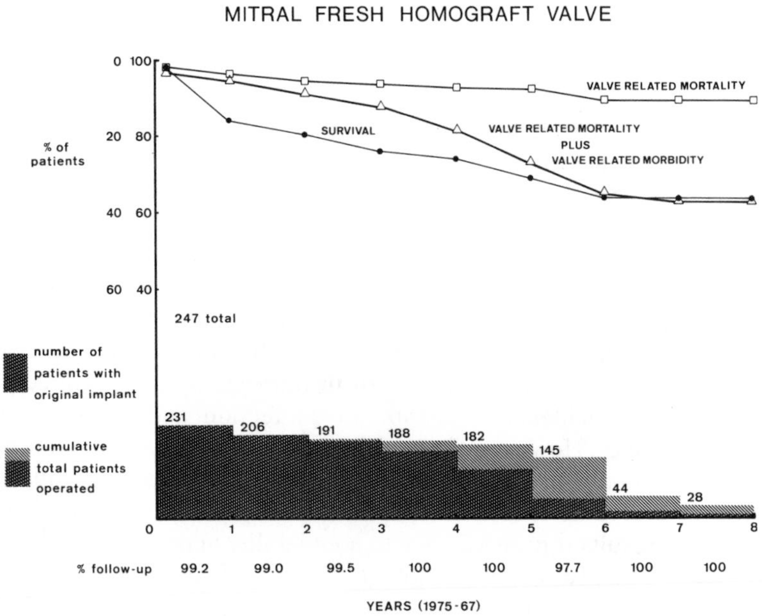

Figure 1. Eight-year actuarial survival rates of patients receiving stented fresh human aortic valves in the mitral position. The value for the "first month" represents hospital mortality rate.

biochemical structure and reactivity of glutaraldehyde with the collagen matrix of the aortic valve. The valve is initially fixed in a 5% glutaraldehyde solution under a pressure of 15 mm Hg. The valves are then examined and selected on the basis of uniformity of cusp size (symmetry), degree of coaptation, and general physical integrity. The preserved valve is then either left free or secured into a support ring which is accurately matched for anatomic detail, including the orifice size, shape, three-dimensional annular pattern, and commissural elevation and support. The ring is flexible and composed of Delrin, a nonreactive, strong, light, and fatigue-resistant plastic. The objective

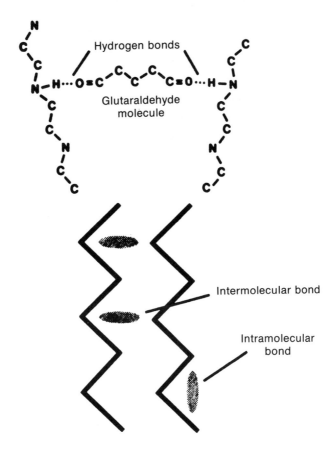

Beta conformation Protein Collagen

Figure 2. Schematic representation of carbonyl group from glutaraldehyde combining with amino group of peptide bond in the chemical interaction between protein and fixative.

is to provide the critical natural leaflet orientation with optimal support and coaptation of its edges. Valves are subsequently stored in 0.5% buffered glutaraldehyde until use.

The functional significance of the anatomical support ring is fivefold.

1. Our initial experience, which involved deforming the valve into a circular, symmetrical, rigid support, showed post implantation fibrous ingrowth continuing to magnify the abnormal stent configuration, and resulting in cusp and valve incompetency. It is, therefore, critical that the orientation of the valve in the support ring be anatomical, thus insuring a valve which will function well not only at the time of implantation, but also after complete healing has occurred.

2. The weak, nonfibrous portion of the valve annulus under the right coronary sinus is permanently supported without decreasing the effective flow orifice.

3. The sinus between commissural supports is wide so as not to crowd the coronary orifices in aortic valve replacement or obstruct the left ventricular outflow tract in mitral replacement. The commissural support posts are exactly positioned and sized to accomplish this.

4. The commissural support posts are slightly inclined along the anatomical lines of the valve. This has the added benefit of lowering the profile and improving the position both in subcoronary and intraventricular positions.

5. The implatation flange is positioned as high on the valve as possible, again, to avoid obstruction of coronary orifices in aortic valve replacement and to minimize the intraventricular portion of the valve for mitral valve replacement. While we were initially fearful of positioning the valve higher in the atrium, we have not seen an increase in left atrial thrombosis or embolism. This higher atrial profile may in fact be responsible for a lack of deleterious pannus growth across the inflow of the valve.

The design and type of fabric covering of the support ring is also of functional significance. While originally made of Teflon, a loose Dacron knit cloth which enhances host incorporation of the implantation flange and encourages host sheathing of the valve cusps is now used. The importance of this sheath is not known; however, it appears that the base of the cusp is less strong than the rest of the leaflet, and thus such ingrowth would be advantageous where it does not cause scarring or cusp retraction. Facilitated host ingrowth at the top of the commissural support serving to anchor valve to stent is a decided advantage, as this is a place where tissue valves tend to fail. The unacceptable incidence of perivalvular leak experienced with Teflon has not been a problem with the Dacron-knit implantation flange. A decrease in fabric thickness on the inner portion of the ring, along with a slimming of the ring profile, has improved the ID-to-OD ratios by one full size (2 mm). This permits use of 24–26 mm valves in the aortic position with a minimal gradient.

Using the methods and techniques described, we have seen no instance of glutaraldehyde tissue deterioration in the 160 patients followed for more than five years (Fig. 3). By contrast, a prospective randomized series of 100 patients comparing the cloth-covered Starr-Edwards valve with the homograft reveals a relatively poor

MITRAL GLUTARALDEHYDE HETEROGRAFT VALVE

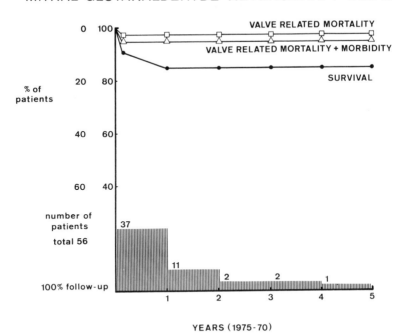

Figure 3. Five-year actuarial survival rates of patients receiving stented glutaraldehyde-preserved porcine aortic valves in the mitral position.

result (Fig. 4). This high incidence of valve-related complications has led us to the conclusion that the prosthetic valve as well as the fresh homograft are unacceptable mitral valve replacements.

The increased hemodynamic function of the anatomical glutaraldehyde valve has resulted in improvement of the NYHA classification and few instances of stenosis. The intense host reaction and/or fibrotic scarring seen in stenotic homografts has not been observed to

STARR-EDWARDS / HOMOGRAFT RANDOMIZED SERIES

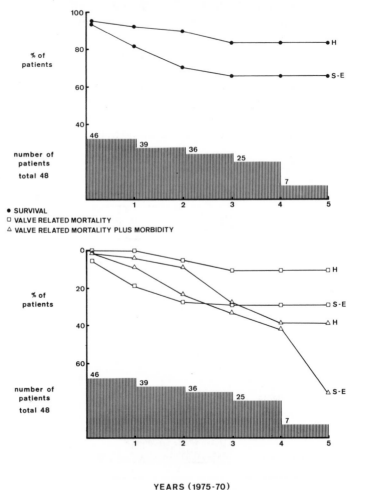

Figure 4. Actuarial comparison of survival among mitral patients receiving either a Starr-Edwards prosthetic valve (S-E) or a fresh human tissue valve (H) in a randomized prospective series.

occur in tanned tissue. Post operative catheterization gradients range from 0 to 9 mm, with an average of 3.5 at rest and 5.5 with exercise.

The thromboembolic incidence in our overall experience with both homograft and heterograft tissue valves used for mitral valve replacement is 0.9%. These instances have always occurred in the first year following implantation, and one half were concomitant with the cessation of Coumadin anticoagulation therapy. This is essentially identical with our experience in surgery not related to valve replacement. Thrombosis is therefore felt to be left atrial in origin. All patients are anticoagulated for three months, and therapy is very gradually stopped over a two- to three-month period.

The post-operative incidence of infection with the glutaraldehyde valve is nonexistent in our present experience. This is thought to be due in part to the surface of the valve which, although it does contain some fibrin deposition, is basically a firm and resistant barrier to circulating microorganisms (Fig. 5). Contrarily, the low, but not optimal, incidence of infection in the fresh homograft is related to the deposition of platelet fibrin on the irregular exposed surfaces.

Virtually the only complication that we have seen with the use of glutaraldehyde-tanned heterografts is asymmetrical opening of the valve under low pressure-low flow conditions. We have seen two valves at post mortem in which one cusp had become immobilized

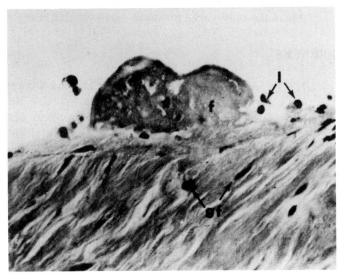

Figure 5. Cross-sectional view of the aortic surface of a porcine aortic valve leaflet, glutaraldehyde-fixed and in orthotopic position for one month. f = fibrin thrombi, l = leukocyte, gf = donor nucleus. H & E × 400.

with fibrin deposition following prolonged post-operative low cardiac outputs. We therefore recommend that valves larger than 34 mm not be used in mitral valve replacement, particularly in low output states, and that only valves of uniform cusp size and symmetry be selected.

In agreement with Carpentier's report,[5] we consider the increase in survival and concomitant decrease in valve-related complications seen in our five-year follow-up adequate to recommend this type of valve. However, this interval is still short for assuring long-term durability. Tissue failure remains the most likely cause of future graft complications. Patients in whom tissue valve replacement is contemplated should be adequately informed of this likely eventuality.

SUMMARY

In our experience, prosthetics have proved inadequate for mitral valve replacement. Deaths and complications occur at an unacceptable rate; complications persist for years after implantation, and no apparent solution has as yet been forthcoming.

The deterioration of fresh tissue valves has seemed to us a much less difficult and dangerous problem, since it is not associated with a myriad of related difficulties. The durability of tissue valves has been markedly enhanced and problems decreased if not solved with the advent of controlled glutaraldehyde fixation. In our surgical unit, this is the only valve presently used for mitral replacement.

REFERENCES

1. Angell, W.W., Wuerflein, R.D., and Shumway, N.D. Mitral valve replacement with the fresh aortic valve homograft: experimental results and clinical applications. *Surgery* 62:807, 1967.

2. Ross, J.K., and Johnson, D.C. Mitral valve replacement with homograft fascia lata and prosthetic valves: A long-term assessment of valve function. *J. Cardiovasc. Surg.* 15:242, 1974.

3. Buch, W.S., Kosek, J.C., Angell, W.W., and Shumway, N.E. Deterioration of formalin-treated aortic valve grafts. *J. Thorac. Cardiovasc. Surg.* 60:673, 1970.

4. Carpentier, A., Lemaigre, G., Robert, L., Carpentier, S., and Dubost, C. Biological factors affecting long term results of valvular heterografts. *Journal of Thor. and Cardiovasc. Surgery* 58:467, 1969.

5. Carpentier, A., Deloche, A., Relland, J., Fabiani, J., and Dubost, C. 6 year follow-up of glutaraldehyde-preserved heterografts. *Journal of Thor. and Cardiovasc. Surgery* 68:771, 1974.

42 Mitral-Valve Replacement Using "Unstented" Antibiotic Sterilized Aortic Valve Homografts

Review of Five and One Half
Years Experience

Magdi H. Yacoub, M.D.

Valve replacement has favorably altered the natural history of patients with advanced mitral-valve disease whose valves are not suitable for reconstructive procedures. The choice of a valve substitute, however, remains a problem. Homograft valves offer the advantages of ideal flow characteristics and freedom from thromboembolic complication; their main disadvantages are infection and mechanical failure. We believe that the long-term function of the grafts depends, to a large extent, on preserving their physical and biological properties, as well as guaranteeing ideal functional conditions at the time of insertion. For sterilization of the grafts, a mixture of antibiotics[1] is used. As most of the antibiotics used have been shown to have a cytotoxic effect directly proportional to the time of contact,[1] the valves are transferred to a tissue-culture medium[1] after 24 hours. The technique for mitral valve replacement in this series[2] consists of fixing the aortic homograft inside a 35 mm Dacron tube, which is then inserted into the left atrium. Two suture lines are used, one to the mitral ring and another in the left atrium. By means of these, a new floor for the left atrium is fashioned using autogenous pericardium

489

(Fig. 1, a, b, c). Anticoagulants were not used routinely. This technique has the following advantages:

1. It preserves the sinuses of Valsalva, which are important for smooth valve function.

2. It prevents distortion of the valve by avoiding fixing the commissures to a rigid stent with equidistant prongs, as the normal distance between commissures is variable.

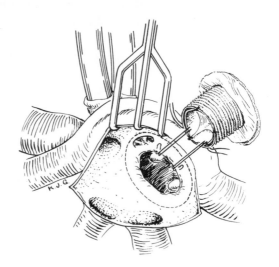

a

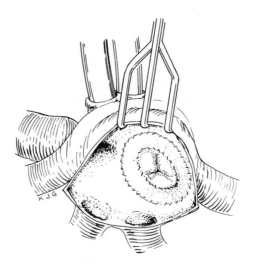

b

3. It allows the valve to alter its shape during the different parts of the cardiac cycle, and thus lowers the stress on the cusps.

4. It prevents torsion between the two suture lines, as the flange attached to the upper suture line allows the valve to take the correct shape when subjected to pressure during ventricular systole.

5. There is no protrusion into the left ventricular cavity or outflow, and thus irritation of the ventricular septum or obstruction of the outflow tract is avoided.

6. It allows smooth flow of blood from the pulmonary veins into the valve without stasis or turbulence.

7. It reduces the size of the abnormally enlarged left atrium and excludes the left atrial appendage from the circulation.

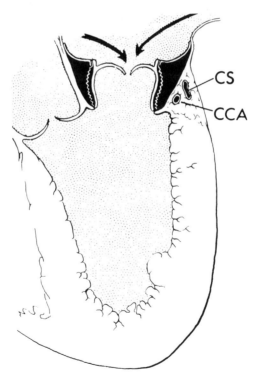

c

Figure 1. Diagrams (a, b, c) illustrating method in insertion of "unstented" aortic homograft in the mitral position. CS = Coronary Sinus; CCA = Circumflex Coronary Artery.

8. It covers all prosthetic material by pericardium or homograft tissue, thus minimizing the risk of thromboembolism.

Between August 1969 and January 1975, 487 patients underwent mitral valve replacement using this technique. The aortic valve was replaced at the same time in 114 patients, and other additional procedures were performed in 69. No patient was considered unsuitable for homograft valve replacement because of age, size of left atrium, degree of heart failure, pulmonary hypertension, or presence of associated valve disease.

The operative mortality (defined as all deaths occurring within the first 4 weeks after operation) was 6.6% for isolated mitral valve replacement (MVR) and 13% for aortic and mitral valve replacement using homografts (DVR). The late mortality was 12.2% for isolated MVR, and 10.3% for DVR. Expressed in the form of an actuarial survival curve, including operative and late deaths, the results are shown in Figure 2. This shows a slow continuous drop in survival; the 60 month survival rate for isolated MVR was 73%. The causes of late deaths are shown in Table 1. The clinical status of 259 patients who were followed up for 1 year or more after isolated MVR was judged to be excellent in 159 (61.5%), good in 92 (35.5%), and fair to poor in 8 (3%).

The valve-related complications are summarized in Table 2. Thromboembolism has occurred in three patients (0.6%), of whom 2 had massive clot removed from the left atrium at the time of operation. Fungal endocarditis has been a problem, particularly after double valve replacement. Several measures have been introduced recently in an attempt to reduce the incidence of this complication.

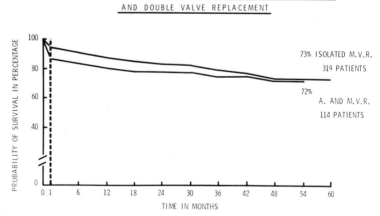

Figure 2. Actuarial survival after aortic homograft replacement of the mitral valve.

Seven patients have been reoperated on for valve failure. In four the valve was affected by endocarditis, and in three mechanical valve failure was secondary to a degenerative process. The hemodynamic response to this form of valve replacement has been good (Figure 3, a, b, and c).

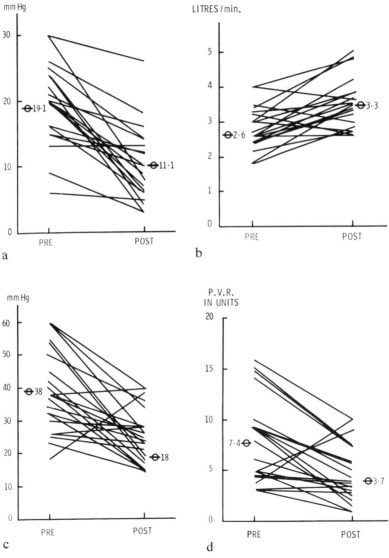

Figure 3. Hemodynamic data before and after homograft replacement of mitral valve. (A) changes in wedge pressure; (B) changes in cardiac output; (C) changes in P.A. pressure; (D) changes in P.V.R.

Table 1

Causes of Late Deaths Following Isolated Mitral Valve Replacement, and Aortic and Mitral Valve Replacement.

Cause	M.V.R.		Ao. and M.V.R.	
	No.	%	No.	%
Cardiac:				
Endocarditis	7	2.2%	4	3.5%
Miliary tuberculosis	2	0.6%	1	0.8%
Coronary thrombosis	7	2.2%	0	0%
Congestive cardiac failure	8	2.5%	0	0%
Arrhythmia	1	0.3%	0	0%
	25	7.8%	5	4.3%
Non cardiac	4	1.2%	3	2.5%
Unknown	10	3.1%	4	3.5%
Total	39	12.1%	12	10.3%

Measurement of instantaneous flow through the valve using computer analysis of changes in left ventricular volume showed a normal pattern (Fig. 4), with most of the flow occurring early in diastole. A definite increase in flow rate late in diastole, presumably due to atrial contraction, was also observed. Echocardiographic examination (Fig. 5) showed the pattern of movement of the anterior cusp of the homograft to be similar to the changes in flow rate, with rapid opening early in diastole followed shortly by partial closure,

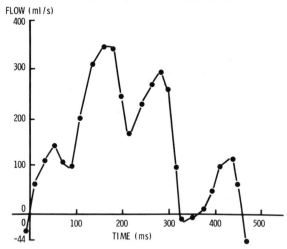

Figure 4. Flow pattern across "unstented" aortic homograft in the mitral position.

Table 2
Total Valve-Related Complications Following Aortic Homograft Replacement of the Mitral Valve in 487 Patients

	Number	%
Endocarditis	12	2.5%
Valve Failure	4	0.8%
Thromboembolism	3	0.6%
Hemolytic Anemia	1	0.2%
Total	20	4.1%

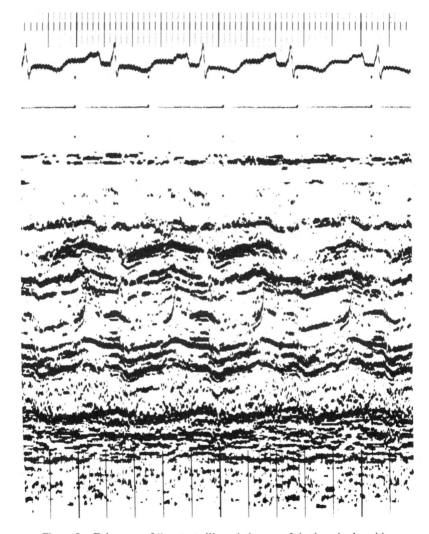

Figure 5. Echogram of "unstented" aortic homograft in the mitral position.

then a small anterior movement late in diastole followed by smooth closure.

In conclusion, experience with the use of aortic valve homografts (without rigid stents) for mitral valve replacement over the past 5½ years has been encouraging.

REFERENCES

1. Yacoub, M., Knight, E., and Towers, M. Aortic valve replacement using fresh unstented homografts. *Thorax Chirurgie* 21:451, 1973.

2. Yacoub, M., and Kittle, C.F. A new technique for replacement of the mitral valve by a semilunar valve homograft. *J. Thorac. Cardiovas. Surg.* 58:859, 1969.

43 Comparative Study of the Björk-Shiley Valve and Aortic Valve Homograft in Mitral-Valve Replacement

F. Fontan, M.D.
E. Baudet, M.D.
J.E. Coqueran, M.D.
A. Chauve, M.D.
P. Ruffié, M.D.
A. Bel Baraka, M.D.

In 1968, encouraged by our results in the use of homografts in aortic valve surgery,[4] we began to use aortic valve homografts in a series of mitral valve replacements; indeed, the results with prosthetic valves had not been satisfactory enough because of thromboembolic and mechanical complications. The first short-term results with homografts were good: patients had a good functional status and did not need anticoagulant therapy. However, valve insufficiency appeared in a later follow-up due to a deterioration of the valves. In 1970 we decided to use the Björk-Shiley valve[2] in the mitral position. The data for these two types of mitral-valve replacement are reported, and a comparative study of the results is presented.

METHOD
Valves

Two types of valve were used for mitral replacement. The first type was an aortic valve homograft sterilized either with beta-propiolactone (29 valves) or antibiotics (5), and stored at 4°C.[1-6] At the

497

498

time of operation, they were mounted on a frame (30) or inserted in a Dacron tube according to Yacoub's technique (4). The second type was the Björk-Shiley prosthetic valve, with a tilting disc of Delrin in the 43 first cases and of pyrolitic carbon in the last 78 cases.

Patients

Among the patients who underwent an isolated mitral valve replacement from 1968 to 1975, 155 (91 males and 64 females) are reported in two comparative groups: the 34 patients of the first group had a mitral valve replacement with an aortic valve homograft, and the 121 patients of the second group had a mitral valve replacement with a Björk-Shiley prosthesis.

They ranged in age from 25 months to 64 years: mean age 39 years and 5 months in the homograft group, 46 years and 5 months in the Björk-Shiley group. There were 146 patients in functional class III or IV (NYHA); 9 patients in class II underwent surgery for either systemic emboli or paroxysmal atrial dysrhythmias (Table 1). There were 80 mitral insufficiencies, 1 congenital mitral stenosis, and 27 mitral restenosis; 47 patients had both a stenotic and incompetent mitral valve (Table 2).

Table 1
Preoperative Functional Status of Patients

Class (NYHA)	Homografts	Björk-Shiley	Total	%
I	—	—		
II	—	9	9	5.8
III	11	61	72	46.4
IV	23	51	74	47.8
Total	34	121	155	

Table 2
Preoperative Mitral Valvular Lesions

Lesions	Homografts	Björk-Shiley	Total	%
M. Insufficiency	13	67	80	51.7
M. stenosis	—	—	—	—
Congenital M.S.	—	1	1	.7
M. Restenosis	4	23	27	17.4
M.I. + M.S.	17	30	47	30.2
Total	34	121	155	

RESULTS
Mortality

Hospital mortality In the homograft group, 2 patients (5.88%) died: one from low cardiac output, the other from acute dysrhythmia. In the Björk-Shiley group, 9 patients (7.4%) died; the death was directly related to the prosthesis in 2 patients: a tear of the myocardium in one, a thrombosis of the prosthesis in the other one 10 days after surgery. The other deaths were due to: low cardiac output (4), heart failure (2), and bleeding (1).

Late mortality (Table 3) Late mortality was observed in patients who were functional class IV preoperatively. In the homograft group with a 7-year maximum follow-up, 18 patients (52.94%) died from the third to the sixty-third post-operative month: bacterial endocarditis in 2 patients, heart failure in 3, sudden death in 1. The majority of deaths (12 patients) was due to an homograft valve incompetence, mostly during the third postoperative year, in relation to valvular lesions in 11, and with a perivalvular leakage in 1.

In the Björk-Shiley group with a 5-year maximum follow-up, 19 patients died (15%) from second to the thirty-sixth postoperative month: thrombosis of the prosthesis in 3 patients, heart failure in 7, pulmonary embolism in 2, sudden death in 3 (no autopsy), extracardiac cause in 4.

The actuarial curves of survival comparing the patients of both groups show an important decrease in the number of survivors in the homograft group, 31.6% seven years postoperatively, which contrasts with the Björk-Shiley group, 74.7% survival at five years (see Figure 1).

Table 3
Late Mortality

Cause of death	Homografts Max. follow-up : 83 months Mean : 66.6 months	Björk-Shiley Max. follow-up : 58 months Mean : 28 months
Disinsertion	1	—
Incompetence	11	—
Thrombosis	—	3
Heart failure	3	7
Bact. endocarditis	2	—
Sudden death	1	3
Pulm. emboli	—	2
Extra-cardiac cause	—	4
Total	18 (52.94%)	19 (15%)

500

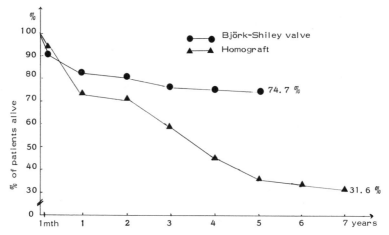

Figure 1. Actuarial curves of survival in the homograft and Björk-Shiley groups.

Morbidity

Late complications (Table 4) In the homograft group, besides the lethal complications, there were 6 patients with homograft incompetence, and 1 with bacterial endocarditis cured by medical treatment. Among the 93 survivors of the Björk-Shiley prosthesis group, there were systemic emboli in 3 patients in spite of anticoagulant therapy, and disinsertion of the prosthesis in 1.

No hemolysis was observed in either group.

Reoperation: Six patients of the homograft group were reoperated upon: for an homograft incompetence in 5 and a tricuspid insuf-

Table 4
Late Complications

Complication	Homografts Max. follow-up : 83 months Mean : 66.6 months	Björk-Shiley Max. follow-up : 58 months Mean : 28 months
Incompetence	6	—
Bact. endocarditis	1	—
Systemic emboli	—	3
Disinsertion	—	1
Total	7	4

ficiency in 1. In all cases, a Björk-Shiley prosthesis was used to replace the homograft. There were 3 hospital deaths and 1 late death from heart failure.

One patient of the Björk-Shiley group was reoperated upon for disinsertion of the prosthesis, with a consequent tricuspid valve insufficiency, 4 months post-operatively; this patient died from heart failure after discharge from the hospital.

Functional status (Table 5) In the homograft group, 7 patients are functional class I and 2 patients are class II, i.e., there was 75% good results among the survivors, but only 25% in the entire group, with a maximum follow-up of 7 years. In the Björk-Shiley group, 73 patients are functional class I and 16 are class II, i.e., 95% good results among the survivors and 73.5% in the entire group, with a maximum follow-up of 5 years.

DISCUSSION

The results of this study of two groups of patients who have undergone a mitral valve replacement with either a frame-mounted aortic valve homograft or a Björk-Shiley prosthesis have demonstrated several points. There was no significant difference between the hospital mortality in both groups. As in other studies,[5-7] the results were poor with the homografts; 21 of the 34 patients (61.7%) developed a valvular insufficiency which was responsible for 11 late deaths and 5 reoperations. In patients reoperated upon, insufficiency was found to be related to anatomical and histological changes: retraction, prolapse, sclerosis of the leaflets, substitution of collagen for normal tissue with few or no fibroblasts. The method of sterilization

Table 5
Functional Status of Patients

Class (NYHA)	Homograft Max. follow-up : 83 months Mean : 66.6 months	Björk-Shiley Max. follow-up : 58 months Mean : 28 months
I	7	73
II	2	16
III	2	3
IV	1	1
Total	12*	93

* 2 patients of the homograft group excluded because their homograft was replaced by a Björk-Shiley prosthesis.

(beta-propiolactone or antibiotics) or the surgical technique (frame-mounted or Dacron tube-mounted homograft) did not seem to modify the onset of the valvular insufficiency. In addition, 3 patients (8.8%) developed a bacterial endocarditis, which resulted in valvular insufficiency in 2 patients who died, and was cured by antibiotics in the other one. So, in spite of the absence of hemolysis and thromboemboli (without anticoagulant therapy), the use of an aortic valve homograft should no longer be recommended as a mitral-valve replacement.

In the Björk-Shiley group, with a shorter follow-up (maximum 5 years, mean 28 months), we observe a stabilization of the actuarial survival curve after 3 years, the majority of the patients operated upon with a poor cardiac function dying within the first 3 years postoperatively. In this group there was no prosthesis dysfunction, no infection, no hemolysis. There were a few cases of thromboembolism when the prosthesis was inserted with the large opening directed towards the anterior leaflet of the mitral valve. Since the prosthesis was put in place with the large opening directed towards the aortic valve and posteriorly to it, no case of thromboembolism was observed. The importance of positioning the prosthesis was mentioned by others.[3]

In conclusion, the Björk-Shiley prosthesis seems to give good results within the limits of the present follow-up, in contrast to the poor long-term results obtained with aortic valve homografts in mitral valve replacement.

SUMMARY

We have reported our experience with isolated mitral valve replacement in 155 patients, aortic valve homografts in 34 patients, and Björk-Shiley prosthesis in 121 patients.

The late results were poor with aortic homografts: 70.5% of the patients presented a dysfunction of the graft. The results were fairly good with the Björk-Shiley prosthesis: there were no dysfunctions of the valve and only 3 systemic thromboemboli.

REFERENCES

1. Baudet, E., Bel Baraka, A., Ruffié, P., and Fontan, F. Résultats éloignés de la chirurgie de remplacement valvulaire aortique par homogreffe. *Coeur no.* spécial 1975. Journées Internationales de Cardiologie consacrées aux remplacements valvulaires, 539.

2. Björk, V.O., Böök, K., Cernigliaro, C., and Holmgren, A. The Björk-Shiley tilting disc valve in isolated mitral lesions. *Scan. J. Thor. Cardiovasc. Surg.* 7:131, 1973.

3. Björk, V.O., Böök, K., and Holmgren, A. Significance of position and opening angle of the Björk-Shiley tilting disc valve in mitral surgery. *Scan. J. Thor. Cardiovasc. Surg.* 7:187, 1973.

4. Fontan, F., Mounicot, F., Ploquin, F., Baudet, E., and Badiola, P. Technique et premiers résultats des homogreffes valvulaires aortiques. *Arch. Mal. Coeur*, 62:527, 1969.

5. Kirklin, J.W., and Pacifico, A.D. Surgery for acquired valvular heart disease. *New England Journal of Medicine*. 288:133, 1973.

6. Ruffié, P., Berjon, J.J., Larrue, J., Baudet, E., Meunier, J.M., and Fontan, F. Aspects biologiques récents des homogreffes valvulaires aortiques. *Coeur* No. spécial 1975. Journées Internationales de Cardiologie consacrées aux remplacements valvulaires, 549.

7. Stinson, E.B., Griepp, R.B., Shumway, N.E. Devenir à long terme des homogreffes aortiques en position mitrale. *Coeur* No. spécial 1975. Journées Internationales de Cardiologie consacrées aux remplacements valvulaires, 533.

44 Valvular Xenograft and Valvular Bioprosthesis: 1965–1975

A. Carpentier, M.D., Ph.D.
A. Deloche, M.D.
J. Relland, M.D.
C. Dubost, M.D.

Tissue valve replacement possesses important advantages: the risk of thromboembolism is decreased, the need for anticoagulation is avoided, and the nature of the occasional valve failure is progressive, thereby permitting elective reoperation under optimal conditions.

The easy availability, large size range, and possibility of long-term storage of heterograft valves stimulated us in early 1965 to begin investigating porcine heterograft valves for cardiac valve replacement. A method for reducing the antigenicity of the graft was developed,[1] permitting the first xenograft valve replacement in the human being.[2] The initial encouraging results were marred by early graft failures occurring from 6 to 24 months after implantation due to immunologic reactions and tissue degeneration. From this early experience, we learned that the most important factor affecting durability was the method of preparation. The theoretical possibility of graft regeneration by host fibroblast infiltration failed to materialize; moreover, cellular ingrowth which did occur proved to be harmful, as the cells invading the graft tissue were most often inflammatory in nature.[3]

It became obvious that the future of xenograft valve replacement would depend upon our capability to develop methods preventing both immunologic reaction and tissue denaturation.

THE CONCEPT OF BIOPROSTHESIS

Since the regeneration of implanted valvular xenografts failed to occur, research was directed towards the possibility of using the valvular tissue as a biomaterial in the construction of a prosthetic valve.[4] The durability of this valve was based on the unfailing stability of the biomaterial, and not on regeneration by host cell ingrowth (Fig. 1). In order to make a clear distinction between this type of valve and the xenograft valve, we coined the term "bioprosthesis," which combines both its biological origin and its role as a prosthesis.[4]

Methods for Conditioning Valvular Tissue

Several chemical methods were investigated to reduce antigenicity of the tissue and to increase long-term stability. Antigenicity was tested by the subcutaneous implantation of the treated tissue in rats and by hemagglutination testing. Stability of the tissue, a

GRAFT-HOST REACTION

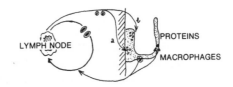

PREVENTION

PROTECTED GRAFT

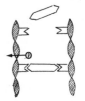

CHEMICAL TREATMENT

Figure 1. Graft-host reaction with cellular ingrowth from tissue host or blood. Prevention by protecting the graft from cellular penetration from tissue, and by chemical treatment: remove soluble proteins and proteo-glycans (P) and introduce crosslinkages (white hexagon) between collagen molecules (////).

function of the number of crosslinkages between the collagen molecules, was tested by heat shrinkage. The higher the temperature initiating retraction of the tissue, the stronger was the crosslinkage. Different chemical treatments were used either to introduce cross-linkages into the tissue (acrolein, succinyldehyde, glyoxal, glutaral-dehyde, formaldehyde, dialdehyde, starch), or to reinforce crosslink-ages[5] (metaperiodate combined with glutaraldehyde), or to stabilize crosslinkages (sodium borohydride).[6] Among these various treat-ments, glutaraldehyde appeared to be the most effective for decreas-ing the antigenicity and increasing the stability of the tissue[3,7] (Fig. 2). Based on these experiments, glutaraldehyde preservation has been adopted as the method of choice in the preparation of tissue valve. The aortic valves, removed from pig hearts, are washed in saline solution for 5 hours to remove soluble proteins and proteoglycans which are highly antigenic. Then the valves, maintained in a closure position by pledgets or physiologic pressure, are placed in a 0.625% glutaraldehyde solution in a 1/15 M phosphate buffer at pH 4. After 24 hours, the valves are trimmed of excess tissue and mounted on a frame according to techniques previously described.[4]

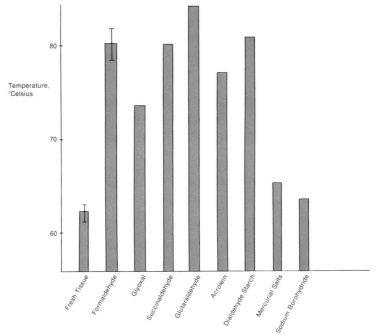

Figure 2. Evaluation of crosslinkage-inducing factors by the heat shrinkage tempera-ture test.

The 1/15 M phosphate buffer used to activate the glutaraldehyde is prepared as follows: 9.07 gm of monobasic potassium phosphate are dissolved in 800 ml distilled water; pH is adjusted to 7.4 using approximately 1N sodium hydroxide; volume is brought to 1000 ml with distilled water; 25 ml of a 25% solution of glutaraldehyde in water is added to 900 ml of the 1/15 M phosphate buffer. The volume is then adjusted to 1000 ml with the phosphate buffer to yield the final buffered solution.

Method for Mounting the Graft

With the aim of preparing a standardized valve, the treated aortic valve xenograft is mounted in a frame designed to preserve its normal function.[1,3] A new, completely flexible frame has been recently developed in order to reduce the loading shock on the valve commissures, the free margin and the base of the leaflets.* The aortic sheath was enveloped in a fabric covering to protect it from cellular penetration from the host aorta.[3,4]

Based on these principles, two laboratories† in the United States began to produce this type of bioprosthesis commercially. They improved the stent design, assured product standardization, and made available various sizes suitable for both adults and children.

CLINICAL MATERIAL

There were 104 patients operated upon at Broussais Hospital between March 1968 through April 1973, with an average follow-up of 39 months (maximum 7 years and minimum 2 years).

Heterografts used in the first 11 patients were preserved in glutaraldehyde solution after the valve had been washed in a balanced salt solution to eliminate the soluble antigenic proteins. Glutaraldehyde solution was prepared according to specifications previously described.

The remainder of the valves were preserved in glutaraldehyde solution after being treated by oxidation, again according to a technique previously described. All valves but one were frame-mounted and protected from cellular ingrowth by covering the aortic cuff with a thin layer of Dacron cloth. A flexible frame was used in the first 12 patients and a rigid frame in the remaining 92 patients. Eighty-

---

* Edwards Laboratories.
† Edwards Laboratories and Hancock Laboratories.

two patients had acquired valvular disease, and the remainder (22) had congenital valvular malformations. A total of 118 valve implantations were required.

In the group that had acquired valvular disease, there were 28 single aortic valve replacements, 15 mitral valve replacements, and 2 tricuspid valve replacements; 37 multiple valve diseases required the insertion of 49 valves in the following positions: aortic 22, mitral 12, tricuspid 15.

In the group of congenital malformations, there were: 8 tricuspid valve replacements, 7 for Ebstein's disease and 1 for agenesis of the anterior tricuspid leaflet; 12 pulmonary valve replacements (8 absent pulmonary valves, 1 truncus type I, 1 Fallot, 2 pulmonary valve stenoses); and 2 mitral valve replacements (1 mitral valve malformation and 1 single ventricle).

RESULTS

This series is heterogeneous due to the various types of patients grouped according to the site of heterograft implantation and the associated lesions. Therefore, actuarial curves could be used only in the aortic valve replacement group, the only group which was sufficiently large to be statistically significant. Mortality rates and incidence of complications in the other groups were analyzed by means of percentage curves.

Acquired Valvular Disease (Table 1)

Aortic Valve Replacement Of the 28 patients in this group, 1 died at operation as a result of a myocardial infarction, for an incidence of 3.5%. An aortic diastolic murmur was noted in another patient prior to discharge from the hospital. Three patients (11%) died during the follow-up period from 1 to 6 years postoperatively. The causes of late deaths were subacute bacterial endocarditis in 1 patient and diabetic coma in another; the cause of death in the third patient is unknown.

The actuarial survival curve shows a relative survival rate of 97% after 1 year, 94% after 2 years, 88% after 3 years, and 80% after 4 to 6 years (Fig. 3).

One patient required reoperation for replacement of the aortic valve after 2 years because of a perivalvular leak. Another required reoperation because of endocarditis. Two patients required reoperation because of valve failures 4 and 5 years postoperatively;

the valves were perforated, and there were scattered areas of calcification. Histology showed collagen degeneration localized at the base of the cusps.

The remaining 21 patients are well, with no thromboembolic complications, and are taking no anticoagulants. All are leading normal lives and are in functional class I (NYHA). The longest follow-up period was 7 years 4 months, and the average follow-up period was 4½ years. Sixteen patients have been followed for more than 4 years. Cardiac catheterization was performed in 2 patients 3 and 4 years postoperatively. The sizes of the heterografts used were 29 and 31 mm in external diameter, and no gradients were present across the valves.

Mitral Valve Replacement   In the group of 15 patients who had mitral valve replacement, there were two hospital deaths due to heart failure, an incidence of 13%. There were three late deaths: two occurred 1 year after operation, and the other occurred 2 years after operation. These patients were among those having massive atrial enlargement with calcification of the atrial wall. The cause of death was atrial thrombosis in 2 patients and mesenteric infarction in the third. One patient was reoperated upon at the end of 5 years for mitral insufficiency; valve morphology was normal, but perforations were found in each of the three cusps. One patient who has been followed for 6 years now has clinical and cardiac catheterization evidence of mitral regurgitation, and will probably require reoperation within the next 6 months.

Eight patients remain well. The longest follow-up period is 7 years, with 6 patients followed for more than 4 years.

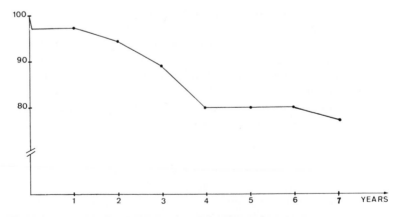

Figure 3.   Actuarial survival curve in aortic valve replacement.

Tricuspid Valve Replacement   The 2 patients in this group were operated upon for tricuspid insufficiency after total correction of tetralogy of Fallot, and have had excellent functional results 4 years and 3 years following the operations. In the absence of clinical evidence of tricuspid insufficiency or stenosis, no intracardiac investigations have been carried out.

Multiple Valve Disease   Among the 21 patients with double valve disease, there were three hospital deaths which were not valve-related, and four late deaths, two of which were valve-related; in the other 2 patients who died, the cause of death is not known. All deaths occurred in the mitral-aortic group. One patient died 3 months postoperatively at reoperation for disinsertion of the valve ring, and the other died after 3 years due to valve failure. Of the 14 survivors, 1 required reoperation after 4 months for recurrent subacute bacterial endocarditis, and 1 has a recurrent murmur. The remaining patients are well; 10 have been followed for more than 3 years.

Among the 16 patients with triple valve disease, there were three hospital deaths and two late deaths. None of the hospital deaths was valve-related. One late death was due to cerebral hemorrhage secondary to anticoagulants; the cause of the other late death is unknown. Of 11 survivors, 2 required reoperation: in 1 patient, thrombosis of the heterograft in the tricuspid position necessitated replacement of the valve graft by a prosthesis 1 year postoperatively. The other was reoperated upon after 4½ years for valve failure. All of the other patients but 1 lost to follow-up are well; 2 of these have been followed for more than 4 years.

Congenital Valvular Diseases (Table 2)

Tricuspid Replacement   Of the 7 patients with Ebstein's disease, 2 died in the hospital due to cardiac failure and arrhythmia, and 1 sustained postoperative atrioventricular block and required pacemaker insertion. Four patients, followed for more than 4 years, have remained well without clinical evidence of either tricuspid stenosis or insufficiency. They have not been taking anticoagulants, and no thromboembolic complications have been observed. One patient had a normal pregnancy. The first patient to be operated upon was recatheterized after 6 years. This study disclosed a 7 mm Hg gradient across the valve and a mean right atrial pressure of 9 mm Hg. The patient operated on for tricuspid agenesis has been followed for 2 years, 3 months.

Table 1
Acquired Valvular Disease

Valve disease	No.	Hospital death	Late death	Valve failure	Good result	Average follow-up
Aortic	28	1	3	3	21	4 years, 3 months
Mitral	15	2	3	2	8	4 years, 5 months
Tricuspid	2				2	3 years, 3 months
Double valve disease	21	3	4*	2	12†	4 years
Triple valve disease	16	3	2	2	8†	3 years, 5 months

* Two deaths were valve-related
† One patient was lost to follow-up

Table 2
Congenital valvular diseases

Valve disease	No.	Hospital death	Late death	Valve failure	Good result	Average follow-up
Ebstein's disease	7	2			5	4 years, 7 months
Agenesis of anterior tricuspid leaflet	1				1	3 years
Absent pulmonary valve	8	1			7	3 years
Pulmonary valve stenosis	2				2	3 years, 7 months
Tetralogy of Fallot plus pulmonary atresia	1					16 months
Truncus arteriosus Type I	1	1				
Mitral valve malformation	1		1	1		
Single ventricle	1		1			4 months

Pulmonary Valve Replacement with Absent Pulmonary Valve
In this group of 8 patients there was one hospital death due to acute right heart failure. The remaining 7 patients were asymptomatic, with regression of right ventricular hypertrophy by electrocardiogram and decrease in heart size by roentgenography. There is no evidence of a diastolic murmur in 6 of these patients, but a moderate diastolic murmur is present in the seventh. Two patients followed for 5 years have had intracardiac investigations, including catheterization and angiography, which showed a 15 to 20 mm Hg gradient across the pulmonary valve. Pulmonary artery pressures were normal and there was no pulmonary insufficiency.

The child with truncus arteriosus Type I died during the operation, but the remaining 3 patients with pulmonary valve replacement were improved. The longest follow-up period in this group was 4 years. One patient was readmitted to the hospital 1 year following the operation because of severe right ventricular failure. Catheterization showed a right ventricular pressure of 135/50 mm Hg and it was impossible for the catheter to cross the pulmonary valve. At operation, the valve exhibited severe calcification and cusp perforations. The patient has remained well following replacement of the defective valve.

Another patient was catheterized 1 year after the operation. There was a 25 mm Hg gradient across the right ventricular outflow tract and no valve insufficiency by angiography.

Mitral Valve Replacement   Both patients with mitral valve replacement died, one of hepatitis and the other of cardiac insufficiency. The valves were normal.

Study of Valve-related Complications

Table 3 summarizes the valve-related complications according to the valve site, irrespective of associated pathology and treatment. Among patients with aortic valve replacment, five of fifty-two valves failed (9.5%). The follow-up period was from 1 to 7 years (average follow-up 4 years 5 months). Two valves failed because of peripheral leaks, a complication which is not specific to this type of valve substitute. The third valve failure was caused by subacute bacterial endocarditis with destruction of the valve leaflets, and the fourth and fifth were due to cusp perforation secondary to tissue degeneration (5 and 6 years).

The incidence of valve failure in the tricuspid position was 3.8% (1 of 26 valves). In this case, the cause was valve destruction secondary to subacute bacterial endocarditis.

One of the twelve valves implanted in the pulmonary position failed, an incidence of 8%. Failure in this case was due to stenosis secondary to calcification of the valve 16 months after implantation. We believe in retrospect that the complication was due to an improperly placed tubular conduit, which was severely kinked and thereby caused excessive turbulence in the pulmonary outflow tract.

The incidence of valve-related complications in the mitral position was higher: 9 of 28 valves (31%). In 2 cases, the complication occurred in previously diseased left atria which had been heavily calcified and thrombotic preoperatively, and which subsequently became thrombotic again; however, the atrial thrombi did not extend to the valves themselves. One case of valve destruction was due to subacute bacterial endocarditis. The remaining 6 cases of valve failure were due to cusp perforation secondary to tissue degeneration, which may have occurred because of the excessive stress on the aortic leaflets implanted in the mitral position. The other 19 valves are still functioning after 4 years, and two of them are operating after 6 years and a half.

Actuarial curves dealing with the durability of valve substitues in the various positions show that glutaraldehyde-perserved heterograft valves maintain good function at 5 years in 72% of cases in the mitral position, 80% of cases in the aortic position, and 83% of cases in the tricuspid position (Fig. 4). Valve failures occurred mainly in valves treated by oxidation plus glutaraldehyde. The incidence of complications was reduced in valves treated by buffered glutaraldehyde alone.

PATHOLOGY

All specimens removed for tissue graft failure displayed similar gross lesions, that is, tears and perforations localized in the central portions of the valve cusps. This is the hinged area of the valve and is

Table 3
Valve Failure

	Aortic N = 52	Mitral N = 28	Tric. N = 26	Pulm. N = 12
Peripheral Leak	2			
Endocarditis	1	1		
Thromboembolism		2	1	
Graft Pathology	2	6		1
	5 (9.5%)	9 (32%)	1 (3.8%)	1 (8%)

that portion which is subjected to the highest pressures. These lesions appear to be induced by fatigue, with high pressures and repeated flexion partially responsible.

Histologic examination revealed that these lesions were of three types:

1. Collagen and elastin degeneration, with areas of hyalinization and fragmentation of connective tissue fibers, were found in all six valves removed because of failure. These lesions were predominantly present in the central portions of the leaflets.

2. Calcium deposition was found in five valves, particularly in those valves treated by oxidation.

3. Inflammatory reactions, characterized by histiocytes, giant cells, and macrophages, were found in three valves in scattered areas on the surface of the cusps.

In addition, three valves were removed from patients who died of non-valve-related causes from 3 years to 6 years and 2 months following implantation (Fig. 5). Grossly, the valves appeared normal. Microscopically, there were slight changes such as elastin fragmentation

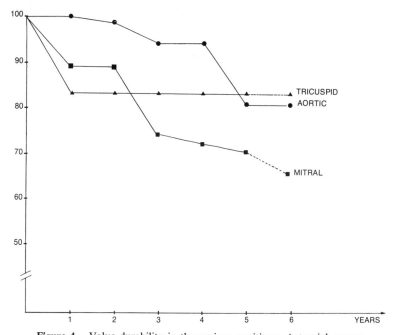

Figure 4. Valve durability in the various positions. Actuarial curves.

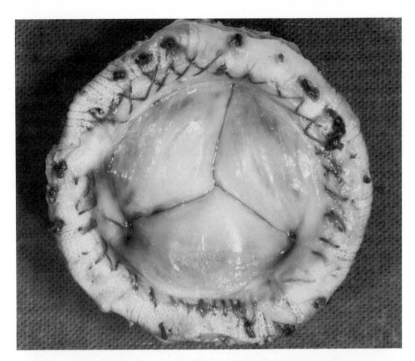

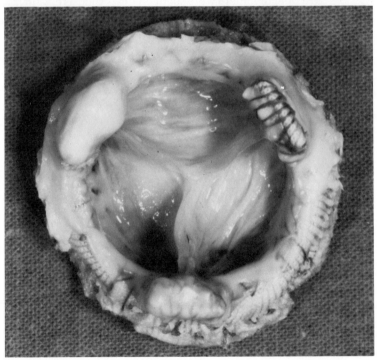

516

Figure 5 (Left). Glutaraldehyde preserved xenograft six years after implantation in the mitral position: normal architecture. (Top) atrial view; (Bottom) ventricular view.

plus areas of collagen hyalinization. There was a thin layer of fibrin (0.1 mm thick) over the cloth-covered portion of the stent, and it extended over the surface of the cusps (Fig. 6). In all specimens this layer contained scattered fibroblasts and collagen fibers which did not penetrate the valvular tissue. This process of "encapsulation" is essentially different from that of cellular ingrowth and could be of critical importance for the long-term durability of these bioprostheses.

CONCLUSIONS

More than 7 years' experience with the glutaraldehyde-treated xenograft allows an evaluation of the present role of this type of valvular substitute in cardiac valve replacement.

The overall mortality was similar to that of prosthetic valve replacement. Thromboembolic complications were exceptional and not related to the bioprosthesis, so that no anticoagulants were required. The incidence of valve failure was 15% at 6 years for the aortic, pulmonary, and tricuspid positions. Production on an industrial scale with accurate selection of the valves and quality controls, as

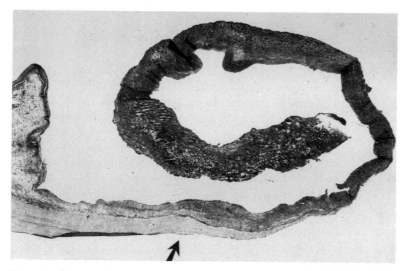

Figure 6. Same specimen as Figure 5. Slight collagen degeneration with areas of hyalinization. Note the layer of fibrin (arrow) extending over the surface of the cusp.

well as recent improvements in stent design and glutaraldehyde preparation, should reduce the already low incidence of valve failure. The process of "encapsulation" observed at 6 years, reinforcing the leaflets, may also play a significant role in the durability of the bioprosthesis.

At the present time, glutaraldehyde-preserved xenograft valves appear to be the best choice for pulmonary and tricuspid valve replacement. This is especially true in the tricuspid position, in which prosthetic valves have a notably high risk of thromboembolism.

In aortic and mitral valve replacement, the ever-present risk of thromboembolic complications with prosthetic valves and the necessity of anticoagulation therapy with its attendant morbidity are factors which confront both the surgeon and his patient. The critical choice between a heterograft valve and a prosthetic valve will depend upon the relative importance of an improved quality of life with a xenograft valve versus a lower risk of reoperation with a prosthesis.

REFERENCES

1. Carpentier, A. Utilisation d'hétérogreffes dans traitement des lésions valvulaires aortiques, *These Med.,* Paris, 1966.

2. Binet, J.P., Carpentier, A., Langlois, J., Duran, C., and Colvez, P. Inplantation de valves hétérogènes dans le traitement des cardiopathies aortiques. *C.R. Acad. Sc. Paris* 261:5773, 1965.

3. Carpentier, A., Lemaigre, G., Robert, L., Carpentier, S., and Dubost, C. Biological factors affecting long-term results of valvular heterografts. *J. Thorac. Cardiovasc. Surg.* 58:467, 1969.

4. Carpentier, A., and Dubost, C. From xenografts to bioprostheses. Ed. by Ionescu, M.I., et al. *Biological Tissue in Heart Valve Replacement,* Butterworth and Co.: London, 1971.

5. Robert, L., and Moczar, E. Personal communication, 1969.

6. Carpentier, A. Le concept de bioprothese—application à la réalisation d'organes artificiels. These Doctorat es Sciences, Paris, 1974.

7. Carpentier, A. Principles of tissue valve transplantation. Ed. by Ionescu, M.I., et al. *Biological Tissue in Heart Valve Replacement,* Butterworth and Co.: London, 1971.

DISCUSSION: PART IX

Mr. Ross: First, one must express admiration for these beautiful results. Having had some experience of mitral valve replacement using unstented aortic valve homografts, I would like to ask Dr. Yacoub two questions. One is—how does he get homografts that are big enough and of sufficiently good quality? My experience is that the larger valves, from older donors, tend to show unacceptable degenerative change. Secondly, we know that chemically or physically sterilized aortic valves in the mitral position have approximately a 50% failure rate at 2½ years. Does he believe that the success he describes in his series depends solely on the method of preparation of the valves?

Dr. Yacoub: In answer to the first question, it is quite true that the valves used for mitral valve replacement are usually or almost always from older donors. If one wants a large valve, it has to be from an older donor. We have been particularly lucky to have a good supply of homografts from people who had died from coronary thrombosis in the age group between 50 and 70, and usually we get enough homografts in that group without calcification.

Dr. Lyngborg: I would like to ask Dr. Yacoub whether he has any histological examination in the patients who died late, as I think it is difficult to evaluate the final results of the homograft operations through a 5-year follow-up study.

Dr. Yacoub: Yes we have had some histological examinations. We are in the process of analyzing these, and the valves look almost acellular but with a definite cellular layer on the aortic wall and at the junction of the pericardium and the homograft. This is a single layer of cells which covers about ¾ of the atrial side of the homograft. There are a few cells in the fibrosa of the graft—but only a few.

Dr. Lyngborg: Dr. Yacoub, I would like to ask a question with respect to reoperating patients with this type of graft. There is presumably a certain masking of the normal anatomy, and a clot of blood is often found under the pericardium. It would seem to me that it might be quite difficult to reoperate such patients.

Dr. Yacoub: Yes. Actually, the amount of clot which usually surrounds the sleeve is absorbed as time goes by, and usually you can open a plane between the graft and the atrium. There is little tissue there, and then one can decorticate that; it is not very difficult to excise it and put in another valve. But the difficulty would be to put in

520

another homograft, because then this tunnel usually fits the valve you have just taken out. So, you cannot put in another one, and you have to put in a prosthetic valve. It is not difficult.

Dr. Silver: Two points. Could Dr. Yacoub tell us why there is such a high incidence of fungal endocarditis in this particular type of valve, and second point, is it any more difficult to treat this type of infected endocarditis with this particular type of graft than with any other sort of prosthesis?

Dr. Yacoub: I do not know the incidence of endocarditis in big series of prosthetic valves, so it is difficult to compare. Regarding treatment, half the patients can be treated effectively, but all of them will come to re-operation.

Dr. Somerville: Dr. Angell, were the heterografts and homografts stented or not?

Dr. Angell: The mitral heterografts and homografts were all stented. The early stents were rigid metal; for 3 years we have used a flexible Delrin plastic.

Dr. Somerville: Do they actually move with systole?

Dr. Angell: The commissural support post will deflect from 1 to 2 millimeters towards the center of the flow orifice with systole.

Dr. Somerville: Is that all?

Dr. Angell: Yes, but Robert Reisat at the N.I.H. showed that a fraction of a millimeter deflection is enough to reduce the tension on the cusp leaflet by tenfold. It takes very little flexion to take the strain off the maximum stress point. In fact, we don't know whether this is important, because we have never seen a glutaraldehyde-treated homograft or heterograft deteriorate at any point along the attachment. We do use a flexible stent because of its theoretical advantage.

Dr. Somerville: This is quite clear if there is a difference between this and the various groups. But I'd like to know why there is a difference.

Dr. Angell: The valve replacement incidence with homografts was 20% at 5 years. About half of those grafts deteriorate from thinning and fenestration due to destruction of the tissue; the other are incompetent for technical reasons or due to fibrous shortening.

Dr. Braimbridge: I think it was Alain Carpentier who said that the technique of insertion had something to do with the long-term function of these valves. Could either he or Dr. Angell tell us about the technique of insertion of the mounted homograft valve in terms of their long-term function?

Dr. Angell: We use exactly the same single-suture line implantation method as you would use for a prosthesis. I like to keep the valve in the atrial side, and out of the functioning ventricle.

Dr. Hancock: This slide clearly shows the marked difference in stability of the collagen cross-links introduced by formalin and glutaraldehyde. The shrink temperature falls very rapidly with time when formalin-fixed tissue is washed in balance electrolyte, whereas the stabilized glutaraldehyde-fixed tissue is quite stable beyond the six year point at this time. Of further interest is the fact that there is a marked difference in the stability of various glutaraldehyde processes.

Dr. Carpentier: In answer to Dr. Hancock, I would like to point out that the heat shrinkage test is only one among the numerous tests necessary for defining the quality of a method of tissue valve preparation. Using this test, we have obtained results which vary significantly from those presented. In-vitro tests must always be approached with great caution in the context of in-vivo tissue implantation.

Dr. Messmer: Dr. Angell, in one of your slides you showed us a histological aspect of a fresh stented homograft three years after implantation, and said that you had there viable donor cells. I can understand they are viable cells, but how do you prove they are donor cells? We had difficulties with fascia-lata valves where we had viable cells too, but we were rarely able to prove they were the same cells as those of the fascia lata.

Dr. Angell: There is a raging argument about the source of these cells. Dr. Barratt Boyes feels strongly that they are recipient cells. I feel that they are donor cells. Our experimental implantation work convinced me that the cell position within the cusp and the rather bizarre morphologic appearance is classic of donor cells. The sex of the chromatin from female donors also documents donor origin. It is only important in that the fresh viable graft cells are alive immediately after implantation, and they lay down collagen that thickens the valve, enough to increase the tensile strength greatly over the non-viable valve. That accounts for the long-term good results.

Dr. Björk: Dr. Yacoub, did you not see any calcification in any of your pathology specimens as was reported in the heterografts? Do you anticoagulate those patients with homo or heterografts during first month, or don't you do anything at all after surgery?

Dr. Yacoub: Histologically we have never seen calcium in the mitral valve position. We have seen calcium in the aortic position, but never in the mitral position. Regarding anticoagulant policy, we do not anticoagulate at all, unless there is a specific indication such as a clot removed from the left atrium, but we give no routine anticoagulant.

Dr. Angell: We anticoagulate for three months with an intensive heparin anticoagulation at the beginning, followed by Coumadin. We have tried acute anticoagulants, chronic anticoagulants, and no anticoagulants. This regimen seems to produce the least incidence of thromboemboli for us. Thromboembolism with these tissue valves originates in the left atrium. The incidence of thromboemboli is the same as with a reconstructive mitral commissurotomy.

Dr. Carpentier: We have adopted the same policy. We give anticoagulants not for reasons linked to the graft, but in order to avoid phlebitis during the post-operative period. We continue this treatment whenever there is a specific risk regarding the left atrium.

Dr. Duran: Just a question to Dr. Angell that might be relevant to the homografts: What sort of pathology did they find in cardiac transplantation patients at the level of the aortic valves? Was there ever rejection?

Dr. Angell: I don't know. All I can say is that we have incidentally seen calcification of mitral homografts. It is rare, but it does happen.

SUMMARY: PART IX

A. Carpentier, M.D.

This session was important in stressing that there is still an interest in tissue valves, and that some surgical groups continue to work to improve this type of valvular substitute. There is good reason for this: valvular prostheses, in spite of recent improvements, continue to be associated with a high thromboembolic risk in the absence of anticoagulants. Tissue valves have a lower risk of thromboembolism and do not require anticoagulation. In addition, the progressive nature of occasional failure permits reoperation under good conditions.

We now have a long-enough followup with the different tissues and the various methods of preservation to select those tissues and those methods which have proven to be the most efficient: fresh pulmonary autograft, fresh allograft, glycerol-preserved dura mater, glutaraldehyde-preserved xenograft. Papers presented by Dr. Fontan, Dr. Angell, Dr. Yacoub, and the Broussais group, among others, were instructive in this regard.

Many of these tissue valves have already been shown to be competitive with the best valvular prostheses.

Valvular prostheses and tissue valves should be considered as alternatives, since they both have advantages which complement each other. Durability favors the prostheses, whereas nonthrombogenicity favors the tissue valves. Our efforts should be directed towards defining the respective indications for each of these two methods. In this respect, tissue valves seem to be preferred for pulmonary and tricuspid valve replacement in all patients, for aortic and mitral valve replacement in women of childbearing age, for patients who may be difficult or dangerous to maintain on anticoagulant therapy, and more generally for those patients who prefer a postoperative course free of anticoagulants and related problems, accepting in counterpart a higher risk of reoperation than with a prosthesis.

PART TEN

CONSERVATIVE VALVE SURGERY

45 Plastic and Reconstructive Mitral Valve Surgery

Alain Carpentier, M.D.

Mitral valve surgery began in 1965 with the attempts of Lillehei, Murray, and others to repair the mitral valve apparatus by a direct approach under extracorporeal circulation.[13] Following these pioneering efforts, several techniques were developed to correct mitral insufficiency either isolated or combined with stenosis. Pure mitral insufficiency was corrected by techniques which reduced the size of the orifice area by commissural plication,[15,17,19] semicircular sutures,[3] or by suturing a pledget of Teflon to the annulus at the mural leaflet.[15] Stenotic lesions were treated by commissurotomy and splitting of the chordae tendineae.[12,15]

These techniques were progressively abandoned for several reasons: first, because they failed to achieve a regular and predictable result,[4,12] second, because they were associated with a high incidence of recurrent mitral insufficiency or stenosis,[2,4] and third, because suitable artificial prostheses became available.

The valvular prostheses, however, still involve thromboembolic problems and a persistent need for anticoagulation, two factors which affect the quality of life of the patient. This should stimulate us to review our policy with regards to mitral valve repair, the more so since progress made in extracorporeal circulation and myocardial protection allows us to perform more sophisticated techniques.

The purpose of this paper is to state the principles which should serve as guidelines for plastic and reconstructive surgery of the mitral valve, and to present techniques which have been developed according to these principles.

FUNDAMENTALS OF CONSERVATIVE MITRAL VALVE SURGERY

The aim of a plastic repair of the mitral valve is to restore valvular function to normal for the longest possible period. The problem therefore is to determine which lesions are suitable for such a repair and which techniques should be used. As we have shown earlier (Chapter 9), mitral insufficiency may be the result of multiple lesions affecting the different structures of the valvular apparatus: annulus, leaflet, tissue, commissures, chordae tendineae, papillary muscles, and the corresponding myocardial wall. Therefore a reconstructive operation should include multiple techniques directed towards all of the different lesions. These techniques were developed according to four basic principles: easy reproducibility, low operative risk, predictability of the result, and stability of the repair.

The reproducibility depends in part upon the complexity of the technique, and in part upon the effort of the surgeon to acquire the necessary experience. It must be accepted that the time required for carrying out the repair be longer than that of a valve replacement, and should not increase the operative risk. This depends upon the excellence of the by-pass technique and of myocardial protection during the operation.

The predictability of the result is one of the most difficult aims to achieve. It means that when leaving the operating room, the surgeon should ascertain that the repair he has performed will assume an excellent hemodynamic function.

Both predictability and long-term stability of the result depend upon the quality of the surgical repair: that is, the ability of the techniques to restore the anatomy and the physiology of the valvular apparatus as close to normal as possible.

TECHNIQUES
Repair of annular lesions

Dilatation of the annulus fibrosis is generally considered to be the major factor in mitral insufficiency. This is partially true, since the deformation of the annulus is at least as important as the dilatation (Fig. 1). The dilatation mainly affects the mural leaflet and the commissure. The anterior leaflet portion of the annulus is not affected in the same way because of its continuity with the aortic root. The deformation may be symmetrical or asymmetrical. In symmetrical dilatation, the anteroposterior diameter of the orifice is greater than the transverse diameter, and both commissures are equally enlarged (Fig. 1). Asymmetrical deformation may result from the enlargement of the anterior commissure or of the posterior commissure. In reconstruction of the mitral valve annulus, not only must the annulus be reduced to its physiologic dimensions, but the commissures must be remodelled as well in order to restore their physiologic curvature. The use of suitably shaped and sized prosthetic rings makes it possible to accomplish each of these corrections accurately and permanently.[6]

The size of the rings and their corresponding interior areas are as follows: 26 mm (3.05 cm²), 28 mm (4.09 cm²), 30 mm (4.85 cm²), 32 mm (5.19 cm²), 34 mm (5.50 cm²), 36 mm (5.78 cm²). Each ring is made of stainless steel and covered with a fine polyester fabric which favors the incorporation of the prosthesis.

The choice of the ring is based on the measurement at the base of the aortic leaflet, which is not affected by the annulus dilatation, and therefore can be used as a guide for the determination of the

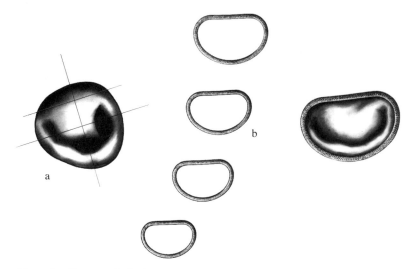

Figure 1. Concept of mitral annulus remodelling. (a) Annulus dilatation is associated with annulus deformation. Dilatation affects mainly the commissures and the annulus at the mural leaflet. Deformation is such that the antero-posterior diameter becomes greater than the transverse diameter. It may be symmetrical or asymmetrical. (b) Suitably shaped and sized prosthetic rings permit the remodelling of the orifice, respecting the normal motion of the leaflet and the commissures.

physiologic dimensions of the mitral orifice. In order to facilitate this measurement, one suture is placed at each commissure (Figure 2a). The distance between these two points is measured with the ob- turators (Figure 2b). Approximately 15 sutures are placed through the annulus along the whole periphery of the mitral ring. These are then passed through the sewing ring of the prosthesis. The same space interval must be maintained between sutures of the aortic leaflet and their point of insertion into the corresponding portion of the pros- thesis. Spacing is reduced for the sutures of the posterior leaflet. If there is an asymmetric dilatation of the annulus with a predominant enlargement of one commissure, the distribution of the sutures must obviously be adapted: the spacing of the sutures must be especially reduced in the corresponding area of the prosthetic ring (Figure 2c). The ring is then brought into position and the sutures tied. This repositions the different annular structures without reducing the normal orifice area or affecting leaflet motion (Figure 2d).

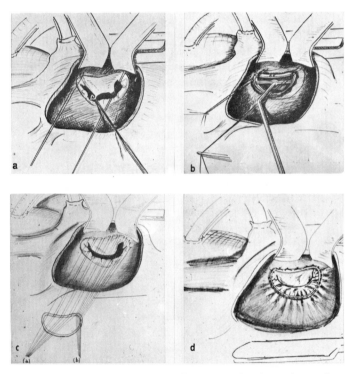

Figure 2. Technique of ring insertion. (a) pilot sutures placed at each commissure; (b) measurement by obturators of distance between commissures; (c) spacing of sutures on prosthetic ring parallel for aortic leaflet sutures, reduced for sutures of the remain- der of the annulus; (d) sutures tied, ring in place.

One criticism which can be leveled at such a repair of the mitral annulus is the rigidity of the prosthetic ring. This is a somewhat theoretical disadvantage, since in mitral insufficiency, the annulus is irreversibly damaged and not capable of contraction during systole. However, a flexible ring has been developed and used in the last year, both in the mitral and the tricuspid areas,[7] to evaluate possible advantages regarding long-term function. The flexibility of the ring is selective: the transverse diameter can be increased but not decreased; the anteroposterior diameter can be decreased 30% of its normal length, but not increased, and the commissures do not modify their shape during systole (Fig. 3). This permits retention of the remodelling effect the mitral annulus.

Repair of commissural fusions

Fusion of the commissures may be divided into three grades as to severity of lesions. Grade I corresponds to partial fusion of the commissures ($\leq$ 5 mm), with preservation of the commissural chordae. The commissurotomy in this case is easy to perform since the commissure is well delineated and the chordae well individualized. The incision is made between two chordae and extends to within no more than 3 mm from the annulus.

Grade II corresponds to complete fusion of the commissures, with a still well defined border appearing as a furrow between the anterior and the mural leaflet. Small calcifications may be present. Chordae may be fused. Because of the still visible commissural line, commissurotomy is not a difficult maneuver, and the result is generally excellent because the edges of the anterior and posterior leaflets still have a surface of coaptation. It may be necessary to remove some

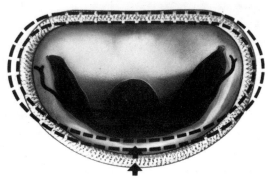

Figure 3. Flexible ring. Dashed line represents the shape of the ring at systole.

calcifications and to split fused chordae to mobilize the leaflets and prevent early refusion of the commissure.

Grade III corresponds to complete fusion of the commissures, with no delineation between the anterior and the posterior leaflets. There is continuity between both leaflets at the level of the commissures. Commissural chordae are often fused, so that it is difficult to know exactly were to perform the commissurotomy. The site and direction of the commissure may be defined as a line joining the attachment of the main chordae of the anterior leaflet to the fibrous trigone.

Repair of valvular lesions

The leaflet tissue may be affected by different lesions such as: perforation, cleft formation, thickening, valve shrinkage, or calcification. A careful analysis of the nature, the site, the extent, and the severity of the lesions leads to a judgment regarding conservation of the valve rather than replacement.

Perforation of the mural leaflet may be treated by cuneiform resection of the leaflet and subsequent suture of the remaining edges. Only small perforations (≤ 5 mm) of the anterior leaflet may be treated by resection and subsequent suture.

Valve thickening, a consequence of rheumatic valve disease, generally does not overly affect the pliability of the leaflets. It may be localized, having the aspect of a fibrous nodule or a fibrous band, which should be either resected or thinned. It may be more extensive and due to hypertrophic intermediary chordae which should be resected. If the pliability of the valve is significantly altered by the fibrous process, the valve should be replaced.

Only *localized calcifications* can be treated by conservative techniques, such as resection of the calcified area and subsequent suture (Fig. 4a).

Repair of subvalvular lesions

The subvalvular apparatus may present different lesions of various etiologies:

Ruptured papillary muscle secondary to myocardial infarction.

Ruptured chordae due to either bacterial endocarditis, degeneration of the chordae, or rheumatic valve disease.

Elongated chordae due to chordae dysplasia or rheumatic process.

Fusion and retraction of the chordae.

In most instances, the three latter types of lesions can be treated by conservative procedures.

Ruptured chordae are treated by resection of the prolapsed part of the valve and suturing of the remaining edges. Resection is preferred to a McGoon type of plication, which may lead to progressive retraction and thickening of the infolded part. A quadrangular resection is preferable in order to avoid excess tension on the free edge of the leaflet, a consequence of triangular resection (Fig. 4 b). Valvular replacement may be necessary if the rupture affects the main chordae of the aortic leaflet.

Elongation of chordae is treated by the following technique: the extremity of the corresponding papillary muscle is longitudinally incised. The excess length of the chordae is firmly attached by closing the papillary muscle around the buried portion of the chordae (Fig. 4 c).

Fused chordae are treated by incision of the chordae or by resection of a triangular portion of the scar tissue in order to completely release the subvalvular stenosis. Those hypertrophic and shortened intermediary chordae arising from the inferior surface of the leaflets and not from their free margins are resected (Fig. 4 d).

CLINICAL EXPERIENCE

These different techniques are the result of an evolution of the author's experience in mitral valve surgery during the past seven years. In the beginning, attention was focused on pure mitral insufficiency due to annular lesions which could accurately be treated by ring valvuloplasty. This group represented only 4% of open heart mitral valve lesions encountered at surgery. Since remodelling of the valve appeared not to reduce the normal orifice area, valvular reconstruction could be extended to the treatment of more complex lesions. These included combined mitral insufficiency and stenosis, which was heretofore considered to be a contraindication to reconstructive procedures. Thus, the great majority of noncalcified mitral valve disease, which accounted for 40% of the open-mitral valve cases in our experience, has been treated by such conservative procedures in the past few years.

Material (Table 1)

Our experience at the Broussais Hospital* between September 1968 to December 1974 consists of 330 mitral valve repairs. Lesions were divided into three groups:

---

* Surgical team: C. Dubost, C. D'Allaines, P. Blondeau, A. Piwnica, R. Soyer, and A. Carpentier

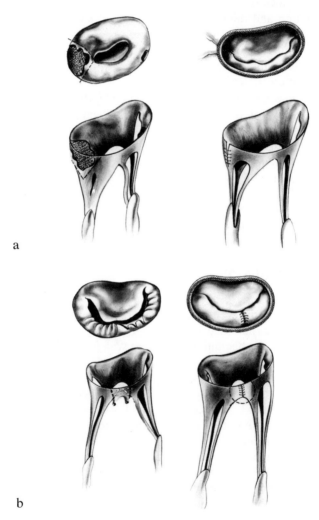

a

b

Figure 4, a and b. (a) Resection of calcification; (b) quadrangular resection of prolapsed portion of posterior leaflet secondary to ruptured chordae tendineae.

Group   I: Pure mitral insufficiency without lesions of subvalvular structures.

Group II: Pure mitral insufficiency with lesions of sub-valvular structures.

Group III: Combined insufficiency and stenosis.

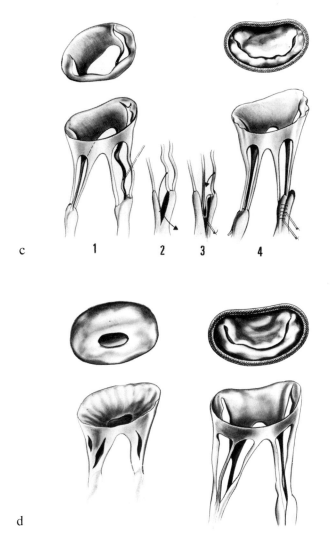

Figure 4, c and d.   (c) Shortening of elongated chordae tendineae: 1, elongated chorda; 2, incision of papillary muscle; 3, extra length of the chorda is buried in the papillary muscle; 4, closure of papillary muscle (d) fenestration of fused chordae tendineae.

Table 1
Material and Surgical Treatment

Group I: pure mitral insufficiency (prosthetic ring): 93

Group II: mitral insufficiency + Sub-valvular lesions: 85
    a) ruptured chordae (ring + Valve resection): 42
    b) elongated chordae (ring + Chordae shortening): 34
    c) fused chordae (ring + chordae fenestration and resection): 9

Group III: mitral insufficiency and mitral stenosis: 152
    a) noncalcified (ring + commissurotomy + chordae fenestration and resection): 136
    b) calcified (ring + commissurotomy + chordae fenestration and resection + Calcium removal): 16

Total: 330

Group I consisted of 93 cases treated by remodelling of the annulus with a prosthetic ring. Group II consisted of 85 cases of which 42 had ruptured chordae treated by valvular resection, and 34 had elongated chordae treated by shortening of the chordae; 9 had both lesions. Group III consisted of 152 cases treated by commissurotomy, annulus remodelling, and treatment of subvalvular lesions: elongated chordae, hypertrophic chordae, fused chordae.

The average age of the patients was 37 years, ranging from 12 to 72 years (mitral valve surgery in children being excluded from this study). Rheumatic disease was responsible for the valvular lesions in 248 patients, bacterial endocarditis in 24, and nonrheumatic dystrophic or degenerative disease in the remaining 58. According to the New York Heart Association Classification, 212 patients (63%) were in Class IV, 110 (35%) in Class III, and 8 in Class II (2%).

Results (Table 2)

There were 29 (9%) operative deaths in the whole series. Operative mortality was somewhat higher in the early period (15.5%) due to technical errors; it has been reduced to 4% in the last 100 patients. Causes of death were: injury to the circumflex artery in our early experience (2), infection (3), myocardial infarction (5), anemia (2), air embolism (2), and low cardiac output (10). Late death occured in 9 patients (3%) followed for 1 to 7 years after the operation (average follow-up 3.2 years). Causes of late death were: persistent or recurrent mitral valve disease (5), cardiac failure (1), noncardiac (2), and unknown (1). The survival curve shows an 87% survival at 6 years (Figure 5).

Table 2
Results for 330 Patients (1968-1974)

Hospital deaths	29	9%
Late deaths*	9	3%
- Valve related - (5-1.5%)		
Reoperations*	10	3.5%
Thromboembolism*	2	0.5%
Poor result*	4	1%
Good result*	260	92%

*Long-term follow up available in 285 patients 1 to 7 years after operation (Average 3.2 years). Percentages based on 285 patients.

Long-term follow-up data are available for 285 patients. Reoperation was necessary in 9 patients (2.7%) because of disinsertion of the ring (3 patients), persistent mitral valve disease (4 patients), and recurrent mitral valve insufficiency (2 patients). Thromboembolic complications occured in 2 patients (0.4%), both of whom had a huge enlargement of the left atrium. Of the patients, 88% were much improved functionally, and 86% had a significant radiologic and electrocardiographic improvement. The best results were observed in groups II and III, followed by patients of group I. In 52% of the cases, auscultation was perfectly normal. In 40% there was a minimal or moderate systolic murmur and/or diastolic murmur. In the remaining 8% there was moderate to severe systolic murmur. These residual valvulopathies were recognized soon after operation and remained unchanged thereafter. Only six patients (0.5%) had a recurrent systolic murmur not heard in the immediate post-operative period.

DISCUSSION AND CONCLUSIONS

The numerous operations proposed between 1957 and 1967 to repair mitral valve insufficiency failed to achieve a predictable result and were associated with a high incidence of recurrent insufficiency.[4, 12, 17] It has been postulated that most of these failures were the result of persistant rheumatic process. In fact, the techniques themselves were to be blamed because of their palliative nature. Narrowing the mitral annulus leads to modification of the anatomy and therefore the physiology of the valve–all the more so since over-correction and even a mild stenosis was considered to be a factor in the success of the technique.[17] Deformation of the annulus and some of the subvalvular lesions which were unrecognized were not treated. The resulting abnormal and limited function of the leaflets led to progressive thick-

538

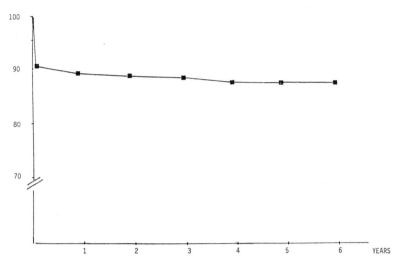

Figure 5. Mitral valvuloplasty survival curve (first 300 cases).

ening and shrinkage. The different techniques presented in this paper and in particular the technique of valvular remodelling using a prosthetic ring[6,7] represent an effort to develop true reconstructive techniques based upon a careful analysis of the lesions and the physiopathology of the orifice.

Several favorable hemodynamic and technical factors become apparent when compared with other techniques: restoration of the normal configuration of mitral annulus, absence of narrowing of the orifice area, respect for the free motion of all the leaflet, prevention of recurrent dilatation of the annulus, accurate treatment of subvalvular lesions.

The clinical results when compared to those obtained with previous methods of valvuloplasty or with valvular replacement are characterized by a low mortality rate, a low complication rate, a good predictability, and stability of the repair.

It must be pointed out that deterioration of an initial good result was exceptional (0.5%), demonstrating the absence of evolution of the rheumatic process. The risk of disinsertion (0.9%) might be reduced in the future by the use of flexible rings.

Thromboembolic complications also were exceptional, in spite of the fact that in most patients anticoagulants were discontinued 3 weeks following operation, the time necessary for the prosthesis to become endothelialized.

The complexity and difficulty of the techniques described above should not be viewed as a deterrent to the surgeon, because they are commensurate with an improved quality of life for the patient.

REFERENCES

1. Acar, J., Caramanian, M., Perrault, M., Luxereau, P. and Arnault, J.C. Les insuffisances mitrales par ruptures de cordages d'origine dégénérative. *Arch. Mal. Coeur* 61:1724, 1968.

2. Anderson, A.M., Cobb, L.A., Bruce, R.A. and Merendino, K.A. Evaluation of mitral annuloplasty for mitral regurgitation: clinical and hemodynamic status four to forty-one months after surgery. *Circulation* 26:26, 1962.

3. Belcher, J.R. The surgical treatment of mitral regurgitation. *Brit. Heart J.* 26:513, 1964.

4. Bigelow, W.G., Kuypers, P.J., Heimbecker, R.O. and Gunton, R.W. Clinical evaluation of the efficiency of mitral annuloplasty. *Ann. Surg.* 154:320, 1961.

5. Björk, V.O. and Malers, E. Annuloplastic procedures for mitral insufficiency: late results. *J. Thor. Cardiovasc. Surg.* 48:251, 1964.

6. Carpentier, A. La valvuloplastie reconstitutive. Une nouvelle technique de valvuloplastie mitrale. *Presse Med.* 77:251, 1969.

7. Carpentier, A., Deloche, A., Dauptain, J., Soyer, R., Prigent, C., Blondeau, P., Piwnica, A., and Dubost, C. A new reconstructive operation for correction of mitral and tricuspid insufficiency. *J. Thor. Cardiovasc. Surg.* 61:1, 1971.

8. Dubost, C. Evaluation of surgery for mitral valve disease. *Am. Heart J.* 82:143, 1971.

9. Ellis, F.H., Jr., Frye, R.L. and McGoon, D.C. Results of reconstructive operations for mitral insufficiency due to ruptured chordae tendineae. *Surgery* 59:165, 1966.

10. Gerbode, F., Kerth, W.J., Osborn, J.J. and Selzer, A. Correction of mitral insufficiency by open operation. *Ann. Surg.* 155:846, 1962.

11. Kahn, D.R., Stern, A.M., Sigmann, J.M., Kirsh, M.M., Lennox, S. and Sloan, J. Long-term results of mitral valvuloplasty in children. *J. Thor. Cardiovasc. Surg.* 53:1, 1967.

12. Kay, J.H., Magidson, O. and Meinaux, J.E. The surgical treatment of mitral insufficiency and combined mitral stenosis and insufficiency using the heart-lung machine. *Amer. J. Cardiol.* 9:300, 1962.

13. Lillehei, C.W., Goot, V.L., De Wall, R.A., and Varco, R.L. Surgical correction of mitral insufficiency by annuloplasty under direct vision. *Lancet,* 77:446, 1957.

14. Mac Goon, D.C. Repair of mitral insufficiency due to ruptured chordae tendineae. *J. Thor. Cardiovasc. Surg.* 39:357, 1960.

15. Merendino, K.A., Thomas, G.I., Jesseph, J.E., Herron, P.W., Winterscheid, L.C. and Vetto, R.A. The open correction of rheumatic mitral regurgitation and/or stenosis. With special reference to regurgitation treated by posteromedial annuloplasty using a pump-oxygenator. *Ann. Surg.* 150:5, 1959.

16. Penther, P. Traitement chirurgical par annuloplastie des insuffisances mitrales. Résultats à long terme. *Presse Med.* 77:1885, 1969.

17. Reed, G.E., Tice, D.A. and Clauss, R.H. Asymmetric exaggerated mitral annuloplasty. Repair of mitral insufficiency with hemodynamic predictability. *J. Thor. Cardiovasc. Surg.* 49:752, 1965.

18. Silverman, M.E. and Hurst, J.W. The mitral complex interaction of anatomy, physiology, and pathology of the central valve. *Amer. Heart J.* 76, 399, 1968.

19. Wooler, G.H., Nixon, P.G.F., Grimshaw, V.A. and Watson, D.A. Experiences with the repair of the mitral valve in mitral incompetence. *Thorax* 17:49, 1962.

46 Indications and Late Results of Reconstructive Mitral Surgery—Hemodynamic Evaluation of the Carpentier Ring

CDR J.H. Oury, M.D.
CDR T.L. Folkerth, MC USN*
CAPT A.D. Hagan, MC USN*
LCDR J.S. Albert, MC USN*
W.W. Angell, M.D.

Prosthetic mitral valves are subject to valve deterioration with failure of the prosthesis, systemic embolization, and a significant incidence of endocarditis. The search for an alternative to valve replacement is therefore warranted and the results subjected to critical hemodynamic evaluation.

Forty-one patients underwent mitral valve reconstruction using the Carpentier ring, a prosthetic device which serves as a framework for annuloplasty and valve reconstruction.[1] These procedures were performed at the Naval Hospital, San Diego, and the Santa Clara Valley Medical Center over a period of 30 months. Twenty-two patients underwent another intracardiac procedure (i.e., coronary artery bypass, valve replacement, etc.). There were two deaths in this series (5%). The mean age of these patients was 51 years with an equal number of males and females. Twenty-four patients were Class III, New York Heart Association Classification, and 16 patients were

---

* The opinions or assertions expressed herein are those of the authors and are not to be construed as official or as reflecting the views of the Navy Department or the naval service at large.

541

Class IV. Only one patient was Class II. The mean follow-up period in this group was 18 months, as summarized in Table 1.

Complete hemodynamic evaluation, including pre- and post-operative right and left heart catheterization, is available in 14 patients. Echocardiographic comparison pre- and postoperatively was analysed in a representative series of seven patients.

The patients were divided into three diagnostic categories similar to the classification outlined by Dr. Carpentier in the *Journal of Thoracic and Cardiovascular Surgery*, January 1971 (Table 2). Type I (6 patients) involved those with pure mitral insufficiency due to lesions of valvular structures. Type II (12 patients) were those in whom the valvular insufficiency was due to lesions of subvalvular structures. The majority of patients (23) were Type III, with mixed mitral stenosis and insufficiency due to rheumatic mitral involvement.

The hemodynamic results in the 14 patients studied pre- and postoperatively were graded as shown in Table 3. An excellent result included those with a transvalvular gradient of 3 mm or less with 0 to 1+ regurgitation. A good result was defined as those with a transvalvular gradient of 4 to 8 mm Hg and with 2+ regurgitation or less. The patient was considered to have had a poor result when the transvalvular gradient exceeded 8 mm of Hg with 3+ mitral regurgitation. It

Table 1
Mitral Valve Reconstruction—Ring Annuloplasty

41 patients with 2 deaths (5%)		
Mean age 51 years (22-70)		
Male: female 21:20		
Functional Class (NYHC)	II:	1 Pt
	III:	24 Pts
	IV:	16 Pts
(Follow-up mean 18 months)		

Table 2
Mitral Valve Reconstruction—Ring Annuloplasty

Patient Category[1]	Anatomic Diagnosis	No. Patients	Mortality
Type I	Pure mitral insufficiency due to lesions of valvular structures	6	1
Type II	Pure mitral insufficiency due to lesions of subvalvular structure	12	0
Type III	Mixed stenosis and insufficiency (Rheumatic)	23	1
	TOTAL	41	2 (5%)

should be emphasized that either the transvalvular gradient or the amount of mitral regurgitation was sufficient to place the patient in the various categories.

Postoperative evaluation of the patients illustrated in Table 4 indicates that the majority (86%) of those undergoing reconstruction for valvular lesions with predominant regurgitation had good results. As shown in the Table, all of the patients who experienced poor results were Type III. The key issue is the therapeutic decision for or against valvular reconstruction in the ''good'' results category. Mitral valve reconstruction may provide more tolerable early and late morbidity than MVR. Careful intraoperative evaluation based on greater operative experience in making the decision for or against reconstruction may also affect this result.

The pre- and postoperative evaluation of a patient with Type II initial regurgitation is illustrated in Figures 1-3. She is a 65-year-old female who presented in congestive failure with 4+ mitral regurgitation secondary to ruptured chordae. Her pre- and postoperative chest x-rays are shown in Figure 1. The presence of a competent valve demonstrated by systolic cineangiogram frames (Figure 2) confirms her excellent clinical result.

Table 3

Mitral Valve Reconstruction—Ring Annuloplasty Postoperative Hemodynamic Evaluation

Result	Transvalvular Gradient	Regurgitation
Excellent	3 mm or less	0-1+
Good	4 mm-8 mm	2+
Poor	8 mm or greater	3+ or greater

Table 4

Mitral Valve Reconstruction—Ring Annuloplasty Hemodynamic Results (14 Patients)

Results	Transvalvular Gradient	Regurgitation	Patients	
Excellent	<3 mm	0-1+	Types I, II:	5
			Type III:	3
			Total	8 (57%)
Good	4-8 mm	2+	Type I:	1
			Type III:	3
			Total	4 (29%)
Poor	>8 mm	3+	Type III:	2 (14%)
	(Follow-up mean 12 months)			

544

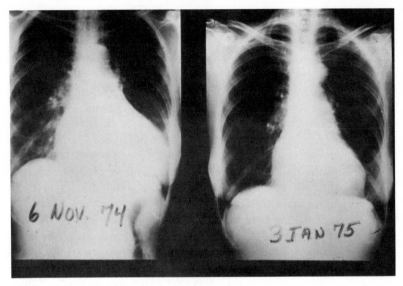

Figure 1. Pre- and post-operative chest X-ray on a 65 year old female who underwent mitral reconstruction for pure mitral regurgitation secondary to ruptured chordae.

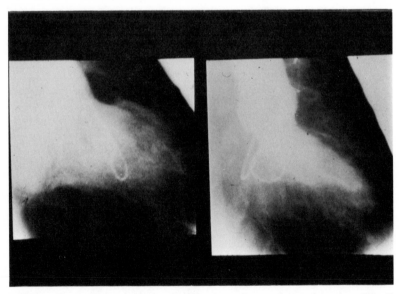

Figure 2. Pre- and post-operative systolic cineangiogram frames in patient (Fig. 1) demonstrating a competent mitral valve.

Figure 3 is a demonstration of pre- and postoperative echocardiograms on the patient with mitral prolapse secondary to ruptured chordae. Note the increased velocity of the anterior leaflet, which is typical of the hyperdynamic state associated with mitral insufficiency. Also illustrated is the flail posterior leaflet due to ruptured chordae. The postoperative echo confirmed the presence of a normal posterior leaflet echo and no change in the anterior leaflet configuration. The echocardiographic evaluation of this patient points out the potential usefulness of this noninvasive technique in evaluating patients before and after mitral reconstruction.

Echocardiograms also proved of particular interest in evaluating the results in seven of the patients having complete studies following their surgery, Table 5. Note that the majority of these patients improved by echocardiographic criteria of anterior leaflet slope. The echocardiographic assessment of left atrial size and ejection fraction parallels the findings of anterior leaflet velocity.

Clinical evaluation of the 14 patients parallels the hemodynamic evaluation with improved functional classification in all but two patients. Figures 4A and 4B are diagrams of the improvement in functional heart classification of all 41 patients. Types I and II diagnostic

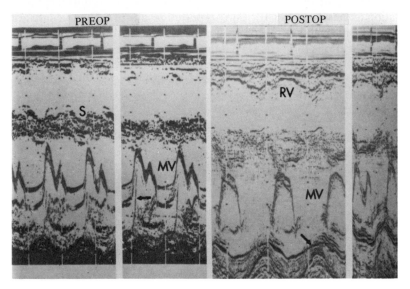

Figure 3. Pre- and post-operative echocardiogram in patient (Figs. 1 and 2) illustrating prolapse of posterior leaflet (arrow in preoperative frame) and normal posterior leaflet motion following repair frame at far right. The arrow in the postoperative frame points to the ring echo.

Table 5
Mitral Valve Reconstruction—Ring Annuloplasty Echocardiographic Evaluation (7 Patients)
(Anterior Leaflet Slope—mm/sec.)*

Patient	Diag. Class	Preop		Postop
A. V.	I	180	⟶	180
E. G.	II	24	⟶	34
L. S.	III	38	⟶	33
S. S.	III	44	⟶	34
			(Reoperation)	
E. W.	III	26	⟶	50
S. B.	III	14	⟶	60
G. N.	III	35	⟶	43
	(Follow-up mean 10 months postop)			

*Normal → 75 mm/sec.

categories with predominant mitral insufficiency are illustrated in Figure 4A, and the Type III category with rheumatic valvular disease with mixed stenosis and insufficiency is illustrated in Figure 4B.

In summary, the Carpentier ring method of mitral valve annuloplasty provides a valuable alternative in the surgical treatment of a selected group of patients whose predominant lesion is mitral regurgitation (either Type I or II). Early reported results of this procedure are reproducible, and an excellent hemodynamic result can be obtained. The indications for its use in patients with mixed lesions secondary to

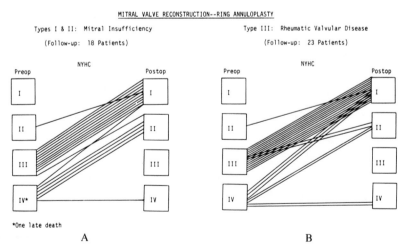

Figure 4. Diagram of functional improvement in types I and II patients (A), and type III patient (B).

rheumatic disease are less clear, and require careful intraoperative evaluation in each case. Patients in this category may also receive superior clinical and hemodynamic results with proper selection.

REFERENCE

1. Carpentier, A., Deloche, A., Dauptain, J., Soyer, R., Prigent, C.L., Blondeau, P., Piwnica, A., Dubost, C., and McGoon, D.C. A new reconstructive operation for correction of mitral and tricuspid insufficiency. *J. Thorac. Cardiovasc. Surg.* 61:1, 1971.

47 Conservative Mitral Valve Surgery: Problems and Developments in the Technique of Prosthetic Ring Annuloplasty

C. G. Duran, M.D.
J. L. M. Ubago, M.D.

Our attitude towards mitral valve surgery has changed considerably in the past five years. From surgery consisting entirely of replacement, we have moved towards a more conservative, more respectful approach to the valvular tissue. While 73% of all open mitral procedures performed in 1970 resulted in valve replacements, in 1975 only 48% of the mitral valves were replaced. This change has been due to the use of Carpentier's method of mitral selective annuloplasty.[1]

Since December 1971 until April 1975 we have placed 202 atrioventricular prosthetic rings in 172 patients, 140 in the mitral position and 62 in the tricuspid valve. In the mitral area 36 rings were placed in patients with mitral stenosis after open commissurotomy, 9 in patients with mitral insufficiencies, and 95 in patients with mitral disease. This experience clearly shows that this procedure is not reserved for cases of pure mitral insufficiency, but is used more often to achieve valve competence after a mitral commissurotomy. It obviously increases the confidence of the surgeon when performing an open commissurotomy, since the presence of a significant residual insufficiency will not necessarily require a prosthetic replacement.

549

In this group of 172 patients, 57% were polyvalvular. There were 52 prosthetic valve replacements, 10 commissurotomies, and 29 non-prosthetic ring plasties. The total hospital mortality was 6.9%, and the late mortality was 4%.

In the group of 140 patients with mitral rings there were 3 patients with thromboembolic phenomena (1.6%). No patients received long-term anticoagulants. This policy is now under review.

There were three mitral-ring dehiscences: one in the immediate postoperative period due to bacterial endocarditis, one in the early postoperative period due to the wrong surgical indication of ring annuloplasty which required a complex mitral valve reconstruction, and one case of progressive mitral insufficiency. The first two cases were reoperated successfully; the mitral valve was replaced with a prosthesis. Sixty-two percent of the patients had no murmurs, 26% a grade I/VI systolic murmur, and 12% a grade III-IV/VI. Twenty-five percent presented a mitral-stenosis type of murmur. These auscultatory findings were present from the moment of surgery and remained stable.

PROBLEMS OF THE PROSTHETIC RING ANNULOPLASTY

However much we feel that the Carpentier ring annuloplasty represents a very useful technique in the mitral area, a number of problems remain to be solved:

Preoperative Mitral Valve Assessment

The preoperative knowledge of whether a particular mitral valve can be repaired is important, since, in some instances, it will determine the indication for surgery. For instance, when the patient is in functional Class II (NYHA) and a valve replacement is anticipated, the patient is turned down for surgery since we consider that only Classes III and IV should be candidates for prosthetic replacement. If, on the other hand, a valve reconstruction seems possible, the same patient is recommended for surgery.

In our Institution, Dr. Ochoteco et al.[2] have devised a mathematical model obtained from left ventricular cine-angiography which predicts which valve needs replacement and which one is amenable to reconstruction (Fig. 1). The formula used to express mitral distensibility is:

$$\text{Elasticity Index} = \frac{\dfrac{\text{Area of mitral ballooning}}{\text{Area of left ventricle}} \times 100}{\text{Diastolic gradient} \times \text{max. ballooning}}$$

In early diastole, due to the atrioventricular gradient, a ballooning of the mitral valve is seen protruding into the left ventricular cavity. The percentage of the left ventricle occupied by this negative area is divided by the instantaneous protodiastolic gradient and by the time taken to achieve maximal ballooning. Obviously a valve will be more

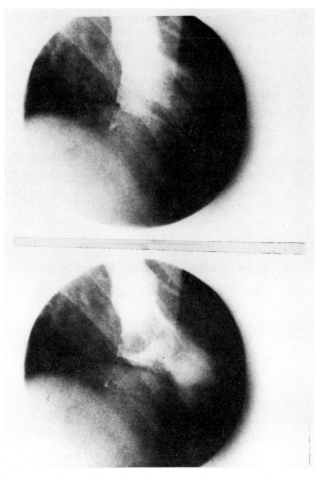

Figure 1. Mitral valve distensibility. Diastolic and systolic frames of a left ventricular cineangiogram showing the ballooning of the anterior cusp of a stenotic mitral valve.

distensible when a large ballooning occurs in a short time and with a low gradient.

Of 22 patients to whom this formula was applied, 9 were considered to have a distensible valve and 13 showed a low figure of elasticity. The first 9 patients were all amenable to a conservative procedure except one, who required a valve replacement. In the 13 patients considered to have a rigid mitral valve, in only two an annuloplasty was performed and in the other 11 the valve was replaced. Echographic studies should also cast some further light on this problem.

Intraoperative Mitral Valve Assessment

It is essential to be able to determine at surgery whether that particular mitral valve can be salvaged. A static and a dynamic assessment is necessary. Thickened, fibrotic, but not calcified leaflets are amenable to reconstruction. Occasionally small calcified nodules can be excised. A good hinge movement is required, and the subvalvular apparatus must be explored and freed if indicated.

To evaluate the dynamics of the mitral valve, we observe it through the open atriotomy with the left vent introduced through the apex and connected to the arterial line. The aorta remains cross-clamped and vented continuously. The left ventricle is blood-filled and often beating, and provided care is taken not to deform the mitral annulus with the retractor, a good dynamic vision of the mitral valve is obtained. The position, direction, and magnitude of a regurgitant jet can be established so as to take the appropriate corrective steps.

Surgical Technique

The surgical technique for the Carpentier annuloplasty has been clearly described by its author,[1] but a number of points must be stressed to avoid some pitfalls. In Figure 2, some of them are diagrammatically illustrated. They are presented in the chronological order they appeared to us. Firstly, the two trigones must be clearly identified, since they determine the size of ring to be used. To avoid malrotation of the ring, the two trigonal stitches must be sutured through the extremities of the straight part of the ring (Fig. 2, IB). At each commissure, we only place one fairly large U stitch, which is passed through a smaller length of the ring, so as to plicate that area of the annulus (Fig. 2, IIb). The remaining area of the annulus, corresponding to the posterior leaflet, is plicated with five or six U stitches;

one must take care to pass them exactly at the point of insertion of the leaflet. Stitches passed through the atrial wall will eventually tear and if passed through the leaflet will decrease the closing surface area. This is particularly significant at the aortic or anterior leaflet where the hinge line is more difficult to identify, and it is often the cause of residual insufficiencies (Fig. 2 III). Occasionally, in spite of a correct surgical technique, a regurgitant jet appears when the valve is tested. This is because the leaflets do not come into proper contact at that point. Once the ring has already been placed, it can be slightly and selectively deformed, so as to decrease its transverse diameter at that point (Fig. 2, IVb). Before the ring is placed, it is more important to recognize that the anterior leaflet protrudes too much into the left atrium. In this case a segmental cuneiform resection of this leaflet will decrease its total length (Fig. 2, Vb). In other cases the posterior leaflet is tethered down and has no full excursion to meet the anterior leaflet. Carpentier[3] has shown that this frequent finding is due to the retraction of secondary chordae at that point, and therefore must be sectioned selectively (Fig. 2, VIb).

It is apparent that this type of conservative surgery is technically more difficult than valve replacement; it calls for the tridimensional vision and imaginative capacity of the surgeon.

Postoperative anti-coagulation

In principle, we do not anticoagulate our annuloplasty patients. However, we feel that those cases with giant left atria, intra-atrial thrombi, and in atrial fibrillation with previous embolic accidents should be anti-coagulated permanently. A long-term study of this problem must be undertaken to establish a clear protocol of therapy.

TECHNICAL PROBLEMS

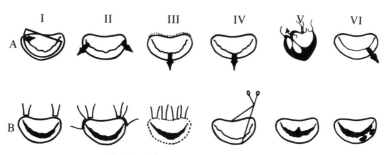

Figure 2. Some technical problems (A) encountered in the placement of mitral prosthetic rings and their surgical solutions (B).

THE FLEXIBLE RING

The experience with the Carpentier ring has led us to develop an entirely flexible, radiologically visible ring, which is easy to insert and can be used for both the mitral and the tricuspid valves. It was felt that a flexible ring would conform more physiologically to the continuous changes of the atrioventricular annulus during the cardiac cycle.[4] There would be less chance of partial disinsertion, and it would interfere less with the normal left ventricular wall movements.

The 3-mm thick, circular ring is made of dacron velour (Fig. 3). It can be deformed in any plane, and due to its elasticity, can increase its circumference by 10%. A radio-opaque thread makes it radiologically visible. The ring is marked at three points, which divide its circumference into three equal parts. The rings are of 78, 84, 90, and 96 mm in circumference. There is no difference between the mitral and tricuspid rings. These rings are placed surgically with the same technique as Carpentier's rigid ring.

Up to April, 1975, 48 flexible rings had been placed in 38 patients: 21 in the mitral position (2 insufficiencies, 2 stenoses, and 17 mixed lesions), and 27 in the tricuspid valve (19 functional and 8 organic diseases). In this group of patients, 20 valves were simultaneously replaced, and 10 aortic or mitral commissurotomies performed. There have been 3 hospital deaths: 1 due to a documented myocardial

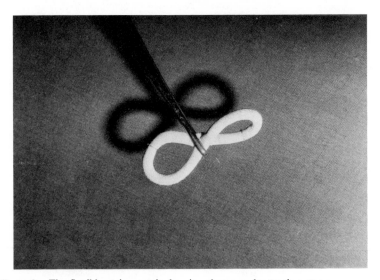

Figure 3. The flexible atrio-ventricular ring shown under torsion stress.

infarction 21 days after surgery, 1 to low cardiac output, and 1 to hemorrhage.

No valve dehiscences have occurred, and no embolic phenomena have appeared in this group of patients. Two patients presented a pansystolic murmur. One of them appeared ten days after surgery for congenital mitral insufficiency and progressed rapidly, needing reoperation. The flexible ring was perfectly placed, but a severe insufficiency had developed due to elongation of chordae tendineae. The valve was successfully replaced. Nineteen patients have been recatheterized, showing a correct functioning of their repaired valves with flexible rings.

Since April, 1975, 20 more flexible rings have been placed without mortality, bringing the total to 68 in 55 patients with a 3.6% hospital mortality and 5.4% total mortality.

In order to assess the theoretical advantages of the flexible ring, we have studied the left ventricular wall motion in a group of patients with mitral xenografts, Carpentier's rigid rings, and flexible rings (Fig. 4). On the telesystolic and telediastolic left ventricular angiogram, a longitudinal axis was traced between the apex and the center of

POSTOPERATIVE LEFT VENTRICULAR DYNAMICS

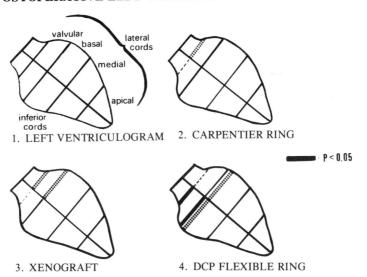

Figure 4. Diagrams of left ventricular cineangiograms divided by cords to calculate the circumferential wall shortening. Dotted lines indicate increased postoperative percent shortening of the wall. Thick lines indicate a statistically significant (p < 0.05) improvement in relation to preoperative wall motion.

the aortic valve. Three perpendicular and equidistant cords were drawn ("basal", "medial," and "apical"). Between the basal cord and the aortic valve plane a fourth cord was traced ("valvular cord"). These cords were divided by the longitudinal axis into four "inferior" and four "lateral" hemiaxes. The percentage shortening of each cord and hemiaxis was calculated. The mean circumferential velocity of shortening between the systolic and diastolic phases was calculated. These data were compared before and after surgery.

Twenty-four patients were studied. Twelve had a mitral commissurotomy performed and a flexible ring sutured. Eight received a prosthetic mounted xenograft and four a Carpentier's ring. All 24 patients had no statistically significant difference in their ventricular function (ejection fraction and volumes), nor in their intrinsic left ventricular contractility. No differences could be found between the basal diastolic gradients in the three groups of patients. After volume load or increase in the cardiac index, there was no difference between the two ring annuloplasties, but a residual gradient was found in the group with xenografts.

The patients with flexible rings showed a significant increase in the percentage shortening of the basal cord, as well as the two inferior basal and inferior valvular hemiaxes. In the patients with Carpentier's ring, only the lateral valvular hemiaxis improved. In the xenograft group, the improvement was seen in the lateral valvular and lateral basal hemiaxes.

This study of the left ventricular wall dynamics clearly shows a difference between the patients with flexible rings and the other two series with rigid rings (Carpentier and mounted xenografts). The flexible-ring patients improve their dynamics by increasing the shortening of the basal hemiaxis next to the valvular plane. Those with a rigid structure improve with the increase in shortening of the lateral hemiaxis next to the aortic valve. It is likely that the difference is due to the fixation of the mitral ring by a rigid structure, so that the post-operative improved shortening of the basal area of the left ventricle is achieved at the expense of the lateral wall. Further studies and experience with this flexible ring are obviously required.

SUMMARY

1. The technique of prosthetic ring annuloplasty described by Carpentier represents a step forward in mitral surgery. It has resulted in a significant reduction in the number of valves replaced at our institution.

2. The immediate and long-term results in our experience with over 200 rings show that this is a stable and non-thrombogenic method of valve repair.

3. A pre-operative hemodynamic and angiographic study to assess the feasibility of ring annuloplasty is suggested.

4. This surgery is technically more difficult to perform correctly than valve replacement. An intra-operative static and dynamic evaluation of the mitral apparatus is mandatory. A number of careful steps must be taken when the ring is placed to achieve valve competence.

5. A new, totally flexible, radiologically visible ring is described. Forty-eight such rings have been placed in 38 patients. The initial results are encouraging. It is felt that a flexible ring will adapt better to the normal mitral closure mechanism and result in a more physiological left ventricular function.

REFERENCES

1. Carpentier, A., Deloche, A., Dauptain, J., Soyer, R., Blondeau, P., Piwnica, A., Dubost, C. A new reconstructive operation for correction of mitral and tricuspid insufficiency. *J. Thor. Cardiovasc. Surg.* 61:1, 1971.

2. Ochoteco, A., Ubago, J.L.M., Colman, T., Pomar, J.L. Mitral valve distensibility. A hemodynamic and cineventriculographic assessment. (To be published.)

3. Carpentier, A. This book, Chapter 9.

4. Tsakiris, A.G., Bernuth, G., Rastelli, G.C., Bourgeois, M.J. Size and motion of the mitral valve annulus in anesthetized intact dogs. *J. App. Physiol.* 30:611, 1971.

48 Surgery for Mitral Stenosis: Comparative Evaluation of the Different Procedures

Interest of pre- and post-operative echocardiography.

J.P. Cachera, M.D.
P. Brun, M.D.
F. Laurent, M.D.
D. Loisance, M.D.
G. Bloch, M.D.
J.J. Galey, M.D.

Surgery for mitral stenosis includes 3 different procedures: 1) closed mitral valvotomy; 2) open-heart commissurotomy and valvuloplasty; and 3) mitral prosthetic replacement. The best surgical procedure can be decided only by an accurate pre-operative analysis of the morphologic components of the mitral apparatus—anterior and posterior leaflet, commissures, chordae tendineae, and papillary muscles—and by a close evaluation of their kinetics. A satisfactory approach for such a pre-operative analysis of both morphologic and kinetic changes is provided today by a non-invasive method: the ultrasonic echography of the mitral apparatus.[4] Better than any other known technique, echography seems valuable to provide the surgeon with satisfactory predictions concerning the severity of the stenosis, thickening of the valves, alterations in the valve's motion, and shortening and fusion of chordae tendineae. According to the data given by the echographic study, the surgeon can choose the optimal method of treatment.

Although closed mitral valvotomy remains the simplest and best procedure in properly selected cases, the natural history of rheumatic

559

disease in our country in the past two decades has deeply modified the balance between recent, pure, non-calcified stenosis and old, severely fibrous, or calcified stenosis; thus, as many other teams, we have observed a progressive shift of the operations for mitral stenosis toward open-heart surgery. For this reason, the selection of patients for closed or open procedures, as well as for conservative or radical techniques, must be supported by a critical and accurate pre-operative evaluation of the pathological and physiological alterations of the mitral valve. The aim of this report is to discuss the present status of the surgery for mitral stenosis by analyzing a recent and continuous series of 100 cases operated upon, with special emphasis on the recent and important contribution of the pre- and post-operative ultrasonic echography.

SUBJECTS AND METHODS

One hundred cases of mitral stenosis have been operated upon, over a period of 3 years. Patients have been routinely submitted to the following pre-operative investigations: 1) right heart catheterization; 2) phonocardiographic analysis of the heart sounds; 3) ultrasonic echography of the heart.

Ultrasonic System

Bom's apparatus* combines a conventional monotransducer with a multiscan transducer made of 20 electronically scanned piezo-crystals on a line array of 8 cm. The display is given on an oscilloscope, with a frame repetition rate of 70 frames/sec, as a two-dimensional direct visualization. Any line in this dynamic mode can be displayed in the M-mode and fed into the Polaroid camera or the line-scan recorder.

Technique of Examination

Combination of both multiscan direct visualization and conventional single element time-motion recordings was used routinely.

Mitral Valve

An attempt was made to develop a rather extensive study of the mitral valve anatomy. In addition to the conventional measurements

---

* Echocardiovisor, Organon Teknika.

of the anterior-valve opening amplitude and diastolic slope, and a rough estimate of the valve thickening, a determination of anatomic and physiologic derangement of the valves was tried. Among these new criteria are to be mentioned the annulus diameter, the loss of elasticity, and localized thickness of the leaflets, including the posterior and, whenever seen, anterior commissural areas, as well as the thickening, shortening, and fusion of the chordae tendineae to their afferent cusp.

Other Cardiac Structures

Apart from the dynamic anatomy of the mitral valve, we studied the enlargement of the left atrium; the size of the left ventricle, and the thickness and motion of its walls; the size of the right ventricle; and the dynamic anatomy of the tricuspid and aortic valves.

According to the data obtained from these investigations, the patients selected for surgery were divided into 3 groups:

A: patients selected for closed mitral commissurotomy;

B: patients selected for open-heart conservative procedure;

C: patients expected to need a prosthetic valvular replacement.

Table I summarizes the 3 groups of patients with respect to the pre-operative predictions as compared with the intra-operative procedure finally achieved. At the post-operative stage, patients who had undergone conservative surgery (i.e., groups A and B) where submitted to echographic evaluation of the surgical repair. In the cases who had been submitted to prosthetic replacement, the specimen of the mitral apparatus was carefully preserved in cold saline; it was then photographed on both sides, and divided for measurements of several

Table 1
Summary of Procedures

	Preoperative indications according to echogram:	Surgical technique actually performed	Operative deaths
GROUP A (closed valvotomy)	38	36	1
GROUP B (open plastic repair)	42	39	2
GROUP C (prosthetic replacement)	20	25	0
TOTAL	100	100	3

parameters. Those morphologic data were compared with the pre-operative information given by the echogram.

RESULTS AND DISCUSSION
Group A: Closed-heart Mitral Commissurotomy

Among 100 cases of mitral stenosis investigated for surgery, 38 were selected for the closed procedure. The selection of patients was made according to the following criteria: 1) aged less than 40; 2) absence of any thromboembolic episode; 3) systolic pulmonary arterial pressures below 50 mm Hg at rest; 4) cardiothoracic ratio less than 0.50; 5) no thickening of the valves, no calcifications, no fibrous shortening and/or thickening of the chordae tendineae, as demonstrated by ultrasonic echography. Among those 38 cases, 36 were successfully treated by the closed procedure, according to the pre-operative investigations. But in two instances, patients had to be re-operated under bypass few days after a first attempt with the closed technique: one had a calcified narrow left appendage and the dilator couldn't be introduced; the second developed a severe mitral insufficiency due to the rupture of a papillary muscle and underwent a valvular replacement.

If it is performed in accord with the above-mentioned criteria, closed mitral valvotomy is usually a safe and effective method. The operative risk is below 1%; the single death we observed among 36 patients was due to septic pulmonary complications, and does not actually express the true mortality rate of this very simple and non-aggressive procedure (Table 1). On the other hand, the long-term results of this technique seem less satisfactory; in all reported series, the rate of "re-stenosis" within 5 post-operative years is approximately 50%.[2]

After a retrospective analysis of such cases, many cardiac surgeons are today convinced that the closed operation as it was performed initially was not actually complete: in most of cases, only one commissure has been divided by the dilator. Fibrous thickening of the commissures resisted, and fused chordae tendineae could not really be separated. Therefore, the selection of patients for the closed operation must be done carefully: each criterion must be discussed with criticism, and the possibilities afforded today by open-heart procedures must be kept in mind.

Group B: Open-heart Conservative Procedures

Forty-two patients were deliberately chosen to be operated under cardio-pulmonary bypass for an open-heart commissurotomy or another conservative procedure. The additional security provided by extracorporeal circulation was judged advisable when the following conditions were present: 1) mitral stenosis "redux"; 2) age over 40; 3) associated valvular disease, namely tricuspid insufficiency; 4) thromboembolism; 5) systolic pulmonary arterial pressure over 50 mm Hg at rest; 6) cardiothoracic ratio over 0.50; 7) data provided by echocardiography consistent with severe sclerotic changes of the valves, thickening of the mitral margins, and marked fibrous modifications of chordae tendineae. Each of these criteria may be present alone or combined in the same patient.

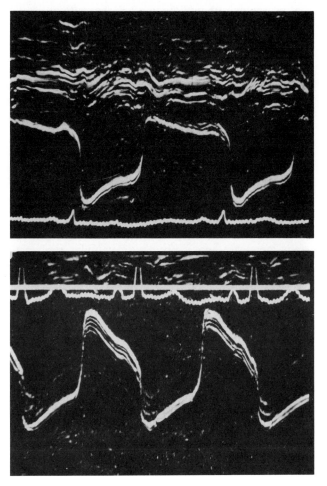

Figure 1. Pre- and postoperative echocardiogram of the anterior mitral leaflet of a patient treated by closed heart commissurotomy. Above: preoperative tracing; below: postoperative tracing.

Among the 42 cases selected for open-heart conservative operations, only 3 finally underwent prosthetic replacement of the mitral valve; in the remaining 39 patients, the previously planned conservative technique was successfully achieved. The conservative operations for mitral stenosis in our own experience involved the following isolated or combined sequences: 1) sharp division with a thin blade of both commissures, which must be fully open; 2) longitudinal separation of the coalescent chordae tendineae; and 3) excision of fibrous or calcified nodules for slicing, and making the valves or their margin thinner. The result of this sequence is immediately tested by filling the left ventricle with saline to judge the competence of the mitral valve after repair. Immediately after the patient is disconnected from bypass, the repair is evaluated by direct measurements of the left atrial and ventricular pressure curves. Before the patient is discharged, a comparative echocardiographic study of the mitral valve is carried out; in these patients the motion of the valves is compared with the preoperative echographic patterns (Fig. 2).

The overall operative mortality in this group was two. One death was due to ventricular fibrillation in a patient with a severe combined aortic stenosis; the second was related to neurologic complications. It is noteworthy that only the second death can be explained by the use of the cardiopulmonary bypass.

Group C: Prosthetic Replacement of the Mitral Valve

The use of the E.C.C. in the management of mitral stenosis does not mean automatic prosthetic valvular replacement in all cases: among 64 patients operated upon with extra-corporeal circulation, only 25 finally received a mitral prosthesis. Among these cases, 2 were done after unsuccessful closed valvulotomy, and 3 after failure of open conservative surgery. In the 20 remaining cases, the valvular replacement was planned according to the pre-operative data consistent with: 1) extremely thickened and/or partially calcified valves shown by echography; 2) severe sclerotic changes of the chordae tendineae with marked limitation in the motion of valves. It is noteworthy that the final decision can be made only by direct vision of the valvular damage, and by intra-operative evaluation by the surgeon himself of the technical conditions. The surgeon today may well try a plastic repair in numerous cases, since valvular replacement remains feasible in case the conservative procedure fails.

The operative results in valvular replacement do not preclude its use in the treatment of severe mitral stenosis, since the overall hospital mortality in this group (0%) is not higher than in closed and open conservative groups. The excised mitral specimens in this group, after photography and measurements, have demonstrated a very close correlation with the echographic data (see Fig. 3, a and b), firmly establishing the value of this non-invasive investigation in the pre-operative analysis of the morphologic changes of the mitral valve.

CONCLUSIONS

In terms of operative mortality, the risk is not statistically different in the different groups considered; 1 death among 36 cases in Group A, 2 deaths among 39 cases in Group B, no deaths among 25

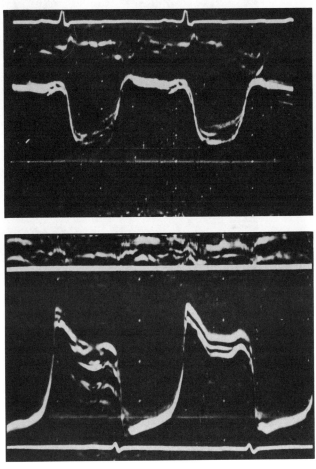

Figure 2. Pre- and postoperative echocardiographic tracings of the anterior mitral valve in a patient treated by open heart commissurotomy. Alterations in the valvular opening and closure are reversed: postoperative (below) diastolic closure speed is within a normal range.

566

cases in Group C. The main question to be discussed is the quality and the durability of the results. The long-term results of the closed valvulotomy are well known, since large series have been reported covering 30 years of experience: 45 to 50% "re-stenosis" occurs after 5 years post-operatively, leading to a second operation.[2]

The long-term results of the valvular replacement with the Starr-Edwards Ball valve No. 6120, which was exclusively employed in this series, are also well known[1]: 3 to 4% thromboembolic non-

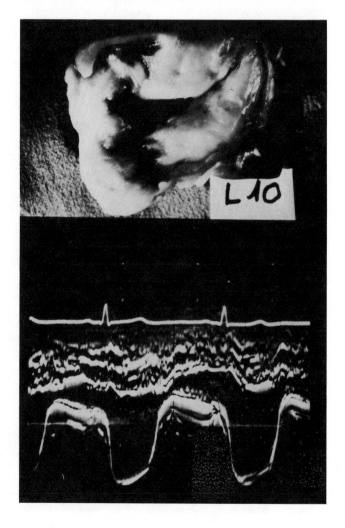

Figure 3. The echocardiographic data of the mitral valve (A) and of its subvalvular apparatus (B) correlate closely with the anatomic findings: the echography suggests a

lethal episodes; 0.5% morbidity due to the prolonged anticoagulant therapy; 1% yearly deaths due to various causes. The results of this prosthesis evaluated now over 12 years after beginning its clinical use are on the whole satisfactory and gratifying. On the other hand, the long-term results of open commissurotomies and valvuloplasties are less well known; some authors are pessimistic,[3] but many others[5] are impressed by the better quality of the morphologic repair in the open methods, leading them to expect better long-term results. In our own

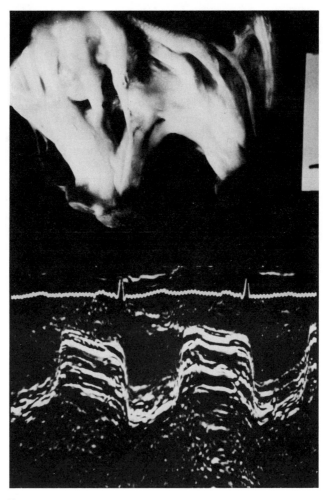

B

severe mitral stenosis, with thickening and calcifications of the anterior leaflet (A); thickening, shortening, and fusion of the chordae tendineae (B).

experience, this impression is confirmed by the echographic analysis of the post-operative results, in closed versus open heart procedures. The total number of cases analyzed is so far too small to draw any firm conclusion, but the benefit in cases treated with open-heart procedures seems more complete and more regular, regarding the motion of the valves (Figs. 1 and 2) as well as the gain in mitral size.

REFERENCES

1. Bonchek, L.I., Starr, A. Prothèse valvulaire à bille. Analyse actuelle de leurs suites lointaines. *Coeur,* No. spécial, p. 365, 1975.

2. Ellis, L.B., Singh, J.B., Morales, D.D. and Harken, D.E. Fifteen to twenty year study of one thousand patients undergoing closed mitral valvuloplasty. *Circulation* 48:357, 1973.

3. Mullin, E.M., Glancy, D.L., Higgs, L., Epstein, S.E. and Morrow, E.G. Amount result of operation for mitral stenosis. Clinical and hemodynamic assessments in 124 consecutive patients treated by closed commissurotomy, open commissurotomy, or valve replacement. *Circulation,* 46:298, 1972.

4. Pernod, J., Servelle, M., Haguenauer, G. and Hermarec, J. Corrélations entre échographie par ultrasons et constatations anatomochirurgicales dans les cardiopathies mitrales (à proposede 140 corrélations). *Arch. Mal. Coeur. Vaiss.* 66:333, 1973.

5. Riviera, R. Chirurgia abierta o cerrada en la estenosis mitral *Rev. Esp. Cardio.* 26:415, 1973.

Dr. Angell: Dr. Cachera, on what percentage of patients do you do open heart commissurotomy?

Dr. Cachera: About 40% of patients referred for mitral stenosis.

Dr. Reid: I would like to ask Dr. Cachera whether he uses the echo intra-operatively to assess his valvuloplasty, and if not, why.

Dr. Cachera: No, we don't use it that way, because we don't have the proper equipment for intra-operative studies.

Dr. Reid: But we have tried it in London and we found it pretty useful to assess the results of the operation.

Dr. Burger: I'd like to congratulate Dr. Cachera on the elegant demonstration of the use of echocardiography. Since he and many other groups have shown that open commissurotomy can be done with no increase in mortality, and little if any in morbidity, and since during the open procedure one does have the opportunity to evaluate the chordae, why should one ever do the procedure closed? Is this perhaps an archaic procedure?

Dr. Cachera: It is clear that mortality following open-heart surgery, even reconstructive surgery, is greater than that of closed-heart commissurotomy, and as for any form of open-heart operation on the left heart, mortality is 3 to 10%. In our experience, open-heart operations are the worst cases; the oldest ones, with the highest pulmonary pressure, and the more severe sclero-retractile lesions.

Dr. Angell: Dr. Starr, what was the average age of your patients for mitral reconstruction?

Dr. Starr: I don't remember the exact figures, but the patients tend to be young. The age will range between 23 and 64 years, with an average around 30.

Dr. Angell: And you are doing about 50% reconstruction?

Dr. Starr: I must admit that we are dealing with a special group, because the cardiologists in the whole region know that we save valves; they therefore send the patients to us rather than to somebody else, so we are getting better patients.

Dr. Dubost: I would like to congratulate Dr. Carpentier for his skill in this reconstruction work he's been doing in my service. The operative indications have gradually increased and broadened, and

most of us have finally been convinced by the quality of this reconstructive surgery, which means that a lot of people don't need the
radical replacement methods. I am in favor of annuloplasty. I use it a
lot. But I operate only on these patients who present either ruptured
cordae, or primary distension of the mitral ring, or pure mitral insufficiency. Carlos Duran goes rather beyond what Carpentier was saying, because he estimates at 50% or more the types of disease which
should be conserved and reconstructed. So these techniques, it seems
to me, have completely changed our concepts in the field of mitral
surgery, and if Carpentier's ring is the answer to tricuspid insufficiency, it is also very interesting in the field of restorative surgery of
the mitral valve.

Dr. Angell: I have a question about the percentage of patients that
you see with mixed type of lesions. What percentage of that group,
with the experience you have had, would you be able to reconstruct,
and what percentage would still have to undergo valve replacement?
Secondly, do you have any four, five, or six-year results with that
group that might give us a comparison with patients who have undergone mitral valve replacement?

Dr. Carpentier: In answer to your first question, of all patients
operated on for mitral valve disease at the Broussais Hospital, 37%
underwent reconstructive surgery. I would like to stress that this
statistic is not a personal one, but rather is representative of the
experience of our entire group. Therefore, it shows the potential
application of the ring valvuloplasty in a large series of patients.

In answer to the second question, comparison between the group
of patients who underwent mitral valve reconstruction and the group
of patients who underwent mitral valve replacement showed a similar
operative mortality in both groups. The late mortality was lower in the
group of reconstructive valve surgery: 6% versus 13% at five years.
The long-term morbidity was significantly less with reconstructive
surgery, with an incidence of thromboembolism of 1.6% at 5 years.

Dr. Cabrol: I would like to congratulate the authors for their
remarkable results. We should be extremely grateful to them for
putting so much emphasis on the value of reconstructive surgery of the
mitral valve. However, I think we should introduce a more realistic
note. I could not be accused of being partial because I have been
practicing this type of surgery for 11 years, but I do believe that these
results are not quite as good as the authors have tried to demonstrate.
That is not a matter of surgical technique. It was well established
many years ago that in the field of reconstructive surgery one can do
anything on any type of valvular lesion: carry out commissurotomy,

remove calcified parts, repair chordae and papillary muscles, or reduce the annulus. The immediate results are usually excellent, but as the years go by those results deteriorate, as can be seen from a group of 180 patients, followed during a mean period of 6 years and a maximum of 11 years. Reasons for the failures were mainly due to sclerosis of all the valvular structures (valves, chordae, papillary muscles), especially on those patients who still had a systolic murmur after the operation. Many of those patients had to be reoperated on, and this is a serious threat to their life expectancy and their social future. Some authors have shown results of a one-year follow-up. This is totally valueless in this specific field.

I would like to make a last comment. The use of the mitral metallic ring had the merit of teaching us how to harmonize reduction of the mitral annulus, but it is not a sound physiologic concept because it hinders the normal contraction of the mitral ring during systole. For that reason, we reduce the mitral annulus with a running suture threaded all along the distensible part of this annulus, i.e., the insertion of the mural leaflet. This semilunar annuloplasty is simple, adaptable, not time-consuming, and very effective.

Dr. Dubost: In our opinion, unfortunately, it does not work.

Dr. Branchini: I wish to express my agreement with Dr. Carpentier's views, and would like to speak up in favor of reconstructive surgery of the mitral valve in small infants. Our experience is based on 9 patients ranging in age between 4 months and 9 years. The congenital malformations involved were as follows: 3 cases of valvular and subvalvular mitral stenosis, 3 cases of parachute valve associated with ventricular septal defect, one case of combined mitral stenosis and regurgitation with endocardial fibroelastosis, one case of dilated mitral ring associated with aortic stenosis, and one case of floppy valve. In five cases we used the Carpentier ring, in 2 cases Wooler's technique, in one case commissurotomy, and in one case we sutured a cleft mitral valve. Actually, we have a clear preference for the Carpentier ring technique, which was in almost all cases preceded by reconstructive surgery of the valve and of the subvalvular apparatus. Results showed 4 operative deaths in patients ranging in age between 4 and 17 months. On the other hand no late death occurred, and excellent results were noted in all other patients.

In order to assess the functional value of the reconstructive surgery, we perfuse the coronary arteries while the aorta is being clamped, a condition which allows a normal cardiac contraction. The left ventricle is filled using a catheter introduced at the apex, and a pressure manometer connected with the intraventricular catheter monitors the left ventricular pressure. Through the atriotomy, it is possible to control the functioning of the valve as well as the eventual occurrence of a residual leak. We conclude that mitral valve reconstructive surgery with the Carpentier ring is a good technique for small infants on account of the excellent results in the long run.

SUMMARY: PART X

A. Carpentier, M.D.

This session clearly showed that changes are occurring in the surgical management of mitral valve disease. Faced with the same mitral valve lesion, some surgeons systematically replace the valve and some try to repair it. Those who still oppose reconstructive surgery cite the unpredictable results, the ease and security of valve replacement, and the small number of cases susceptible to being corrected by conservative techniques. These arguments seem to be no longer valid. New techniques based on the anatomy and physiology of the mitral valve have attained a high level of predictability. Using these techniques, various groups from Pamplona, Bergamo, San Diego, Palo Alto, and Paris have reported excellent long-term results. Dr. Oury's and Dr. Angell's reports have shown that the types of disease observed in the United States are quite similar to those observed in Europe, and that they were able to repair more than 40% of the mitral valve lesions. It is true that calcified valvular disease is being seen with increasing frequency in European and North American countries, but this is largely due to advances in medical therapy which allow the patient to go for a prolonged period before operation. This is done, of course, at the expense of the myocardium, which has sustained relatively greater damage during this period. An earlier reconstructive procedure prior to the advent of valvular calcification and irreversible myocardial damage might be advanced as an alternative. It is our present policy to operate mitral valvular disease as soon as atrial fibrillation occurs, if the patient has a noncalcified valvular lesion as demonstrated by image intensification. Recent atrial fibrillation may be easily converted after mitral valve repair, allowing the patient to lead an absolutely normal life.

Reconstructive valvular surgery is even more important in children and infants. Dr. Branchini's report on our common experience has shown that the first results are encouraging and already superior to valvular replacement.

Both in adults and in children, the increased technical difficulties of valvular reconstruction, the length of time required to carry out the procedure, and the additional effort on the part of the surgeon are no longer sufficient factors when weighed against the added benefit to the patient. As a reward for his efforts, the surgeon will enjoy the satisfaction of being able to offer his patients a superior quality of life following operation.

CREDITS FOR ILLUSTRATIONS

Chapter 1: Figures 1 and 3 courtesy of the American Heart Association, Inc., reproduced with permission from *Circulation* 41:459, 1970. Figures 2, 4, and 5 courtesy of the American Heart Association, Inc., reproduced with permission from *Circulation* 41:449, 1970.

Chapter 3: Figures 1 and 2 courtesy of the American Physiological Society from Tsakiris, A.G., von Bernuth, G., Rastelli, G.C., Bourgeois, M.J., Titus, J.L., Wood, E.H. Size and motion of the mitral valve annulus in anesthetized intact dogs. *Journal of Applied Physiology* 30:611, 1971.

Chapter 5: Figures 1 and 2 courtesy of Perloff, J.K., and Roberts, W.C., *Circulation* 46:227, 1972.

Chapter 6: Figure 1 courtesy of Dr. J.B. Walker. Figure 4 courtesy of Dr. S. Ritchie.

Chapter 9: Selected figures from *Cardiovascular Research* 6:199, 1972.

Chapter 11: Figure 1 courtesy of J.A. Shercliff, *The Theory of Electromagnetic Flow Measurement*. London: Cambridge University Press, 1962.

Chapter 13: Selected figures courtesy of Nolan, S.P., Dixon, Jr., S.H., Fisher, R.D., and Morrow, A.G. The influence of atrial contraction and mitral valve mechanics on ventricular filling. *American Heart Journal* 77:784, 1969.

Chapter 18: Figure 3 courtesy of Yellin, et al., The Application of the Gorlin Equation to the Stenotic Mitral Valve. *1975 Advances in Bioengineering* ed. A.C. Bell and R.M. Nerem, ASME, New York.

Chapter 19: Figure 4 courtesy of Nolan, S.P., Fisher, R.D., Dixon, Jr., S.H., Williams, W.H., and Morrow, A.G. Alterations in left atrial transport and mitral valve blood flow resulting from aortic regurgitation. *American Heart Journal* 79:688, 1970.

Chapter 20: Selected figures courtesy of Kalmanson, D., Veyrat, C., Bernier, A., Savier, C.H., Chiche, P., and Witchitz. S. Diagnosis and evaluation of mitral valve disease using transseptal Doppler ultrasound catheterization. *British Heart Journal* 37:257, ed. W. Somerville.

Chapter 25: Figures 1, 2, and 3 courtesy of Nolan, S.P., Stewart, S., Fogarty, T.J., Dixon, S.H., and Morrow, A.G. In vivo studies of instantaneous blood flow across mitral valve prostheses: the effects of cardiac output and heart rate on transvalvular energy loss. *Ann. Surg.* 169:551, 1969.

Chapter 29: Figures 1 and 2 courtesy of Roelandt. J. Current applications of echotechniques in cardiology. *Hart Bulletin* 6:9, 1975. Figure 3 courtesy of Roelandt, J., van Dorp, W.G., van Zeller, P. Echocardiology: present possibilities of ultrasound applications to the heart. *Schweizerische Medizinische Wochenschrift* 105:1407, 1975.

Chapter 30: Figure 1 courtesy of Gramiak and Waag, *Cardiac Ultrasound*, St. Louis, Mo.: C.V. Mosby Co. Figure 2 courtesy of Grune and Stratton, *Seminars in Roentgenology*, New York, N. Y., October 1975.

Chapter 32: Figure 1 courtesy of Rutishauser, *Kreislaufanalyse mit Roentgendensitometrie*. Bern, Switzerland: Huber, 1969.

Chapter 33: Figure 1 courtesy of Lewis, B.S., Gotsman, M.S. Left ventricular function during systole and diastole in mitral incompetence. *American Journal of Cardiology* 34:635, 1974.

Chapter 36: Figure 1 courtesy of Cabrol, C. Une nouvelle methode de valvuloplastie. *Presse Medicale* 1:1366, 1972; Masson et Cie, Editeurs, Paris.

Chapter 42: Figures 1a and b courtesy of Yacoub, M.H., Towers, M.K., and Somerville, W. Results of mitral valve replacement using unstented fresh semilunar
valve homografts. *Circulation* 45, Suppl. 1:44, 1972. Figure 1c: courtesy of Yacoub,
M.H., and Kittle, C.F. A new technique for replacement of the mitral valve by
semilunar valve homograft. *Journal of Thoracic and Cardiovascular Surgery* 58:859,
1969.